CLINICS IN DEVELOPMENTAL MEDICINE NO. 119
CHILDREN WITH SPECIFIC SPEECH AND LANGUAGE IMPAIRMENT

Clinics in Developmental Medicine No. 119

CHILDREN WITH SPECIFIC SPEECH AND LANGUAGE IMPAIRMENT

CORINNE HAYNES, MSc, MCST
Head Speech and Language Therapist

SANDHYA NAIDOO, MA
Headmistress (1974–1983)
Educational Psychologist (1984–1990)

Dawn House School
Helmsley Road, Rainworth
Nottinghamshire NG21 0DQ

1991
Mac Keith Press
OXFORD: Blackwell Scientific Publications Ltd.
NEW YORK: Cambridge University Press

©1991 Mac Keith Press
5a Netherhall Gardens, London NW3 5RN

First published 1991

British Library Cataloguing in Publication Data

Haynes, Corinne

Children with specific speech and language impairment.
  1. Children. Speech disorders.
  I. Title. II. Naidoo, Sandhya. III. Series

  618.92855

ISBN (UK) 0 901260 88 6
   (USA) 0 521 41275 7

Printed in Great Britain at The Lavenham Press Ltd., Lavenham, Suffolk
Mac Keith Press is supported by **The Spastics Society, London, England**

CONTENTS

FOREWORD

It gives me very great pleasure to see the publication of *Children with Specific Speech and Language Impairment*, and I am delighted to have been asked to write a Foreword to this important work.

I first met the authors nearly 20 years ago, when as a green research student interested in comprehension problems I visited Dawn House to study some of their pupils. Since that time, I have returned to the school on several occasions and have been pleased to see it grow to accommodate older children, whose needs were not previously met.

Throughout this period, I have come to appreciate the breadth and depth of knowledge of those who worked with language-impaired children on a daily basis. I personally owe a great debt to staff at the special schools, who not only made me welcome, but were also keen to discuss my research and offer advice and suggestions, and to draw my attention to the crucial questions that practitioners wanted answered.

The problem is that the expertise of the practitioners seldom makes any impact on the scientific community. Most people who are involved in therapy or education of children with specific language impairment lack the research training, the confidence and the time to conduct systematic studies and to organise their knowledge into a coherent form. Hence my delight to see this book. Corinne Haynes and Sandhya Naidoo have drawn together their mass of data about pupils at Dawn House, and used it to elucidate the antecedents, correlates and prognosis of specific language impairment. Each section is put into theoretical context and related to existing research questions. The authors are not afraid occasionally to state personal opinions based on their experience, but they maintain a clear distinction between conclusions that follow from the data, and interpretations that await further evaluation. No other study has offered such a comprehensive picture of a large sample of language-impaired children seen over a period of time. Nevertheless, while considering the broader issues, the authors manage to keep the reader aware of the nature and variability of individual children. The result is a book that will have an unusually wide appeal. Researchers will find it an invaluable source of basic information about children with specific speech and language impairment. Those concerned with investigating causes of disorder as well as those interested in pinpointing the underlying cognitive basis of developmental language difficulties will find this a mine of useful information. The book will also appeal to those with a more practical interest in language-impaired children. It provides helpful accounts of the range of disorders encountered, giving information on long-term outcome of children with different types of language problem. Relationships between language and literacy problems are given particular attention.

As well as informing other practitioners, this book should also inspire some of them, by demonstrating that the gulf between research and practice can be crossed. It would be foolish to suggest that this is easy. Teachers and therapists do not have ready access to control groups of children, and their training emphasises an individual approach to each child which does not mesh easily with the collection of uniform and systematic observations on large groups of children. It is necessary to plan ahead, and to collect data with a specific research aim in mind, rather than hoping just to make use of information that happens to be on file. As the authors note, even when one does this, there will be frequent and frustrating instances when one finds one lacks crucial information. Yet despite such limitations, this book shows that educators and therapists can make a lasting contribution to the scientific study of language disorder. *Children with Specific Speech and Language Impairment* should be required reading for others wishing to follow this path.

My own understanding of specific language impairment has been enriched by conversations with Corinne Haynes and Sandhya Naidoo. It is gratifying that, with the publication of this book, their insights and experience can now be shared with a wider audience.

DOROTHY BISHOP
Department of Psychology
University of Manchester

PREFACE

When Dawn House School opened in the autumn of 1974, it soon became obvious to both authors that the information routinely collected and necessary for the care and education of children in a boarding school presented a unique opportunity to carry out a comprehensive study of the whole child with a specific speech and language impairment. Increased interest and research in SLI had been, and largely continues to be, concentrated on particular aspects of the impairment and on fairly small samples. Children remain in school for years, giving us the opportunity to build up a large sample. Here, too, was a chance to examine problems longitudinally. There were other reasons for embarking on the project. In the mid-seventies, and sadly still today, there are two major obstacles to meeting the needs of these children. One is the continuing lack of awareness of this disability, which is too rarely recognised and even more rarely understood. Linked to this is inadequate and often inappropriate provision, as the I CAN survey *Adequate Provision* (Hutt and Donlan 1987) has demonstrated.

The sample and data relating to it were collected over a period of 13 years during the normal day-to-day running of the school. The primary concern of staff, including ourselves, is the welfare of the children in our care. The major adverse effect on the project has been a variation in numbers in several items of information. We could not limit the school to a uniform battery of tests during such a long time. Some tests were improved or revised, and naturally the original versions were dropped. Some tests were not available when the school opened. Another complication has been the age range of our sample and the limitations this has imposed on the selection of test material. Although record-keeping procedures were agreed with staff, inevitably some data are missing.

We are fortunate to have had, throughout the five years of the project, the encouragement and financial support of I CAN who administer the school. We are indebted to school staff, both past and present, who have cheerfully accepted the disruption of our comings and goings, and without whom there would have been no data to analyse. Particular thanks must go to Mrs Eunice Bardsley, the school's social worker, who collaborated in planning and was responsible for collecting the developmental and social histories. Ms Kim Grundy and Mrs Bridget Tempest both read and made useful comments on part of the manuscript, and Mrs Eva Grauberg also gave an ever-ready ear and tongue in discussion and contributed to the delineation of subgroups. Much of the preparation of the data prior to analysis was carried out by our efficient, interested and cheerful research assistants, Cindy Wells, Stephen North and Caroline Lowe. We are grateful also to academic researchers who generously found time to discuss issues and suggest ways forward.

These include Dr Susan Gathercole, Professor Pamela Grunwell, Professor Elizabeth Newson and Professor David Wood.

We owe special votes of thanks to two people. Without the continuous advice and support in using the computer database and statistical programmes given by Mr Paddy Riley at Nottingham Cripps Computing Centre it is doubtful whether our results would ever have seen the light of day. We are equally indebted to Dr Dorothy Bishop, who began by warning us of the perils and pitfalls of retrogressive research, and then was unstinting in offering us every assistance and guidance.

We owe much to the warm support of our families who adjusted to living with our almost constant preoccupation elsewhere, and most of all to the Dawn House children and their parents, who told us in so many ways what it means to be a language-impaired child.

CORINNE HAYNES
SANDHYA NAIDOO
April 1991

1
INTRODUCTION

What is specific language impairment?

There are probably as many communicative styles as there are human beings who use them. Whether brilliant, ponderous, witty, ironic or gently persuasive, styles of communication richly reflect the abilities and personalities of the speakers. However, some people are not endowed with those skills which the majority use so naturally. Although they have a wide range of personalities and non-verbal abilities, these are not reflected in their use of language, which is often halting and impoverished. Particularly in childhood, these language-impaired individuals are unable to understand and express themselves in the same effortless way as their peers.

This book is concerned with such people, particularly those whose impaired language skills cannot easily be ascribed to a known primary condition such as deafness or mental subnormality, and who are therefore often described as having a specific language impairment (SLI). The book describes the background, development, language characteristics and progress of one such group of children attending a special school in the Midlands of England for pupils with severe SLI.

Historically, interest in speech and language problems has moved from a concern with overt difficulties of speech production (Demosthenes was said to have a stammer, Mendelssohn a speech impediment) to more analytical accounts of the subtle, complex and pervasive nature of language disabilities (*e.g.* Fletcher 1986). Not only is recognition of the complexities of language impairment gradually developing, but the focus of interest in normal language is also changing. During the last 30 years this focus has moved from vocabulary, to syntax and to a current preoccupation with pragmatics. Under such changing conditions, the aspects of language selected for assessment in language-impaired populations have also changed.

Although a considerable body of knowledge about SLI has been derived from clinical studies, the growth of precise knowledge has been hampered by the absence of any agreed criteria for defining language impairment. When criteria are defined they are particular to the study in question rather than universal. Stark and Tallal (1981) sought to define language impairment more precisely and improve upon the usual definition which is one of exclusion (*i.e.* language impairment not secondary to hearing impairment, mental subnormality or emotional disturbance). They proposed the positive criterion of measured language age at least one year below chronological age or performance mental age, whichever was lower. This produced a relatively homogeneous subject group, but selection of a different assessment procedure from the multifarious measures available to compute a language age

1

could produce a rather different population of impaired children, even when the criterion gap between language and cognitive function is retained. Most language assessments measure only one specific area of linguistic function such as comprehension of grammar (Bishop 1983) or word-finding skills (German 1986). More global language assessments may have a disputed theoretical basis (Kirk *et al.* 1968) or a low age ceiling (Reynell 1969, 1977) and are not universally used, even in the English-speaking world. Some studies use a variety of local assessments (Hall and Tomblin 1978) or put together their own language composite from a test battery (Schery 1985). Until assessments have some known degree of comparability, the subjects in each study must be considered individually and conclusions reached with caution.

Given the changing foci of interest and the wide range of instruments of measurement, longitudinal studies such as this one (which covers a period of 13 years) will almost invariably find that both what is measured and the instruments used for measurement change during the course of the study, with subsequent problems for the comparison of findings and the building up of a precise body of knowledge.

A further problem stems from the variation in subject groups. Most studies have proceeded from an already established population attending a particular clinic (Allen and Rapin 1980, Aram and Nation 1980), special classes (Luick *et al.* 1982, Schery 1985) or a special school (Griffiths 1969), who meet the local eligibility conditions required, although not all studies describe precisely the measures upon which the diagnosis of language disorder has been based (*e.g.* Garvey and Gordon 1973, King *et al.* 1982). The present study is retrospective and comprises children meeting the selection criteria of one particular school.

Instead of clinical groups, some studies have identified speech- and language-disordered groups within normal populations (Morley 1965, Sheridan and Peckham 1973, Fundudis *et al.* 1979, Silva *et al.* 1987) but such groups are generally less tightly defined than in the smaller clinic or school studies. In the study by Morley (1965), and that of Sheridan and Peckham (1973) which used data from the 1958 National Child Development Study (Davie *et al.* 1972), the emphasis was on speech defects rather than on language impairment, in line with the model of communication problems current at that time. The studies by Fundudis *et al.* (1979) and Silva *et al.* (1987) included children with more global handicaps than are usual in smaller clinic studies.

One hotly debated topic of the 1960s—whether language impairment is a question of delay or deviance (Menyuk 1964, Leonard 1972)—has become a less central concern of researchers and clinicians in the 1970s and 1980s, as the quest for a unitary disorder with a single aetiology has given way to the acceptance of language impairment as a relatively heterogeneous set of disorders with multiple and possibly synergistic aetiologies (Rapin and Allen 1983, Bishop and Rosenbloom 1987). Certainly the concept of language *delay* as a developmental imbalance, in which verbal skills lag a year or two behind other aspects of

2

development and then 'catch up' to normal, does not apply to the seven- and eight-year-olds being admitted to special units and schools, whose problems persist in varying degrees into adult life. This is not to deny that there are children with a language *delay*, possibly due to an environmental or physical setback, but such children are not the subject of this book.

The acceptance of a variety of conditions and multifactorial aetiologies, under the umbrella title of language impairment, has also taken the heat out of the other debate of the 1960s: whether SLI is a discrete phenomenon or shades into the continuum of normal language skills. It now seems entirely possible that while there exists a continuum of language *behaviours* ranging from the highly articulate to the barely verbal, some children with extremely poor language skills may have some as yet undescribed variation of cerebral organisation, or some other discrete basis of their handicap which is abnormal. There has currently been no research to indicate that language impairment of pathological origin, and language at the bottom end of the normal distribution curve, have differences of development or outcome which merit different treatment.

Antecedents
Although SLI is popularly defined as language impairment *of unknown origin*, there have been many attempts to uncover possible antecedent factors. The best supported finding, a familial concentration of language problems (Neils and Aram 1986a, Tallal *et al.* 1989a, Tomblin 1989), suggests the strong possibility of a genetic link. There are also relatively rare but significant findings of chromosome abormality in SLI children (Friedrich *et al.* 1982, Mutton 1982, Ratcliffe 1982).

More debatable is the contribution of prenatal and perinatal problems, the incidence of which is often raised in language disordered populations in demographic studies (Fundudis *et al.* 1979, Paterson and Golding 1986) where perinatal factors may be confounded by socioeconomic factors such as family size and low birthweight, or associated with more global handicaps. There are contradictory reports in smaller clinical studies, many finding no effect of perinatal factors, and others lacking consistency in the significant features they report.

Even more controversial are the studies into factors such as early otitis media or environmental disadvantage. Some report significant effects but with no cross-study consistency. Several writers have concluded that while single-factor aetiologies are rare, congenitally predisposed children may be edged into overt handicap in the presence of an additional penalising factor (Rapin and Allen 1983, Bishop 1987).

Possible antecedent factors in Dawn House children will be discussed in relation to other research in Chapter 3.

Correlates
A number of studies have considered the correlates (possibly causally associated) of SLI. The most frequently investigated of these has been intelligence, usually

employing a non-verbal measure of ability. Where language impairment has been examined within demographic surveys, criteria for inclusion are usually broad. Children with low IQ were included by Fundudis *et al.* (1979) and Silva *et al.* (1987), who found more long-term low intelligence in children diagnosed as having a language delay. In a clinical follow-up study of four- to eight-year-olds, Stark *et al.* (1984) found that, four years on, IQ (and particularly verbal IQ) had improved with language skills, possibly an indication of delayed maturation in this particular group. However, in their follow-up study of somewhat older children (four to 11 at first, then seven to 13 years old), Ajuriaguerra *et al.* (1976) commented on the stability of IQ levels. As with the discussion of antecedent factors, the conclusions have not been concordant, and confounding factors such as social class and age have not always been satisfactorily excluded.

There is some convincing evidence relating auditory perceptual abilities to SLI, Tallal and colleagues have repeatedly demonstrated abnormalities of auditory perception in the language-impaired population (Tallal and Piercy 1973, 1978; Tallal *et al.* 1980). However, their identification of a specific perceptual difficulty with rapidly changing acoustic phenomena has yet to be related precisely to the nature of impaired language skills, or to the wider range of auditory perceptual abilities. Research into the importance of auditory discrimination in language impairment has been particularly unsatisfactory, marred by the variety of stimuli selected and the nature of the discrimination task which might be instantaneous or sequential, linguistic or non-linguistic. Auditory short-term memory (ASTM) is a much stronger contender for a significant role in the complex relationship of language impairment and associated skills, and has figured in the research literature of specific language and specific reading impairment for at least 40 years. In the related fields of spoken and written language, ASTM has become particularly associated with the skills of phonological coding and storage, and some current theories will be discussed in relation to Dawn House data in later chapters.

Behavioural correlates of language impairment have been the particular concern of three major studies, the Waltham Forest study (Richman *et al.* 1982), the Dunedin study (Silva *et al.* 1984) and the Los Angeles study (Cantwell *et al.* 1979). Language impairment is generally agreed to be frequently accompanied and followed by problems of social adjustment, and it seems reasonable to assume that the social problems are sometimes the result of the communication problems. There is less agreement about whether behavioural problems may also precede specific language difficulties, or whether language impairment which is subsequent to emotional difficulty can truly be described as specific.

Motor clumsiness is frequently reported as a correlate of language impairment (Gubbay 1975), though there is little hard evidence. Like language impairment, the term 'clumsiness' is not objectively defined. Historically, but also controversially, there has been an association between late establishment of laterality, or mixed laterality, and spoken and written language disorder (Naidoo 1972, Zangwill 1978). Both motor problems and abnormal lateralisation suggest some overt or 'soft' neurological dysfunction. Johnston *et al.* (1981) identified a number of neurologically modulated tasks which successfully demarcated SLI children from a control group, but could draw no firm conclusions about causality or specificity with regard to this particular disabled population.

The possible association between abnormalities of intelligence, auditory perceptual skills, behaviour, lateralisation, neurological development, motor skills and the language impairment of Dawn House pupils will be discussed in Chapter 5.

Subgroups
As the characterisation of language impairment has become increasingly complex, so the descriptions of subgroups (patterns of language disability within the general concept of impairment) have become more diverse, developing from the early dichotomies of language *vs* speech (Eisenson 1984) or receptive *vs* expressive (Reynell 1969) to fuller taxonomies of linguistic impairment (Rapin and Allen 1983). There is currently no completely satisfactory classification of SLI into subgroups, partly due to the imprecise definition of SLI and the heterogeneity of subjects, and partly due to the variety of ways of measuring language ability. Quantitative groupings based on specific psychometric measures and statistical analysis (Aram and Nation 1975, Wolfus *et al.* 1980) are often limited to particular test availability or appropriateness, or are inapplicable to all age groups; and more clinical measures (Martin 1980) may be hard to replicate. Perhaps the most useful classification to date has been that of Rapin and Allen (1983, 1988), who delineated syndromes of language disorder, combining clinical observations with formal investigations of syntax, phonology and pragmatics. Wilson and Risucci (1986) also stressed the need for an alliance between clinical consensus and quantitative data, and this is an alliance which we have sought to attain.

Longitudinal studies
Follow-up studies of language-impaired populations are relatively recent and scarce. Their main concerns have been with the nature of persistent difficulties and the prediction of outcome (Griffiths 1969, Hall and Tomblin 1978, Paul *et al.* 1983, Aram *et al.* 1984, Schery 1985). Weiner (1985) compared the 17 studies produced since the seminal study of Ajuriaguerra *et al.* (1976). In spite of the methodological variations and somewhat arbitrary selection of data reported, he found a surprising degree of agreement in all their reports of communicative, academic and social-adjustment problems, which sometimes continued into adult life. He found less agreement regarding the factors which accurately predict outcome: hardly surprising, considering the wide variation in age, subject and severity of impairment, and indeed in the variation of possible predictors selected for examination. Thus vocabulary level was found to predict outcome in two-year-olds (Fischel *et al.* 1989), play, social interaction and comprehension in 2½- to 3½-year-olds (Allen and Rapin 1980), while non-verbal intelligence predicted language and educational outcome 10 years later in preschoolers between 3½ and seven years

(Aram *et al.* 1984). Bishop and Edmundson (1987*a*), with a narrower age range (3.9 to 4.2), also found a non-verbal intelligence measure a valuable predictor of outcome, but less good than a language test involving a story-retelling task. However, in a large study of over 700 children between three and 16 years, Schery (1985) found intelligence only a weak predictor of improvement compared with the major factor of initial language status.

Why another study?
Each of the studies referred to above contributes in some degree to our knowledge of SLI. Many methodological deficiencies have been indicated (Kamhi 1985), and Weiner (1985) suggested that the problems of such investigations are currently insuperable. Many of these methodological flaws, notably the lack of strictly defined objective criteria to select subjects, the changing nature of assessments and the low ceilings of many language measures, will be apparent in this book. The retrospective use of data which was not collected for research purposes presents many problems with comparability and missing data. But our study of 156 subjects uses a broad database. The longitudinal nature of the data allows us to relate the difficulties of the children at school entry to background variables, and to examine which demographic or linguistic features (or a combination of these) may predict outcome at school-leaving age. Some data are also available on the career and social development of 34 ex-pupils, now young adults. Both authors have been closely involved with all the children throughout the period of the study. This personal daily involvement with a large group of children over a long period is, to the best of our knowledge, unique among studies of SLI. We have combined our individual clinical insights (as speech and language therapist and psychologist) with a large dataset of demographic, psychometric and linguistic variables in order to describe the children, and to delineate subgroups with some objective and clinical coherence. This study cannot resolve theoretical issues or draw universally applicable conclusions, but we hope it will contribute to the knowledge of the natural history of specific language impairment.

Description of sample and data
The school
Dawn House School was opened in 1974 to provide intensive speech and language therapy and education for children with severe specific language disorders. It is a special residential and day school recognised by the Department of Education and Science and administered by a charitable body, Invalid Children's Aid Nationwide (I CAN). I CAN (formerly ICAA) is particularly interested and experienced in this field, and administers two other language schools in the south of England, the first of which has been catering for young SLI children since 1958. Pupils at Dawn House are sponsored by their local education authorities, if there is no suitable local provision. The original establishment was for 54 children, 48 of whom were boarders and six were day pupils. Places have increased with demand, and there are

6

TABLE 1.I
Children excluded from the sample

N	Reason for exclusion
25	Intellectual grounds
11	Hearing problems
3	Behavioral problems
3	Short stay at Dawn House
1	Missing file
Total 43	

TABLE 1.II
Children included in the sample

	Boarders	Day pupils	Total
Boys	108	21	129
Girls	23	4	27
Total	131	25	156

currently (1991) 68 boarding and 20 day places. Most of the boarders go home weekly or fortnightly. At the time of the study pupils were mainly admitted between the ages of five and 10, with a top age of 13. A secondary department was opened in 1987, and pupils with long-term needs can now remain at Dawn House until they reach school-leaving age. Because of this, some children over the age of 11 were admitted as pupils.

Children are taught a normal school curriculum, adapted to their special language needs, in small classes of between six and 12 pupils. Because their individual capabilities vary enormously, they require individual programmes of work, planned by the speech and language therapist and specialist teacher working together. Individual therapy is provided for all children, daily or according to need, and each speech and language therapist has responsibility for 10 or 11 children. Dawn House also employs a part-time educational psychologist, a part-time social worker and a part-time physiotherapist. After school hours the children are cared for by a separate care staff in small family units of eight in the junior school, moving up into a senior residential house with a wider range of facilities suitable for adolescents when they are about 12 years old.

The aim of the school is to enable children to attain their full communicative and educational potential, allowing as many as possible to return to mainstream education, and providing a comprehensive alternative education for those who cannot.

The children

SELECTION CRITERIA

Children attending Dawn House have a primary language problem which prevents them from fulfilling their potential in mainstream education. We do not accept children with global cognitive retardation, significant hearing loss or psychiatric disorder.

Some children who do not strictly meet these criteria have occasionally been admitted to the school, either as special cases, or because of the difficulty of making an accurate assessment given the fundamental and pervasive nature of language disorder. In order to make the sample reasonaby homogeneous, such children have not been included in this study (Table 1.I). This leaves 156 children, admitted to

TABLE 1.III

Specific language problems of Dawn House children

Input problems
Perception and interpretation of individual speech sounds
Understanding word meanings because of failure to develop concepts
Understanding word meanings because of failure to associate label with meaning
Storing word labels in mental lexicon
Understanding semantic relationships within sentence or clause
Understanding grammatical relationships within sentence or clause

Output problems
Relating conceptual meaning to production of spoken word
Accessing word labels from mental lexicon
Formulation of sentences based on semantic relationships
Formulation of rule-governed grammatical sentences
Relating sequences of logical ideas to sequences of coherent sentences
Production of individual and sequenced speech sounds associated with failure to develop internal
    model of phonological system
Voluntary programming of sound sequences (words) and/or word sequences
Neuromotor production of sound and word sequences

Problems of use
Using language in functionally effective way
Using language which is appropriate to context

TABLE 1.IV

Geographical origins of the sample

East Midlands	75
West Midlands	28
South East	23
Yorkshire and Humberside	21
North West	5
South West	2
East Anglia	1
Scotland	1

Regions defined by Office of
Population Censuses and Surveys
1970.

TABLE 1.V

Age of admission and discharge

Age (yrs)	Admission N	Admission %	Discharge N	Discharge %
5.0– 5.11	18	11.5	0	0
6.0– 6.11	33	21.2	1	0.8
7.0– 7.11	32	20.5	1	0.8
8.0– 8.11	36	23	7	6
9.0– 9.11	31	19.9	6	5
10.0–10.11	4	2.6	11	9
11.0–11.11	0	0	21	18
12.0–12.11	2	1.3	48	41
13.0–13.11	0	0	23	20
Total	156	100	118*	100

*4 children, removed from school for family
reasons, are excluded

TABLE I.VI

Height and weight centiles at entry

Centiles	Percentage of children Height (N 128)	Percentage of children Weight (N 146)
<3	13	10
4–10	17	7
11–25	17	15
26–50	22	20
51–75	14	15
76–90	8	10
91–97	8	22
	100	100

school between 1974 and 1987, who make up our sample. All studies of developmental language disorders report more boys than girls, *e.g.* 3.8:1 by Robinson (1987), and 2.6:1 by Schery (1985). The male-to-female ratio in this study is particularly high at 4.8:1 (Table 1.II).

Children included in the study have:

(1) a severe language or speech-language impairment which is deemed to be primarily responsible for failure to attain those communicative, educational and social accomplishments which might reasonably be expected in the absence of such impairment (Table 1.III)*

(2) a desire to communicate, using whatever means are available, and the ability to participate in and benefit from the education, therapy and care available at Dawn House

(3) non-verbal intelligence within or above 1SD of the mean (127 children) or within 1SD of the mean on three subtests of one of the Wechsler Scales of intelligence (29 children)

(4) a mean hearing loss in the better ear no greater than 30dB, measured at frequencies of 500HZ, and 1,2 and 4kHZ

(5) no primary psychiatric, emotional or behavioural problem.

REGIONAL ORIGIN

Children are sent from local education authorities in many parts of the UK, with the largest number coming from the East Midlands (Table 1.IV). There are no private pupils.

AGE

Children in the study range in age from 5.2 to 13.10. They were admitted as pupils between the ages of 5.2 and 12.11 (mean 7.10), and left the junior department of Dawn House between the ages of 6.10 and 13.10 (mean 11.9). One hundred children left to go to other schools; 22 pupils went into the senior department of Dawn House after it opened in 1987. The length of stay at Dawn House (junior department) varied from 11 months to 6.11 (mean 3.9). Table 1.V shows the ages at which children were admitted to and discharged from Dawn House junior department.

PHYSICAL DESCRIPTION

Table 1.VI compares the available heights and weights of the children at the time of admission to Dawn House, with a normal population using the centiles provided by the Institute of Child Health (Tanner 1958). The Dawn House entrants are physically rather small, with 17 children (13 per cent) at or below the third centile,

---

*It is currently impossible to define SLI succinctly. Those language problems which contribute to our definition of SLI, singly or in combination, are listed in Table 1.III. These are no standard assessments for diagnosing each of these language problems in a population ranging in age from five to 13 years. The diagnosis is arrived at by a mixture of standard, age-appropriate assessments, and clinical observation.

and 40 (30 per cent) at or below the 10th centile. Weight for age is distributed more normally, although with an increase in underweight children (predictable because of the small heights recorded), and with a more unexpected increase at the other end of the scale, with 32 overweight children (22 per cent) above the 90th centile.

Structural physical abnormalities in the sample comprised three children with repaired cleft palates, one with unilateral atresia of the external auditory meatus, one with bilateral narrowing of the auditory meatus, one with bilateral talipes equino-valgus and one with a heart defect.

Data

The data are taken from school files and include some preschool and post-school reports. Some of the data are longitudinal.

Sources of information are:

1. *School case history.* Before any child is admitted to Dawn House, the school social worker visits the home and takes a detailed case history from one or both parents. This includes information on family history of language disorders and other relevant conditions; birth and developmental history; health, and physical and emotional factors; and school and speech therapy experience.

2. *Application reports.* Further information in the above areas is taken from the medical, psychological, school, speech therapy and parental reports, which are sent at the time of application as part of the Statement of Special Educational Needs or, prior to 1981, the Special Education Procedure.

3. *Dawn House speech therapy records.* In the first term at school the child's speech and language therapist assesses hearing acuity, ASTM, speech discrimination, comprehension and use of vocabulary and syntax, language content, articulatory and phonological skills, and the communicative value of language in use. The actual assessment procedures are selected individually for each child and include clinical-observational and in-house tests as well as standardised procedures. Reassessment in relevant areas is undertaken at six-monthly intervals.

4. *Dawn House psychological records.* These contain information about verbal and performance IQ, laterality, visuo-spatial and visuo-motor skills, and the measures are selected as appropriate for each child. The frequency of reassessment relates to the level of an individual child's progress.

5. *Dawn House educational records.* Class teachers keep records of reading, spelling and numerical ability. Biannual school reports include comments on all aspects of educational attainment, patterns of learning, motor skills, personality and behaviour.

6. *Dawn House child-care records.* These records are maintained by the houseparents for residential pupils. They contain information about the child's physical state (height, weight and vision) and health (eating habits, illnesses, vaccinations, medication, accidents, and clinic and hospital visits). Biannual reports contain comments on self-confidence, sociability, emotional development, behaviour problems and communicative behaviour.

7. *Medical records*. School files contain reports of medical investigations and visits to consultants made while the child is a pupil. The school's honorary paediatric neurologist maintains his own records of children examined (see Chapter 5).

8. *Follow-up questionnaire*. A questionnaire has been completed by telephone interview with 34 ex-pupils aged over 18. Questions were asked about living conditions, further education, employment, leisure activities and social life.

Longtitudinal data comprised speech therapy, educational and psychological records. These were taken from initial assessments during the first three months after school entry, and also from the final reports on discharge from Dawn House. For those pupils whose stay at Dawn House was four years or longer, interim educational and speech therapy data from assessments at the end of the second year were entered.*

Synopsis

Chapter 2 of this book describes the assessment measures which were used when subjects entered school, and the resultant linguistic and educational profiles. From these profiles, nine subgroups of language impairment form a basis for comparative analysis throughout the study.

Antecedent factors proposed as causes of SLI are considered in Chapter 3. We compare our findings with those of other studies, and examine the interactive and individual effects of familial language problems, perinatal risks and neurologically threatening conditions, environmental factors and early middle-ear disease.

Chapter 4 deals with the developmental factors which may be associated with SLI, and relates the age of walking and talking, and the development of oromotor skills in our sample to their later language proficiency.

In Chapter 5 we consider several factors which have long been associated with SLI, although the exact nature of the relationship has yet to be established: auditory processing, cognitive functioning, laterality, behaviour and neurological function. We look at these factors within our sample in terms of the background factors, current language abilities and subgroup profiles.

Chapter 6 is devoted to reading ability, and the relationship between oral language proficiency and written language proficiency. We discuss the difficulties encountered by SLI children in learning to read phonically and semantically.

The final language and educational profiles of 118 school-leavers are compared with those at entry in Chapter 7. We derive a final outcome measure from language, speech and reading performance and consider the final status of our subgroups of SLI. We discuss the possibility of predicting outcome from antecedent, associated and entry language measures, and look at the educational, career and social achievements and problems of those youngsters aged 18 or more at the time of the study.

*Data were entered on to an ICL 3980 computer at the University of Nottingham, using the Scientific Information Retrieval (SIR) database management system.

2
PROFILE OF LANGUAGE ABILITIES AND IMPAIRMENT

When Dawn House opened in 1974, profiles of linguistic abilities in areas such as syntax and phonology were only just beginning to emerge from the field of applied linguistics. Language assessments were still based mainly on the medical model of adult acquired aphasia, in which language is divided into two general areas, comprehension and production. Reading and spelling difficulties, although often associated with SLI, were generally considered to be separate from oral language handicap and to have a different aetiology. Because our data are largely drawn from tests devised within this framework, the description of the language abilities of the Dawn House children will be presented under four headings: comprehension, expressive language, speech and written language.

A uniform test battery has not been used at Dawn House. Every attempt is made to examine the scope of linguistic and learning abilities for each child, so different assessments are selected according to suitability and current practice. The assessments available for disorders of language vary considerably in their degree of standardisation and in the age range for which they are suitable. Because a high level of language competence is achieved at an early age by normal children, many of the test ceilings are low, although Dawn House pupils still generally score under that ceiling. For these reasons, the number of data is not consistent from test to test and the only available comparison of performance across tests is age equivalence, shown here as a lag behind chronological age. Data are presented from test results and reports at the time of admission to school for up to 156 children.

Comprehension
Comprehension of vocabulary
ENGLISH PICTURE VOCABULARY TEST AND BRITISH PICTURE VOCABULARY SCALE

Some assessments measure specific aspects of comprehension and some are more holistic. Both the English Picture Vocabulary Test (EPVT Tests 1 and 2), with an age range of 5.0 to 11.11 (Brimer and Dunn 1962), and the British Picture Vocabulary Scale (BPVS), with an age range of 3.0 to 19.0 (Dunn *et al.* 1982), specifically measure receptive vocabulary and are derived from the original and revised versions of the American Peabody Picture Vocabulary Test respectively. Both tests are administered in a similar way. The child is presented with arrays of pictures, four to a page, and has to indicate which one represents the word spoken by the examiner. Arrays of increasing difficulty are presented until the child reaches a ceiling. The EPVT was used at Dawn House until 1982 when it was replaced by the

TABLE 2.I		
Vocabulary scores at first assessment (EPVT and BPVS) in SD bands		
SD	*N*	*%*
+1 to 2	2	1
0 to +1	16	11
0 to −1	61	41
−1 to −2	54	37
−2 and below	15	10
Total	148	100

Mean standard score = 84.8, with a standard deviation of 13.4

TABLE 2.II		
Vocabulary age lag at first assessment (age range 7.3 to 12.7)		
Chronological age minus vocabulary age	*N*	*%*
No gap	9	7
Up to 1 yr	27	21
1–2 yrs	43	34
Over 2 yrs	48	38
Total	127	100

Excluding children below 7 years of age tested on the EPVT, which has a 5-year basal. Mean lag = 17.8 mths, with a standard deviation of 15 mths

BPVS. Both tests produce standardised scores with a mean of 100 and a standard deviation of 15.

Of the 151 children given a vocabulary test, standard scores could be computed for 148. Ninety-eight EPVT standard scores and 50 BPVS standard scores are combined in Table 2.I. There is a wide range of standard scores from 127 down to 50, with 88 per cent falling below the normal mean. The mean standard score at entry is 84.8, with a standard deviation of 13.4.

Both EPVT and BPVS allow the calculation of a vocabulary age. Table 2.II shows the lag of vocabulary age behind chronological age at entry for 127 children. It excludes children below seven years of age who were assessed on the EPVT, as the base age of five years for that test would eradicate the possibility of age lags of more than two years. The mean age lag at entry was 17.8 months, with a standard deviation of 15 months.

In subsequent chapters a standard set of language measures will be repeatedly used for statistical analyses. The 148 available standard scores of EPVT and BPVS are used as the measure of *comprehension of vocabulary*.

Comprehension of grammar
TROG
The Test for Reception of Grammar (TROG) also deals with a particular aspect of comprehension (Bishop 1983). Dawn House had early access to an experimental version of this test (1976), since some of the pupils contributed to its development, but the final published version has been in use since 1982. Both versions assess the understanding of selected aspects of grammar in childen aged four to 13 years plus, using a picture pointing response format which eliminates the need for expressive language ability. Both use a limited vocabulary which can be pretested in order to eliminate deficits in vocabulary as a cause of errors. In the current edition, the child hears a sentence and indicates which of four pictures is described by the sentence (*e.g.* 'he is sitting in the tree'), as opposed to the grammatical distractor ('*she is*

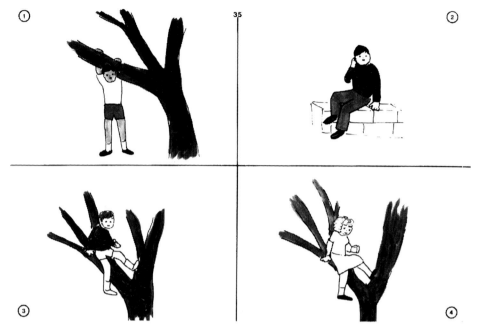

Fig. 2.1. Array from the TROG assessment for selecting 'He is sitting in the tree'.

sitting in the tree') or lexical distractors ('he is sitting on a *wall*, he is *hanging* from a tree') (Fig. 2.1). The earlier version had variable numbers of distractors per page. The grammatical items examined also differ in the original and final versions, and there are no data relating performance in the two versions. The experimental version was concerned with the understanding of four structures: word inflections ('the dogs', 'long*est*'), function words ('*her* ball' '*not* pushing'), word combinations ('the girl with the big black box') and reversible structures ('the boy chasing the dog is spotty'). The final version tests understanding of parts of speech, simple and complex sentences, active, passive and comparative sentences, pronouns, word inflections, relative clauses, post-modification and embedding.

Although different grammatical items are tested, we consider both versions to be a good over-all indication of grammatical decoding ability, and have used data from both in the computation of z-scores*.

The results of initial TROG tests are presented in Table 2.III in bands of z-scores. Early pupils could have been in school for two years before TROG came into general use in 1976. The percentages of children within each band from the two TROG versions do not differ significantly, and have been combined. TROG ages and the lag behind chronological age could be computed for 93 children (Table 2.IV). The mean lag at entry was 18.1 months, with a standard deviation of 27 months.

*We are indebted to Dr Dorothy Bishop for providing formulae for converting scores from both versions of TROG to Z-scores.

TABLE 2.III		
TROG scores at first assessment in Z-score bands		

Z-scores	N	%
Over 1	4	4
0 to 1	24	24
0 to −1	31	31
−1 to −2	22	22
−2 to −3	19	19
Total	100	100

Z-scores from 45 children using original version and 55 children using final version

TABLE 2.IV		
TROG grammar age lag at first assessment (age range 5.10 to 12.7)		

Chronological age minus TROG age	N	%
No gap	22	24
Up to 1 yr	15	16
1–2 yrs	17	18
Over 2 yrs	39	42
Total	93	100

Mean lag = 18.1 mths, with a standard deviation of 27 mths

TROG z-scores will be used as the measure of *comprehension of grammar* in subsequent analyses.

General comprehension

REYNELL SCALES

The Reynell Developmental Language Scales (RDLS) (Reynell 1969, 1977) use the polarised comprehension-expression model of language ability, with separate scales for comprehension and expression, each assessing a number of developmental language skills. The age range of the revised version is between one and seven years, and between six months and six years for the provisional version, but because of their very severe language difficulties, most entrants to Dawn House scored within the range of the test. The 1977 revision of the test kept the original format and materials as far as possible, expanding some of the sections and removing some anomalies. It also increased the difficulty at the top end to give a higher ceiling. The RDLS comprehension scale assesses understanding of a wide range of verbal input, comprising verbal preconcepts (words or phrases with situational significance), noun labels of real objects (*e.g.* ball, spoon), symbolic representations using inanimate (table) and animate (dog) toy models, the relationship of two named objects ('put the doll on the chair'), association of objects with a subjective function ('which one do we sleep in?') and an externalised function ('which one shoots the rabbits?'), longer instructions involving negatives and attributive terms as well as nouns and verbs ('which red pencil has not been put away?'), increasingly complex relationships between a number of concepts ('put all the animals except the black pig into the box') and inferential questions ('Mary and Bobby go to school. Who stays with mother?').

It is thus a general rather than a specific comprehension test. Thirty-six children were assessed at entry with the provisional version of the scale, and 74 with the revised version. Because of the limited age range of the test, a standard score could be computed for only 43 children, and these results are given in Table 2.V. It was possible to establish an equivalent Reynell comprehension age, and thus an age

15

TABLE 2.V

Standard scores of Reynell comprehension scale at first assessment in SD bands

Standard scores		N	%
1.1 and over		3	7
−1 to 1		16	37
−1 to −2		9	21
−2.1 and below		15	35
	Total	43	100

TABLE 2.VI

Reynell comprehension age lag at first assessment (chronological age 5.5 to 10.5)

Chronological age minus comprehension age		N	%
No gap		4	4
Up to 1 yr		16	17
1–2 yrs		32	33
Over 2 yrs		45	46
	Total	97	100

Mean lag = 24 mths, with a standard deviation of 15.7 mths

TABLE 2.VII

TACL age lag at first assessment (chronological age 5.6 to 12.4)

Chronological age minus comprehension age		N	%
No gap		7	10
Up to 1 yr		16	24
1–2 yrs		16	24
Over 2 yrs		28	42
	Total	67	100

Mean lag = 20 mths, with a standard deviation of 14.1 mths

lag, for 97 children (Table 2.VI). The mean gap at entry was 24 months, with a standard deviation of 15 months.

TEST FOR AUDITORY COMPREHENSION OF LANGUAGE

A further test of comprehension, the Test for Auditory Comprehension of Language (TACL), was developed in the USA (Carrow 1973). The child tries to select the appropriate picture from an array of three pictures in response to a spoken word, phrase or sentence. The age range of the test is from 3.0 to 6.11, and the 101 items test parts of speech (nouns, verbs, adjectives, adverbs, pronouns), spatial and numerical concepts ('in' 'on the left' 'find the middle car' 'some' 'four'), morphological inflections ('sleeps' 'painter') and syntactic structures (passive sentences, question forms, conditional clauses). TACL was designed to test understanding of spoken vocabulary and grammar. In fact the inclusion of several abstract or inferential concepts ('alike' 'go!') and sentences requiring verbal reasoning ('find the one that is neither the ball nor the table', 'look at the third picture, then point to the baby of this animal'), make its inclusion as a test of general language comprehension more appropriate.

This test was sometimes used as an alternative to the Reynell Scales at school entry (for example if the RDLS had been recently administered in a local clinic), but it was also sometimes used in addition to RDLS. There is a strong positive correlation of 0.7 between raw scores for 55 children who performed both tests.

Seventy children were assessed with TACL but standard scores could be measured for only 24 because of the age ceiling. Equivalent ages were found for 67 children and the lag behind chronological age computed (Table 2.VII). The mean lag at entry was 20 months, with a standard deviation of 14.1 months.

Because of the small number of standard scores available for either the RDLS or TACL, the gap between chronological age and Reynell comprehension age (available for 97 children) will be used as the language measure of *general comprehension* in subsequent chapters.

Comprehension tests compared with evaluations
The results of these four assessments are remarkably similar. Only 4 to 10 per cent of children scored at or above chronological age, while between 38 and 45 per cent were at least two years behind chronological age. Such results do not support the view that SLI is a predominantly expressive disorder, with only a minority group also having difficulty with comprehension. Comprehension problems are a common feature of the severely handicapped Dawn House population. There are quite consistent results from scales which aim to assess different aspects of understanding. This opens up the question of whether comprehension deficiencies in vocabulary, grammar, concepts and reasoning co-occur, or whether they all relate to some other underlying skill. Formal assessments of this kind are fairly gross measures to apply to the subtle and complex skills of language. They do not take proper account of attention, listening skills, motivation or auditory memory. They are also administered in intrinsically unreal situations, being specifically devised to assess oral comprehension out of context.

When teachers and house-parents at Dawn House write reports for parents and local education authorities, they comment on the functional level of a child's understanding in the classroom and residential unit. These comments have been collated into four categories—good, qualified, poor and tangential (where 'qualified' indicates a weakness in some areas only, and 'tangential' indicates apparent understanding of the literal force of a remark, but not its underlying meaning—see Appendix 2.A). Using these staff reports as a basis, 47 children (30 per cent) had good functional comprehension, 55 (35 per cent) had problems in some areas ('qualified'), 48 (31 per cent) were poor, and six (4 per cent) tangential. These evaluations are relative to the school population, not a normal one. Figures 2.2 to 2.5 compare staff evaluations with the results of formal assessments, at school entry. Children categorised as 'tangential' have been subsumed into the poor comprehension group as their numbers were small, and this type of comprehension error is very damaging to communication. Chi-squares were used to compare staff evaluations of good, qualified or poor with measured age gaps of up to one year, one to two years, and over two years on formal tests with the following results:

vocabulary (N 127, chi-square 21.6, df 4, p = 0.0002)
RDLS comprehension (N 97, chi-square 21.2, df 4, p = 0.0003)

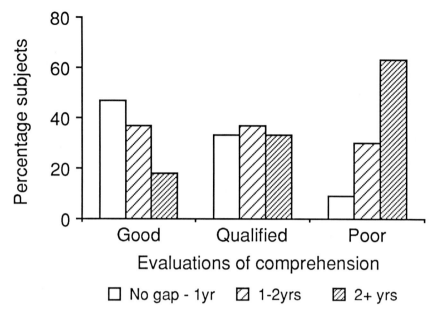

Fig. 2.2. Vocabulary age lag at entry and staff evaluations.

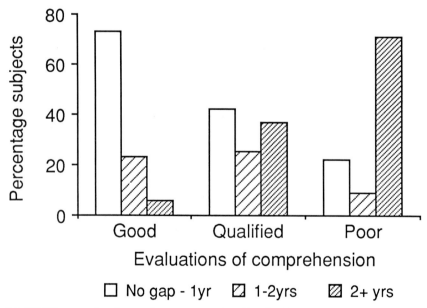

Fig. 2.3. TROG comprehension age lag at entry and staff evaluations.

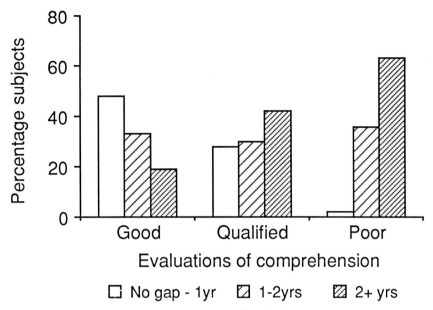

Fig. 2.4. RDLS comprehension age lag at entry and staff evaluations.

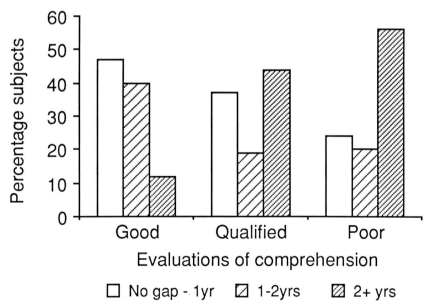

Fig. 2.5. TACL comprehension age lag at entry and staff evaluations.

19

TROG (N 93, chi-square 23, df 4, p = 0.0001)

TACL (N 67, chi-square 6.8, df 4, NS)

There is a good measure of agreement between the formal measures and functional performance judged in real situations. In particular the test of grammatical comprehension (TROG) and the general measure (RDLS) seem to reflect the difficulties noted by staff in communicating with the children.

In summary, at least two thirds of children with SLI coming to Dawn House have marked comprehension problems which adversely affect their functional communication. All measured aspects of comprehension are affected, and to similar degrees. The disability measured by the tests equates with the difficulties noted by staff, providing some sort of validity for formal and informal assessment procedures.

Expressive language

The production of language depends upon the possession and co-ordination of a number of skills, not all of them linguistic. The linguistic skills include the ability to represent the world symbolically using words, the development of concepts wherein one word (such as 'container' or 'book') refers to a cluster of features and can therefore represent innumerable objects or ideas, the relationships of words to each other (*e.g.* 'bird' subsumes 'duck', 'large' excludes 'tiny'), the ability to string words together meaningfully and grammatically, the ability to inflect words to change their grammatical value (*e.g.* past tense and plural forms), and the use of language which is contextually relevant and socially appropriate. Most assessments deal with those skills which can be measured most easily, rather than with those which are most important to communication, although currently (1991) there are some preliminary attempts to measure communication value in a more systematic way, and to profile the interrelationship of linguistic skills. Our assessments dating from the 1970s are limited to the measurement of vocabulary, grammar (syntax and morphology), and content.

Expressive vocabulary

WORD-FINDING VOCABULARY SCALE

The Renfrew Word-Finding Vocabulary Scale (WFVS) is one of a series of early assessments devised by a speech therapist in the 1960s, when almost no formal and standardised measures were available to assess developmental speech and language difficulties (Renfrew 1972). The stated purpose of the test is to assess word-finding, that is the child's ability to produce the correct word label when given an appropriate stimulus. The age range of the test is three to eight years. It consists of 59 line-drawings of objects, which are presented to the child to name individually. Speechless children who use a manual sign system can sign their responses. The words range from simple and common objects such as 'cup' and 'table', to rarer words such as 'hinge' and 'castor'. Errors can be separated into those resulting from failure to recognise the picture or object, and those resulting from inability to

TABLE 2.VIII				TABLE 2.IX		
Expressive vocabulary age lag at first assessment				Age lag in content (Bus Story) at entry		

Gap (Age minus vocabulary age)	N	%	Gap	N	%
			No gap	1	1
No gap	6	4	Up to 1 yr	4	5
Up to 1 yr	22	16	1–2 yrs	8	10
1–2 yrs	46	34	Over 2 yrs	67	84
Over 2 yrs	61	45	Total 80		100
Total 135		100			

Age range 5.4–12.11. Mean lag was 2.1 yrs with a standard deviation of 16 mths

Age range 5.5–12.10. Mean lag was 3.5 yrs with a standard deviation of 18 mths

produce the correct name. Renfrew considered that a high number of the second type of error, and increased response latency, indicated a specific word-finding difficulty. It is not always possible to make this distinction with the Dawn House children, who sometimes have insufficient language to indicate knowledge of the function of an object, so for all children both types of error were totalled together. For this reason, and also because there is no indication whether or not the selected words are part of the child's receptive vocabulary, we consider this test to be a measure of expressive vocabulary, and not specifically of word-finding ability within our population. There are no standard scores for the Word-Finding Test but it is possible to establish age equivalence. Of the 146 children assessed at entry, 135 scored within the age range of the test. The lag of expressive vocabulary age behind chronological age is shown in Table 2.VIII. The mean age lag at entry was 2.1 years, with a standard deviation of 16 months. The gap between chronological age and Renfrew word-finding age will be used as the measure of *expressive vocabulary* in subsequent chapters.

Content
BUS STORY TEST
Another test devised by Catherine Renfrew is concerned with the amount of relevant information that a child can relay to a listener. The Bus Story Test (Renfrew 1969) consists of a short story which is read aloud by the examiner to the child while s/he follows the events in comic-strip form. The child then uses the picture strip to retell the story, which is tape-recorded, transcribed and scored. Relevant details of the story are not all recoverable from the pictures but rely on an understanding of the spoken text. More points are awarded for items of information which carry the narrative forward than for those which enumerate details. The score is totalled and used to produce an information age within the age range of the test, three to eight years. Although this test does measure the child's ability to offer relevant information, it also depends upon a number of other abilities being intact, including listening, understanding of grammar, co-ordination

of visual and auditory input, memory, sentence formulation and narrative coherence. It is not surprising that the Dawn House children find this test and related tasks (more age-appropriate material is used with older children) very difficult. The broad nature of skills required may mean that the story-retelling paradigm is a better probe of language impairment than more narrowly specific measures. Bishop and Edmundson (1987*a*) certainly found that the Bus Story was the single best test to predict whether language impairment in four-year-olds was persistent or transient.

An information age lag behind chronological age could be computed for 80 of the 117 Dawn House children who were assessed with the Bus Story. These results are shown in Table 2.IX. The mean age lag at first assessment for these 80 subjects was 3.5 years, with a standard deviation of 18 months. This age gap will be used as the measure of *content* in language production in ensuing analyses.

Grammar

LARSP

The most commonly used assessment of grammatical abilities at Dawn House is LARSP, the Language Assessment and Remediation Screening Procedure (LARSP) (Crystal *et al.* 1976). This is not a test producing raw and standard scores, although it can be used to indicate developmental levels in a general way. Rather it sets out to describe the patterns of grammatical structures employed by any individual and, by comparing these with a profile of normal grammatical development, to pinpoint strengths and weaknesses which can then be used as a basis for remediation. The process has been evolving since 1970 with the most recent amendments prior to this study being produced in 1981. The procedure consists of a half-hour tape-recording of the child communicating in one or more situations which are made as spontaneous and natural as possible. This recording is transcribed and then grammatically analysed. The analysis is recorded on a profile chart which is preprinted with the clause, phrase and word developments which may be expected of normal children between the ages of one and five years, divided into seven stages of development. A prototype chart was in use at Dawn House prior to publication of the profile chart in 1976. Stages I to IV correspond approximately to the ability to produce structures (sentences or phrases) of one to four words, and last until about the age of 3.0 in normal development. Stage V marks the beginning of recursion—that is the use of more than one clause in complex sentences—which normally occurs between the ages of 3.0 and 3.6. Stage VI is the system completion period, developmentally occurring from 3.6 to 4.6, when residual errors are eradicated in such syntactic systems as pronouns, irregular verbs and determiners; and Stage VII is characterised for normal children of 4.6 and over by developments in linguistic style and skills in discourse. Word-level development (*e.g.* plural forms, comparative forms, tense markers) is charted from Stage II to Stage V. Eleven of the sample were not profiled at entry, three of these had insufficient language to analyse and eight had no, or very minor, problems with language

TABLE 2.X

Clause and phrase development stages (LARSP) at first assessment

	LARSP stage		Children tested	
	Clause	Phrase	N	%
Group 1. Competent				
	VII		12	8
	VI		31	21
			43	29
Group 2. Productive				
	V	V	13	9
	V	IV	19	13
	V	III	3	2
	V	II	1	1
	IV	V	3	2
			39	27
Group 3. Limited				
	IV	IV	20	14
	IV	III	9	6
	III	IV	5	3
			34	23
Group 4. Basic				
	III	III	12	8
	III	II	6	4
	II	III	1	1
	II	II	5	3
	II	I	1	1
	I	II	3	2
	I	I	1	1
			29	20
		Total	145	100

structure. The speech of 30 children was too unintelligible to permit accurate transcription of spontaneous language, so these children were administered an imitated version of LARSP, developed at Dawn House and tried out with local nursery children. In the imitated version, children are asked to repeat examples of every structure on the profile chart. Because they are unable to repeat structures beyond their productive capacity, a reasonable approximation of their LARSP level can be obtained.

Profiling has an advantage over tests which are scored for the presence or absence of selected features, because it enables individual patterns of language use to be detected. Thus not only can the developmental level of SLI children be estimated, but their idiosyncratic language behaviour can be examined and individual remedial programmes planned. Interpretation of the profile is a very important part of the LARSP process, and Crystal (1979) demonstrated how pattern analysis could be used to plot the most potentially effective remedial path. Our study also demonstrates the disadvantage of profiling, with 145 children having 145 different results! By imposing some rather arbitrary parameters, we have been able to sort the children into groups which have some clinical validity. Each stage of

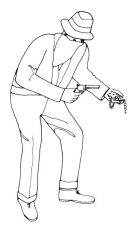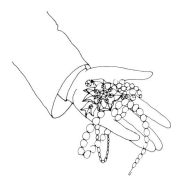

Fig. 2.6. From the Grammatic Closure subtest of the ITPA.

clause and phrase development has a number of syntactic structures listed, which are expected to emerge at this stage. Appendix 2.B gives the criteria by which children were deemed to have entered each stage. Four groups have been derived from the clause and phrase levels, and these are clinically interpreted as important stages of syntactic advance (Table 2.X). Group 1 (N 43) are reasonably competent language users with some minor structural and morphological errors. Group 2 (N 39) are still acquiring basic structural rules but have reached the important stage of clause connection, giving them productive flexibility. Group 3 (N 34) can string words together in the correct order and meaningfully, but are very limited in their ability to express themselves; and Group 4 (N 29) are at a basic and inadequate level of language structure. These LARSP groupings will constitute the measure of productive language *structure* in subsequent analyses.

ITPA GRAMMATIC CLOSURE

The Illinois Test of Psycholinguistic Abilities (ITPA) (Kirk *et al.* 1968) was designed to assess a variety of skills and abilities thought to underlie proficient language. One of its 12 subtests, Grammatic Closure, deals mainly with the ability to use word inflections according to grammatical rules, the linguistic term for which is morphology. It tests knowledge of regular and irregular forms of nouns, verbs, adjectives, pronouns, and prepositions. There are 33 items. For each item the examiner shows the child pictures and describes them in two sentences, the second of which is left for the child to complete using the grammatically appropriate word: *e.g.* 'Here is a child. Here are three ———' (children). 'The thief is stealing the jewels. These are the jewels that he ———' (stole) (Fig. 2.6). The ITPA has been standardised on children aged 2.8 to 10.3. Each subtest has a mean of 36 and a standard deviation of 6. Age equivalents and scaled scores can be computed. Whereas LARSP charts the word inflections *selected* for use by a child, the ITPA Grammatic Closure demonstrates his or her abillity to produce the correct

24

TABLE 2.XI				TABLE 2.XII			
ITPA Grammatic Closure scaled scores at first assessment				Grammatic closure age lag at first assessment			
SD	*N*	*%*		*Gap*		*N*	*%*
+1SD or above	1	1		No gap		4	4
−1 to +1	20	21		Up to 1 yr		19	18
−1 to −2	20	21		1–2 yrs		24	23
−2 to −3	17	18		Over 2 yrs		57	55
Below −3	39	40			Total	104	100
Total	97	100					

Mean lag was 2.5 yrs with a standard deviation of 19 mths

inflection in a compulsory context. Mastery of such skills is not expected until the child reaches LARSP Stage VI, although some inflections are used from Stage II onwards. The Grammatic Closure scaled scores for 97 children and age lags for 104 children are presented in Tables 2.XI and 2.XII. Mean age lag at the first assessment was 2.5 years, with a standard deviation of 19 months. The Grammatic Closure scaled scores will provide the language measure of *morphology* in later statistical analyses.

The three aspects of expressive language which were measured are positively correlated. Using raw scores and Spearman's rho, correlation coefficients were 0.6 between vocabulary and content (N 113, $p<0.001$), 0.3 between vocabulary and grammar (N 99, $p=0.004$) and 0.5 between content and grammar (N 78, $p<0.001$).

Discussion of language production test results
Probably the classic presenting feature of SLI is abnormal and impoverished oral expression. It is therefore to be expected that children selected for special education because of SLI will have severe problems with every aspect of expressive language: inadequate vocabulary, halting limited sentence structure and general impoverishment of content. For many Dawn House pupils this is the area of greatest handicap, but smaller numbers of children admitted because of major problems of comprehension or speech production almost without exception have additional problems in this area. The extent of their expressive language disabilities goes beyond those presented here and interacts with problems in other linguistic and cognitive domains. This is exemplified to some extent by the very poor results obtained for the Bus Story Test, which relies on the co-ordination of language abilities, and in which over 80 per cent of pupils tested lagged more than two years behind chronological age. Although there were individual patterns of strengths and weaknesses, on the whole expressive disabilities in one area were echoed by poor performance in another. We did not find that an inability to form sentences might mask a good vocabulary, or that pupils could give a high level of information in spite of ungrammatical sentences. The most disabled children expressively were likely to be disabled in every expressive function.

The structural patterns revealed by the LARSP analysis are informative. Half of the 102 children who are still developing language structure (our Groups 2 to 4) show an unbalanced profile with either a clause or a phrase bias. Both of these patterns are described as common in language-disordered children by Crystal *et al.* (1976) with the phrase level bias being the most common pattern of language delay. In the Dawn House sample, 39 (77 per cent) of the 51 children who showed an unbalanced profile were biased in the other direction, with clause level development ahead of phrase and word level. In practice this indicates the prevalence of the kind of language sometimes described as 'telegraphic', in which each element of clause structure (subject, verb, object, adverb) is represented by a single word and not developed into phrases, *e.g.* 'boy get present Christmas' instead of 'that boy will get some nice presents at Christmas'. Given that there are severe limitations both in the numbers of words available and in the knowledge of how to connect them, and that there is also a deficient ability to hold and sequence ideas mentally, then adoption of this language pattern can be seen as an efficient and intelligent use of limited resources to convey the main items of information. The four groups which we have labelled *competent, productive, basic,* and *limited,* are based on level rather than balance, and have been so divided because they seem to represent definite stages of structural expansion. They will be referred to again in the discussion of subgroups of language impairment at the end of this chapter.

To summarise the pattern of expressive language difficulties (excluding phonological problems) at school entry—any language impairment normally includes expressive deficit. Many children who were referred to Dawn House predominantly because of comprehension problems or phonological problems, demonstrated expressive difficulties on assessment. Of 154 children who were able to participate in assessments of expressive oral or manually signed language, only four showed no deficit in the functions that were tested. A further 10 had minor problems in one aspect of expressive language only.

The degree of impairment in one expressive function was usually repeated in other areas, so that profiles of expressive functions are relatively flat.

More difficult tasks such as story retelling, which require the co-ordination of language skills, may be useful screening devices.

Speech
Over 95 per cent of Dawn House pupils have abnormal-sounding speech which ranges from the use of a few immature speech sounds to complete unintelligibility. For strangers, unusual sounding speech is often the first indication that the child has a problem, and the children themselves frequently regard their disordered speech as the major and most distressing feature of their impairment. Just as SLI itself has been recognised to be heterogeneous and multicausal, so the patterns of speech abnormality are known to vary considerably relative to a number of factors, principally aetiology.

Since the spoken word is the end-product of the process of communication, it can be affected at any stage from thought to utterance. Deficient knowledge of the systemic *rules* by which speech sounds have particular qualities, both intrinsically and in relation to each other, and inability to apply these rules to the production of single or sequenced words, are considered to be disorders of language rather than speech. Such disorders are currently termed *phonological disabilities*, or more properly *language impairment at the phonological level*. Before the 1970s these conditions were frequently termed *dyslalia* or *functional articulation disorders*. Currently *articulation disorder* is a term only applied when the problem is one of speech production and not of the linguistic system which underlies speech. Structural abnormalities of the vocal tract such as cleft palate, and pathology of the central or peripheral nervous system, can cause articulation disorders. In this study, *speech disorders* include both phonological and articulatory impairments.

Disorders of phonology and articulation sometimes co-exist and may interact. Children at Dawn House are assessed in order to estimate the contribution of each to impaired speech pronunciation. Articulation is assessed by reference to the medical and neurological history, by examination of the structure and function of the articulatory organs, and by consideration of the child's ability to produce the sounds of speech singly, in sequences and while speaking. Assessments of phonology examine the patterns of speech sounds in communicative use. They provide information which is not established by articulation tests, concerning the possibility of perceptual mismatch (see also Chapter 5), the limitations of the child's working phonological system and his or her productive immaturity. Phonological assessments have become part of normal clinical practice only during the last decade. Prior to that the assessments of speech disorders were really tests of articulation, although some phonological and developmental information could be derived from them.

Edinburgh Articulation Test
The test in general use at Dawn House since 1974 has been the Edinburgh Articulation Test (EAT) (Anthony *et al.* 1971). The EAT is a test of single word production, standardised on 500 normal Scottish children aged from three to six years. A selected sample of speech consonants and consonant clusters is elicited, in varying syllable positions, in a picture-naming task. As well as producing a standard score (for children younger than 6.0) and an articulation age, the EAT provides useful qualitative information by analysing the production errors and assigning a developmental level (almost mature, very immature, *etc.*) or an *atypical* categorisation of them. A total of 152 children were tested at entry, but one of these children had no atypical score recorded. Of the four children who were not tested, two had no speech and two had normal sounding speech.

Neither the standard score nor the articulation age are useful measures for the Dawn House children, most of whom (63 per cent) enter school with articulation performance below the three-year floor of the test. Instead we have divided the raw scores into four bands with cut-off points—out of a total possible raw score of

TABLE 2.XIII

TABLE 2.XIII

EAT raw scores by age at first assessment

Age	Over 50		34–50		16–33		Under 16		Total	
	N	%	N	%	N	%	N	%	N	%
5.0–6.11	4	9	9	21	11	26	19	44	43	100
7.0–8.11	11	16	11	16	27	39	20	29	69	100
9 yrs and over	12	30	10	25	8	20	10	25	40	100
Total	27	18	30	20	46	30	49	32	152	100

TABLE 2.XIV

EAT mean scores by age at first assessment

Age	N	Mean score	SD
5.0–5.11	13	17	14
6.0–6.11	30	27	17
7.0–7.11	35	25	18
8.0–8.11	34	30	17
9.0–9.11	31	34	20
10 yrs and over	9	37	19

Chi-square 12.6, df 6, $p < 0.05$

68—at 50, 34 and 16 (see Table 2.XIII). These scores have been selected because they approximate to levels of articulatory efficiency. Thus a child entering school with a score of 50 will generally be producing most single consonants with the exception of /r/ and /th/, and many but not all consonant clusters. This is the level of a normal child aged 4.6, considered by Anthony *et al.* (1971) to have reached 85 per cent articulation efficiency. The speech of such children sounds immature but is usually intelligible.

The next cut-off point of 34 is just above the three-year floor of the test. An example of a child attaining this score is one who has yet to develop /r/ and /th/ as above, and also the affricates /ch/ and /j/, the palato-alveolar /sh/ sound, and consonant clusters incorporating /s/ and /l/. At Dawn House a child who was developing speech normally but very late might have this kind of pattern and an EAT raw score in the 30s, although children with abnormal speech development can reach this level too. Speech would typically be intelligible in context but difficult to understand generally, although intelligibility would vary according to the individual child's particular phonological system and which sounds were used contrastively.

The final cut-off point of 16 was chosen after reflecting on the speech at school entry of the subjects, all of whom were known to both authors, as no developmental information below three years is supplied by Anthony *et al.* (1971). Children with scores below 16 were severely impaired and unintelligible. A child with a score around this level, but with normally developing speech, would probably be using only a few single sounds such as the lip sounds /p/ /b/ /m/ /f/ and /w/ and tongue-tip sounds such as /n/ /t/ and /d/, a level of development reached by

TABLE 2.XV

EAT atypical scores by age at first assessment

Age	Atypical 0–4		Atypical 5–21		Atypical 22–47		Total	
	N	%	N	%	N	%	N	%
5.0–6.11	6	14	18	42	19	44	43	100
7.0–8.11	20	29	27	39	22	32	69	100
9 yrs and over	16	41	12	31	11	28	39	100
Total	42	28	57	38	52	34	151	100

the normal child at about the age of 2.0 (Grunwell 1985). Many of the Dawn House children with scores of 16 or less had more abnormal patterns of speech production.

A basic question regarding the speech of language-impaired children is whether it is truly deviant or merely considerably delayed. In order to address this, it is important to consider the effect of age, and also the nature of the speech produced. The mean raw scores of the EAT by age are given in Table 2.XIV. There is a developmental improvement which just reaches significance (chi-square 12.6, df 6, $p<0.05$).

Deviance in speech production is indicated in a number of ways, including the use of non-English sounds, the use of sounds which do not occur in a particular context during normal phonological development, prosodic abnormality, phonotactic (word-structural) abnormality, idiosyncratic methods of signalling speech contrasts and an unbalanced development of any of these features. The first two of these deviations are counted in the *atypical* score of the EAT. Since there can be no developmental information about something essentially aberrant from normal development, the scores selected to indicate levels of abnormality have again been based on clinical assessment of children's difficulties. Sixty-five items can be graded *atypical* and the examiner, who must be a qualified phonetician, is allowed some flexibility in the interpretation of dialectal variations. The atypical score bands which best seem to demarcate impairment in the Dawn House population are 0 to 4, 5 to 21, and above. Numbers of subjects by age in each band are presented in Table 2.XV.

Only 28 per cent of the 151 children fell in the relatively normal 0 to 4 band. Although there is a decrease in atypical scores with age, it is not statistically significant. Mean scores for age are shown in Table 2.XVI.

In the battery of language measures used in the statistical analyses, the raw score of the EAT is used as a measure of speech *maturity*, and the atypical scale is used as a measure of *deviance*.

Dawn House Speech Assessment

The Dawn House Speech Assessment developed from the need to record more systematically some of the clinical observations which were routinely made, and from a desire to incorporate some of the new insights from linguistics into our practice. When it was produced by two therapists working at Dawn House, there

29

Fig. 2.7. Dawn House Speech Assessment.
Picture used to elicit the phoneme /t/.

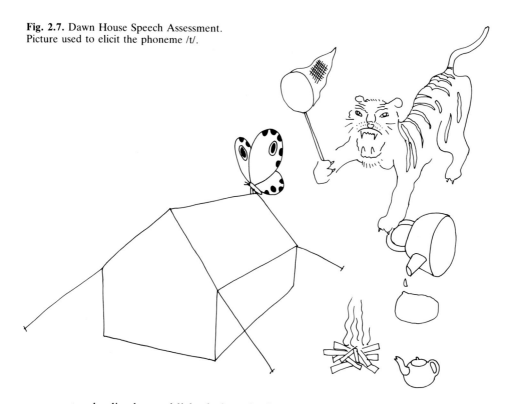

was no standardised or published phonological assessment available and the Dawn House assessment was intended to be an informal and flexible tool, used according to individual need as a basis for planning remediation. It seeks to examine a child's normal use of continuous speech in a natural context. This is done by presenting the child with 21 large composite pictures of amusing or bizarre events. The child is then invited to comment on the picture, and if possible to converse about it. Structure is imposed by the representation in each picture of objects and actions using a particular phoneme or set of consonant clusters, so that any description will include some use of the target phoneme (Fig. 2.7), but the child is not asked to name objects or repeat words and the conversation is maintained at a natural level. For example the picture used to elicit the speech sound /sh/ is of a train in a sta*ti*on. On the platform are an open box of *sh*oes and a box of fi*sh*. A man sits on the train roof fi*sh*ing from the box of fi*sh*. Behind a railway worker who is bru*sh*ing the train down with a large sweeping bru*sh*, some *sh*eep are walking on to the platform. Words which include the target phoneme together with the preceding and following word are transcribed with stress and intonation marking by the speech therapist from the taped recording and then analysed. The following information derived from the analysis is recorded:

(1) a phonetic inventory of all the sounds—consonants and vowels—used in any way during speech

30

TABLE 2.XVI			
EAT mean atypical scores at first assessment			
Age	N	Mean	SD
5.0–5.11	13	24	12
6.0–6.11	30	18	13
7.0–7.11	35	18	15
8.0–8.11	34	14	13
9.0–9.11	30	14	16
10 yrs and over	9	11	13

No significant difference

TABLE 2.XVII		
Range of place of articulation at first assessment		
	N	%
Uses all places of articulation	68	83
No velar or palatal	8	10
No apical or laminal	4	5
No apical, laminal or velar	2	2
Total	82	100

(2) phonotactic information about the structure of words (possible combinations of consonants and vowels)

(3) a contrastive assessment of what may be signalled by each sound used by the child in his or her individual phonological system, and

(4) a count of the phonological simplification processes operating.

Optionally information can be recorded concerning the structure and function of the articulators, the speed of articulation and any abnormalities of prosody or voice quality. Additional observations are made of children who appear to have problems with volitional motor programming for speech, for whom comparison between performance on this analysis of continuous speech and performance on a single word response task, such as the EAT described above, can be very illuminating. Finally speech therapists summarise the analysed and observed features of a child's speech pattern and list remedial aims and plans. From this information is derived an evaluation of the nature of the speech disability. The Dawn House assessment of speech yields descriptive information rather than test scores or developmental ages. Not all of this information can be summarised across groups, but some general observations can be made. Eighty-five pupils were given some part of the Dawn House speech assessment soon after entry.

Phonetic inventory

The inventory is essentially a list of all the sounds the child uses for speech: consonant and vowel, normal and abnormal, appropriate or inappropriate (in adult terms). Thus if 'cigarette' is pronounced 'tidi', the three sound /t/ /d/ and /i/ are added to the phonetic inventory. The information derived from the phonetic inventory is not phonological, but phonetic, *i.e.* it lists the sounds that can be produced and are used without reference to their function. Any difficulty with a particular *place* of articulation (*e.g.* labial, velar) or *manner* of articulation (*e.g.* plosive, fricative) is apparent from consideration of the phonetic inventory. It provides valuable information about the nature of the speech difficulty and about motor ability. Table 2.XVII presents information about the range of possible place of articulation, including labial and labio-dental (p,b,m,f,v), apical and laminal (t,d,l,n,s,z,sh,ch,dg) and velar and palatal (k,g,ng,y).

31

TABLE 2.XVIII
Range of manner of articulation at first assessment

	N	%
Uses nasals fricatives, plosives, approximants	71	88
No fricatives, approximants	3	4
No fricatives	1	1
No approximants	2	2
Other	4	5
Total	81	100

TABLE 2.XIX
Phonotactic structure at first assessment

	N	%
Using more than 1 C, final C and clusters	42	54
No clusters	15	19
No initial clusters	11	14
No final C or clusters	2	3
Other	8	10
Total	78	100

C=any consonant

Table 2.XVIII presents information about the same speech sounds categorised according to manner of articulation. The categories included here are nasal (m,n,ng), plosive (p,b,t,d,k,g), fricative (f,v,th,s,z,sh) and approximant (w,y). Our interest was in whether some language-impaired children would have a complete inability to use particular articulatory modes or positions. Ability was credited if a child produced four tokens of two types in any category. Thus, a comment such as 'uses all places of articulation' does not necessarily indicate an intelligible speaker, but merely one who is capable of making some labial, alveolar and velar sounds.

Relatively few children had complete articulatory lacunae. Seventeen per cent had failed to develop use of one or more places of articulation, and 12 per cent lacked one or more articulatory modes.

Phonotactic structure
Further information can be derived from a consideration of phonotactic structure. If consonants and vowels are considered to be the two basic building blocks of syllables, phonotactics is concerned with the possible sequences of these blocks in the spoken output. In English the longest possible sequence in one syllable is cccvcccc (as in some pronounciations of *strengths*). We noted use of syllable-final consonants (u*p*), two consonants in one syllable ('ca*t*'), and two consonant clusters initially ('*bl*ue') or finally ('te*nt*'). The consonants and vowels do not have to be accurately realised. Phonotactic limitations can result from motor or kinaesthetic problems, but may also be symptomatic of perceptual or linguistic impairment. Table 2.XIX shows the phonotactic limitations observed in children at first

assessment. In all cases the absence of a particular feature means that it did not occur during a sample of approximately half an hour, which is very unlikely in an unimpaired child.

Contrastive assessment
The relationship of the sound system used by the child to the target adult system is analysed in the contrastive analysis. A child who describes 'two cups of coffee' as 'two tup ob tossee' has a phonological system in which /t/ may represent /t/ or /k/; /b/ may represent /v/ word finally and preceding /t/; and /s/ may represent /f/ between vowels. This potentially most useful part of the assessment does not lend itself easily to conversion to numerical data for research purposes. Since the children are encouraged to talk naturally about the drawings, making comments at their own level of competence and interest, the amount and quality of available data are very variable. This allows the therapist to explore individual systems and plan specific intervention, but does not permit clear comparisons between children, as we cannot use any recognised research measure such as percentage of correctly realised targets (Shriberg *et al.* 1986). Various attempts to compute a level of achievement in the contrastive system failed to produce meaningful grades of ability and were abandoned. No further reference is made to this part of the assessment.

Phonological simplification processes
Both normal and impaired children acquire speech gradually and in a systematic manner. As perceptual and motor capabilities develop, skills in one have to be married to skills in the other, so that the child steadily acquires phonological and articulatory prowess. Unlike the apocryphal child who, when asked why he had suddenly begun speaking in full sentences after four years of silence, replied that he had never had anything interesting to say before, real children will communicate by whatever means are at their command, and simplify the structure of words and sentences to the level of their competence. These simplifications, which have been described and categorised by a number of linguists (Ingram 1976, 1981; Abberton 1980; Grunwell 1982) affect whole classes of sounds and the structure of words. This approach has changed our understanding of speech development from a process of acquiring individual sounds, to one in which general systemic phonological abilities are acquired. As the child becomes more able, perceptually, motorially or both, the simplification processes cease to operate. Developmental norms have been proposed for this progression, particularly by Grunwell (1981, 1985).

The phonological simplification processes noted in the Dawn House Speech Assessment are listed in Table 2.XX with the numbers of children in whom they were found to be operating. An explanation of the terms is given in Appendix 2.C. They are listed in approximately developmental order (Grunwell 1975, Ingram 1976), that is to say that reduplication (of syllables) is a very early process normally

TABLE 2.XX

Phonological simplification processes operating at first assessment

Process	Children	
	N	%
Reduplication	11	16
Final consonant deletion	20	29*
Neutralisation of vowels	7	10
Diphthong reduction	13	19
Glottalisation final consonant	35	51
Consonant harmony	22	32**
Stopping	42	61*
Palatalling of velars	6	9
Fronting of velars	29	42*
Weak syllable deletion	31	45*
Confusion of liquids and glides	40	58*
Context-sensitive voicing	24	35
Cluster reduction	62	90*
Fronting—palatal, alveolar, dental	24	35†
Lengthening and epenthesis	4	6
Metathesis	3	4
Idiosyncratic processes	34	49
Rule-free variation	21	30
Total	69	100

*One of 8 sound processes responsible for 90% of errors in Shriberg *et al.*
(1986)
**Shriberg's category of assimilation is wider than this
†Shriberg uses the smaller category of palatal fronting only

ceasing in babies around 15 to 18 months ('bibi' for 'biscuit', 'popo' for 'potty') whereas cluster reduction ('bed' for 'bread', 'top' for 'stop') may be a normal feature of the speech of three- and four-year-olds. All processes may persist very much longer in retarded or disordered speech development, and there may be some additional and unusual processes operating. In the Dawn House assessment a process is counted as operative if the therapist records two or more occurrences during the assessment. Grading children according to number of simplification processes is not meaningful for similar reasons to those given for the omission of the contrastive analysis, but it is possible to consider the over-all balance of processes operating.

Discussion of results of speech articulation and phonology
Although children were referred to Dawn House with a variety of language problems, not always thought to include problems of speech, none of the children assessed at entry to school had mature phonology (although it is possible that two of the four unassessed children did). Children with SLI all had some impairment at the phonological level. Since language-impaired children are known to be delayed in their acquisition of speech, and since many also have slow motor development, could they be following the normal route to speech at a slower rate? There was a significant effect of age on the raw scores of the EAT with particularly low scores

from the 13 five-year-olds. However, if the five-year-olds are excluded from the analysis, age is no longer significant. Nor is age a significant factor in the number of atypical realisations scored on the EAT. Although low atypical scores are more likely to be found in the older group (chi-square 7.5, df 2, p<0.05), high atypical scores of 22 and more are fairly evenly distributed with no age effect. The higher scores of the younger children may not be truly atypical at all. Anthony *et al.* (1971) suggested that as there is no information for children at a speech developmental stage below three years, many of the utterances they have classified as atypical may merely indicate extreme retardation.

The phonetic inventory of our in-house assessment was scanned for evidence of deviant speech patterns. Over 80 per cent of children assessed were able to produce a wide range of manners and places of articulation. The greatest single difficulty was with the production of velar and palatal sounds, which were absent in 10 per cent of those assessed. This is abnormal in children over the age of 2.6. Rather more children had a problem with phonotactics, about a third of them having a problem with sequencing consonants, a skill normally achieved between 3.6 and 4.6. These difficulties in children of 9.0 and 10.0 must be considered deviant.

The same mixture of extreme delay and abnormality is suggested by the phonological simplification processes which are still operating. Shriberg *et al.* (1986) concluded that eight such processes were responsible for 90 per cent of the errors in the speech of both normally developing and speech-delayed children of three years and above. These processes (marked with an asterisk in Table 2.XX) all occur quite frequently in the speech of Dawn House entrants but there are also many unclassified patterns which have been included as *idiosyncratic processes* and other variants which do not appear to conform to any rules (see Appendix 2.C).

Language impairment at any linguistic level affects phonology. In the youngest children, the picture is one of extreme retardation of speech development. A different pattern emerges with children over six years of age, and it becomes clear that for some children speech is deviant as well as severely delayed. The characteristics of children with persisting abnormalities of speech will be explored further in Chapter 7.

Comment on oral language tests
A major problem in this study, as in others which attempt to encompass a wide age range, is the limitation of current instruments for measuring different aspects of language. Many language tests are standardised on different populations, on small numbers of children or not at all. No common model of language informs the assessment procedures. Many problems are known to exist among the older children, but because of the low age ceilings of most tests, they cannot be quantified: nor can rates of progress be reported beyond a fairly low level. At the other end of the scale, there is a need for tests to have lower floors which would help to identify the balance of relative strengths and deficits in the most severely

impaired children. The availability of improved, professionalised tools of measurement would greatly enhance the value of future investigations.

Language measures

In subsequent chapters we shall be examining a range of speech and language functions in relation to antecedent, developmental, auditory perceptual and cognitive factors. The tests and the scores derived from them are described fully below. Here, they are briefly summarised under headings which are used in all analyses which include 'language measures'.

COMPREHENSION

Vocabulary—standard score on English Picture Vocabulary test (EPVT) or British Picture Vocabulary Scale (BPVS)

Grammar—z-scores on the Test for Reception of Grammar (TROG)

General—gap between chronological and Reynell Developmental Language Scale (RDLS) Comprehension ages

LANGUAGE PRODUCTION

Vocabulary—gap between chronological and Word-Finding Vocabulary Scale (WFVS) ages

Structure—clause/phrase group of LARSP

Morphology—ITPA Grammatic Closure standard score

Content—gap between chronological and Renfrew Bus Story ages

SPEECH

Maturity—Edinburgh Articulation Test (EAT) raw score

Deviance—EAT atypical score

WRITTEN LANGUAGE

Reading—reading age at entry.

Of the 30 children who were non-readers at entry, those aged six years and above (18 children) have been given a nominal reading age of 60 months.

Written language at entry

Reading

When children learn to read, they learn how to transform a visually displayed code into the language which it represents. They must be able to recognise and remember visual patterns including letters, strings of letters, syllables and words, and the punctuation marks which symbolise spoken language. The symbols are based on the sounds which make up speech. The correspondence between sounds and letters is a loose one, encompassing irregularities and exceptions as well as alternatives (*e.g.* the sound *k* may be represented by *c,k,ck* or *ch*). Rules govern many of the phonographical pairs. Although visually displayed, reading is essentially a linguistic skill which demands much more than the mere decoding of visual pattern to oral word, although this is a crucial skill especially in the early stages of learning. To read is to comprehend the messages and ideas conveyed by the text. This requires a knowledge of the vocabulary, concepts and syntax of the language which has been coded. Young children use their knowledge of semantics to deduce from contextual clues words which they do not recognise immediately or are unable phonically to decode, and also draw unconsciously upon their own understanding and use of syntax to find the most probable class of word, *e.g.* noun, verb or adjective (Beardsley 1982, Murray and Maliphant 1982, Potter 1982). When learning letter/sound associations, children must be able to perceive sounds sufficiently accurately to form an auditory image which approximates the adult form, and be able to recall this. It helps if the auditory feedback from their own production of the sound corresponds to and reinforces the desired target. Children need phonological awareness, at first implicit and later explicit, to understand that words can be broken down into their constituent syllables and phonetic units, and also that these units can be blended together to reconstitute the whole word.

We have seen above that there are widespread deficits in a broad range of articulatory, phonological and language functions in groups of children and in individual children. It is hardly surprising then that children with speech and language disorders should find learning to read so inordinately difficult (Morley 1965, Griffiths 1969, Hall and Tomblin 1978, Fundudis *et al.* 1979, Levi *et al.* 1982, Aram *et al.* 1984, Stark *et al.* 1984).

Reading levels at Dawn House
As one aspect of language, information about reading was evaluated along with information on speech and language when children were considered for admission. Levels of reading did not themselves determine admission but severe reading difficulties (not uncommon among older applicants) increased the urgency for admission. A few children were admitted with speech and/or language disorders which were less handicapping educationally than the immense difficulties they had experienced in trying to acquire written language skills.

The school has established a programme of regular testing. The first examination, by the remedial teacher or the educational psychologist, is part of the initial assessment procedure and takes place shortly after a child's admission. This establishes whether a child can read at all and at what level. Some of the skills and subskills used in reading are also explored. Thereafter the class teacher administers a standardised test twice a year as an approximate measure of progress. Since the school aims to return as many children as possible to mainstream schools, it is important to know how children compare with others of similar age, so that appropriate recommendations can be made about future schooling and about further help after they leave.

Most tests fall into one of two categories: word recognition tests, comprising lists of words which yield a measure of mechanical decoding ability, and tests involving an understanding of single sentences or longer prose passages. The results are expressed in centiles or, more commonly, in reading ages. The reading age into which a raw score is transformed corresponds to the average level of a child of that age. Like reading schemes, reading tests assume normal language development. A test was needed that would not unduly penalise the SLI child and which would avoid problems of scoring because of unintelligible speech. Most entrants were below nine years of age and not expected to be much beyond the stage of acquiring a sight vocabulary. A low test floor was required. Since regular retesting was intended, a test with parallel forms was thought to be advantageous.

The Southgate Group Reading Tests 1 and 2 (Southgate 1976) met the most important requirements. In Test 1, the Word Selection Test, the child responds not verbally but by circling the word believed to correspond to the word spoken by the tester. Each of its 30 words is embedded in a shortlist of five, each list being enclosed in a separate box. Sixteen of these are accompanied by a simple outline drawing of the target word. The test was intended for average children aged between six and 7½ years, and for backward readers up to 14 years. Reading ages range from 5.9 to 7.9. Although designed as a group test, we administer it individually.

Test 2, the Sentence Completion Test, is used when a reading age of about 7½ years is reached. The reading ages range from 7.0 to 9.7 years, by which level the basic reading skills are expected to have been acquired. No oral response is called for. The test comprises 42 sentences, each of which ends in five underlined words. One of these correctly completes a sentence such as 'Daddy is a ———— (boy, girl, mat, woman, man)'. The child has to read and understand the sentence, then circle the correct word. There are two parallel forms.

Sixteen of the children for whom a reading age could be obtained (generally older and possibly competent readers) had been given either Schonell's Graded Word Reading Test (Schonell and Schonell 1970) or Burt's Word Reading Test, 1974 Revision (Scottish Council for Research in Education 1976) with ceilings of 15 and 12 years respectively. Each is a word reading test and employs the traditional procedure whereby a child utters each word. Reading ages on all tests have been combined in the results presented below.

A child's reading ability in relation to age has been evaluated by subtracting reading from chronological age. This is unsatisfactory when the aim is to select children who are retarded in reading from a normal population, since on the whole the bright child learns faster and the dull child more slowly. To overcome problems of age and IQ bias, a child's reading age can be evaluated by comparison with a prediction derived from a regression equation calculated from age, IQ and reading age. In this study the aim is not to select those who have reading difficulties. Indeed, our exceptions are the children who read reasonably well. Chapter 6 explores relationships between reading and other language variables and IQ, verbal and performance. The IQ will be considered as only one of several possible contributory or associated factors.

TABLE 2.XXI

Reading age at entry of 156 children aged 5.4 to 12.10

Age (yrs)	Non-readers N	Reading age				Total N
		≤6.11 N	7–7.11 N	8–8.11 N	≥9 yrs N	
5	12	3	1			16
6	11	18	3			32
7	5	16	5			26
8	2	29	12	2		45
9		14	12	3	1	30
10		3	2			5
12			1		1	2
Total	30	83	36	5	2	156

TABLE 2.XXII

Difference between reading and chronological ages (CA-RA) 126 children aged 5.9 to 12.10

Age (yrs)	Difference				Total
	≥CA	<2 yrs	2–2.11	≥3 yrs	
5	4				4
6	8	13			21
7	3	17	1		21
8		32	9	2	43
9	1	10	12	7	30
10			2	3	5
12			1	1	2
Total	16	72	25	13	126

Results

Thirty children were unable to read at all (non-readers). Reading age is generally linked to age and most of the 30 non-readers (77 per cent) were under seven years of age. Reading ages between 5.1 and 11.4 were obtained for 126 children aged 5.4 to 12.10 (Table 2.XXI).

All but 16 children were reading below age level (Table 2.XXII). Differences between reading and chronological ages ranged from 67 to −20 months, a negative value representing a higher reading than chronological age. Children of five or six years are almost evenly divided between those who were reading at or above age and those who had not reached age level. At seven years and above, the proportion of children reading at age level decreases sharply while the difference between reading and chronological age increases. The most severely retarded reader was a girl of 12.10 with a reading age of 7.3.

The greater frequency of differences of two years and more among children of nine years and over is due at least partly to age itself. A gap of two years or more is not possible until a child reaches an age of between seven and eight. Moreover, gaps tend to widen with age. Every year, to keep pace with their increasing age, children must also increase their reading skills by one year. The child of eight years with a reading age of six has acquired one year's skill in three years at school. Even if the pace of learning subsequently doubles, itself quite a feat, the gap between age and reading age inexorably widens.

Initially most children, including our pupils, learn and are taught by a whole-word method, whereby a printed word is linked to its verbal counterpart. A sight vocabulary is built up. There is evidence that at this stage a child may go straight from the visual pattern of a word to its meaning (Barron and Baron 1977). The visual pattern which is recognised may not be the whole word but some of its elements, letters, or features such as shape and length. When reading prose, unknown words are guessed from context, and syntactic cues take precedence over semantic ones (Murray and Maliphant 1982). There need be little explicit awareness of the sound structure of words at this stage. Guesses are unlikely to bear a phonological relation to the unknown word (Marsh *et al.* 1980). While acquiring a sight vocabulary, children are introduced to individual letters and their sounds and the normal child begins to use partial phonic cues, mostly from the first or last letters, as well as contextual cues. The transition from a reliance on whole-word recognition and contextual cues takes place gradually.

Observation of children as they read suggests that at around a reading age of seven years on the tests employed here most begin to demonstrate an incipient ability to work from letters to sounds: the beginnings of the phonological awareness which assumes a major role for continual success in reading (Ellis and Large 1988). Despite the fact that before school entry these children had been receiving speech therapy, almost certainly including work on their phonological sound systems, 69 (64 per cent) of the 108 children aged seven years and over had not reached this stage in reading.

Spelling
Children begin to learn to read and write at the same time. While early reading generally focuses on the decoding of whole word patterns, the basic skill required in spelling is the reproduction of those strings of letters which encode the words they represent. The processes involved at the beginning of acquiring these two aspects of written language are thought to be dissimilar. Bryant and Bradley (1980) showed that reading and spelling are learned independently of each other, at least initially. In the first stages of reading, the use of visual recognition and syntactic and semantic cues predominate. In the case of spelling, phonological cues are very important from the beginning. A child must attend to and consider the sound of speech, his/her own and that of others, as opposed to the meaning of speech. S/he must be able phonically to segment speech.

This early specialisation declines as reading increasingly demands explicit phonological awareness and spelling requires visual recall for irregular spellings and for chunks such as *-ing*, *-ed*, *-ful*. Differences remain. There is a greater predictability in transforming letters to sounds (reading) than sounds to letters (spelling). For example, the sound of the letter *f* is more predictable than the graphemes which represent it: *f*, *ph*, *gh*. Again, reading can be accomplished by a partial processing of orthographic information whereas a word's complete orthographic structure is required for spelling.

The dynamics in the development of visual and phonological skills, of short-term memory, reading and spelling in normal children aged five to seven years, have been tracked by Cataldo and Ellis (1988, 1989) who demonstrated that the experience of spelling itself promotes the use of a phonological strategy in reading. Arriving at a similar conclusion but by a different route, Francis (1984) found that in their first year at school, normal children began to deduce orthographic information—especially related to initial letter sounds—before they received any phonic teaching, just by reading aloud regularly. Spelling generally lags behind reading, partly because reading involves the easier transformation route, from the unfamiliar (print) to the familiar (speech). But perhaps it is more likely to be due to the necessity in spelling for phonological skills which develop from reading as well as contributing to it.

Spelling ability at Dawn House
At entry, the aim of investigating a child's ability to spell was not so much to obtain a spelling age as to discover whether or not there was any capacity for reproducing the written form of selected words. Spellings and errors were scrutinised for evidence of the use of phonic analysis, information which is more likely to come from watching and listening as a child attempts to spell a word than from looking at the finished spellings.

While testing the spelling of 6½- to 7½-year-old children in normal schools it is common to see and/or hear them spontaneously repeat the dictated word, aloud or sub-vocally. As they do so, they write the letters which they believe correspond to the sounds they are making. Such children demonstrate that they have reached the stage of being able to break a word into a string of phonemes and that they understand that these phonemes can be graphically represented. This accomplishment is rarely displayed by the SLI children at Dawn House regardless of age. Very few will repeat a word, let alone use its string of sounds as a clue to its spelling. Many words, notably those of high frequency, are irregularly spelled and require the storing and recall of all or part of the visual word pattern. Spellings were scanned for evidence of this ability. Abilities and disabilities were discussed with the class teacher so that tuition would take these into account, but unfortunately they were not recorded in a form which could be quantified.

However, spelling ages can themselves provide some information about the children's skills. The two most commonly used tests were Burt's (Revised) Spelling Test and Schonell's Graded Word Spelling Test A. Both have a spelling age range of five to 15 years. Burt spelling ages, expressed in whole and decimal years, were converted to years and months in the manner recommended for a similar conversion for Schonell ages (Schonell and Schonell 1970). The first 10 words of the

TABLE 2.XXIII
Spelling age at entry 155 children aged 5.4 to 12.10

Age (yrs)	N	Non-speller N	≤6.11 N	7–7.11 N	8–8.11 N	≥9 yrs N
5	16	15	1			
6	30	21	9			
7	29	12	13	3	1	
8	43	7	31	5		
9	30	4	15	10	1	
10	5	1	3	1		
12	2		1			1
Total	155	60	73	19	2	1

Burt test range from single letter ('*a*') to three-letter words at least some of which (*e.g.* 'the', 'and') are likely to have been learned as visual wholes. The second 10 words are largely composed of phonically regular three-letter words. On the other hand the Schonell test begins with phonically regular words, followed by some which include features like a double final consonant more likely to be reproduced at that early stage from visual memory than by phonic rule. Recently Vernon's Spelling Test (1977) has been used within the school for retesting, and it has also been given to 12 children at entry. Vernon spelling ages range from 5.7 to 15.10, and 12 correctly spelled words would yield a spelling age of seven years. Its first 15 words include many which are short and phonically regular. If a spelling age of seven years has been reached on any of the tests, some ability to segment a word phonically can be assumed.

Results
A spelling age could not be achieved by 60 children, of whom 36 (60 per cent) were aged five or six years. The total inability to spell decreases with age but is present at all ages up to and including 10 years. A further 50 children could write too few words to reach a spelling age of six years. Only 22 children aged 7.3 to 12.10 achieved a spelling age of seven years or above, the level at which some ability for phonic analysis might be assumed (Table 2.XXIII).

Reading and spelling
Normal children of average ability can be expected to be reading and spelling at around age level. In normal populations, differences between mean reading and spelling ages tend to be small. Among dyslexic children and others with severe reading difficulties, however, the gap between reading and spelling is very much wider, with spelling most commonly lagging behind reading (Rutter *et al.* 1970, Naidoo 1972). Reading and spelling have been compared in this sample of SLI children. Reading age has been tabulated with spelling age, including non-readers and non-spellers (Table 2.XXIV).

Nearly all of the children unable to read were also unable to spell. The

TABLE 2.XXIV

Reading age by spelling age 155 children aged 5.4 to 12.10 at entry

Spelling age		Reading age			
	Non-readers	≤6.11	7–7.11	8–8.11	≥9yrs
Non-spellers	29	31			
Under 7 yrs	1	51	21		
7–7.11			14	4	1
8–8.11			1	1	
9 yrs and over					1
Total	30	82	36	5	2

Correlation reading age and spelling age (94 children)
Spearman rho 0.85, p<0.001

TABLE 2.XXV

Difference between reading and spelling 94 children aged 5.11 to 12.10 at entry

Age (yrs)	Spelling at or above reading N	Reading ahead of spelling			
		1–5mths N	6–11mths N	12–17mths N	18–22mths N
5				1	
6		1	3	6	1
7	2	5	3	5	
8	1	2	12	17	3
9	1	5	10	6	3
10	2		1	2	
12	1		1		
Total	7	13	30	37	7

Mean difference between reading and spelling 10.2mths, with a standard deviation of 6.2mths

majority of these, 23 out of 29, were only five or six years old and at the first stages of learning to read and write. A further 31 with a wider age range had some slight reading ability but were unable to achieve any success on a spelling test. There is one exception, a child of eight years unable to read but able to achieve a meagre spelling age of 5.4 after much help in his previous school. Ninety-four children had obtained both reading and spelling ages and these were correlated using a rank correlation procedure. Despite the low levels of attainment generally, it can be said that the reading and spelling ages of individual children are more likely than not to occupy similar rank order positions.

However, this does not tell us whether reading and spelling are developing at the same rate, *i.e.* whether similar levels have been achieved in each. Table 2.XXV suggests that this is not so. The difference between reading and spelling ages has been calculated by subtracting the gap between age and reading age from the gap between age and spelling age for the 94 children with the necessary data. Differences ranges from −14m (spelling ahead by 14 months), to 22m (spelling lagging behind reading by 22 months). Reading was in advance of spelling by an average of 10.2 months, with a standard deviation of 6.2. Unusually, seven children were spelling at the same level or ahead of reading. All had attained a reading age of at least seven years and could be said to have acquired at least the rudiments of phonics. A further 13 children were spelling less than six months below reading, a small and unexceptional difference.

It is often thought that the ability to read is a major influence upon learning to spell. However, in a longitudinal study of normal five- to seven-year-old children, Cataldo and Ellis (1988) found striking evidence that spelling had a greater effect on reading than *vice versa*. It was noted above (see Table 2.XXII) that 16 children were reading at or above age level. Were these children also spelling well? Since 12 were aged only five or six years, both age range and numbers were extended by adding those children lagging behind age by less than a year, a gap which is not regarded as abnormal.

This produced a group of 40 relatively 'good' readers. Three of these (7.5 per cent) were spelling at or above age level, and a further seven (17.5 per cent) were spelling less than a year behind age. Thus 10 of the 40 'good' readers (25 per cent) could spell at a level comparable with reading.

If now spelling is treated in similar fashion, there are 11 relatively 'good' spellers. Of these, eight are reading at or above age level and a further two, reading within a year of age. These are of course, the same 10 children identified above among the 'good' readers. The difference is that they form a much greater proportion of spellers than of good readers.

As Cataldo and Ellis (1988) found among normal children, in the early stages of learning to read and write, spelling in this sample of SLI children is more strongly associated with good reading than *vice versa*.

Summary
The general picture is one of low proficiency in reading and spelling at entry.

Thirty children were unable to read but most of these, 23, were only five or six years old. Of greater concern are the low levels achieved by children aged seven or above, nearly two thirds of whom had not managed to reach a seven-year reading level and 35 per cent of whom were retarded by at least two years. Only seven of the 82 children aged eight or above could be said to have acquired the useful reading skills of an eight-year level or above.

On the whole, spelling, as might be expected, was even more poorly developed than reading. Sixty children (38.7 per cent) were still non-spellers and a further 50 spelled below a six-year level. Of 107 children aged seven or above, only 22 (20.5 per cent) were able to spell at or over a seven-year level. Of the 95 with a spelling age, 76 per cent were retarded in spelling by at least two years.

For the 94 children with both reading and spelling ages, a correlation, rho 0.85, indicated that reading and spelling held similar rank order positions for most children. Spelling lagged behind reading by an average of 10 months. Of 11 relatively good spellers, eight were reading at or above age level. Good spelling is

TABLE 2.XXVI

Criteria for grading impairment in comprehension, expression and speech

	Severe	Impairment Moderate	Minor
Comprehension			
RDLS SS*	<−2	−2 to −1	>−1
TROG Z	<−2	−2 to −1	>−1
EPVT/BPVS SS*	<84	85–89	≥90
TACL RS*	<75	75–89	≥90
BTBC RS*	<30	30–37	≥38
Staff evaluation	Poor	Qualified	
Expression			
LARSP	IV or below	V	VI or better
GC SS*	<9	9–29	≥30
APT G	<20	20–29	≥30
RDLS RS*	<36		
Speech			
EAT RS*	<34	34–50	≥51
Evaluation	Dysarthric		Normal
			Minor problem

*RS = raw score; SS = standard score (or scaled score ITPA)

more strongly associated with good reading than is good reading with good spelling. Despite their general low performance, the children were not uniformly poor. Within the sample there existed a range of levels. A few children, the exception rather than the rule, were both reading and spelling normally or well.

So far it is the mechanical word decoding and encoding aspects of reading and writing which have been reported. As the children progressed through the school and their reading skills improved, most were given, at least once, Neale's Analysis of Reading Ability. Prose reading accuracy and comprehension are examined in Chapter 6.

Subgroups of language impairment

Although language-impaired children are acknowledged to comprise a hetero-geneous population, some patterns of disabilities become recognisable to those who work closely with them. We have used tests of linguistic variables supplemented by staff reports, to group the children in a way that most nearly conforms to our intuitions about subgroups of language impairment. This has been achieved by establishing three levels of impairment, in oral language comprehen-sion, oral language production and speech production, and then grouping children according to their profiles of disabilities in these areas.

All measures refer to assessment made at entry and reports during the first term at school. Oral comprehension was graded using the Reynell Developmental Comprehension Language Scale (RDLS-C) for pupils under seven years of age, and the TROG for pupils of seven and over. Cut-off points for grading severe, moderate and minor impairment were standard scores (RDLS) or z-scores (TROG) of −2, −1 and above. For 39 pupils for whom these results were missing, scores from available

TABLE 2.XXVII

Criteria for subgroup membership

Language subgroup (N)		Impairment	
	Comprehension	Expression	Speech
1. Speech (19)	Minor	Minor	Severe
2. Speech Plus (23)	Minor/moderate	Moderate	Severe
3. Classic (46)	Minor/moderate	Severe	Severe/moderate
4. Semantic (30)	Severe/moderate	Severe/moderate/minor	Moderate/minor
5. Residual (10)	Moderate/minor	Moderate/minor	Moderate/minor
6. Moderate (13)	Moderate/minor	Moderate/minor	Moderate/minor
7. No Language (6)	Severe	Severe	Severe
8. Young Unclassified (6)	Severe	Severe	Severe
9. Severe (3)	Severe	Severe	Severe
Total 156			

tests were used. The tests were the EPVT, the BPVS, the TACL and a further test not described here, the Boehm Test of Basic Concepts (BTBC) (Boehm 1971). Evaluations from staff reports (good, qualified, poor or tangential) were used in combination with test results. The selection of cut-off points was necessarily arbitrary, based on our personal acquaintance with the subjects' functional comprehension, so that the three resulting groups with severe, moderate or minor impairments of comprehension seemed to have some clinical comparability. Details of cut-off points are given in Table 2.XXVI. Although we have categorised the least disabled group in each language domain as 'minor', this term is relative to the difficulties of a very disabled population, and in absolute terms can represent a considerable degree of impairment.

Language production was graded according to LARSP stage (see p.22). Eleven children who lacked LARSP analyses were graded by using scores from the Grammatic Closure subtest of the ITPA (GC), or two further tests, the scores of which have not been reported because of the small number of data available, the Renfrew Action Picture Test Grammar Score (APT G) (Renfrew 1966) and the Reynell Developmental Expressive Language Scale (RDLS-E).

The speech production measure was the raw score of the EAT, for which most data are available. Four children did not have an EAT score. Two of these had been evaluated as dysarthic by speech therapists at their first assessment, and these were graded as severely impaired. One child was evaluated as having normal phonology and one as having a minor phonological problem; both of these were given the highest grading.

Subgroup profiles

The balance between these oral language impairments was used to delineate subgroups of the disorder. Permutations of three levels of three categories created 27 potential groups, although in practice only 25 groups contained subjects. We began by looking at the children within these 25 groups to see which divisions had clinical significance in terms of our knowledge of the children's language behaviour. Some clearly recognisable patterns of disability seemed to emerge from the divisions, although some distinctions did not seem clinically meaningful, and some contained only one or two children. We also had to consider age. As many of the assessments had ceilings below the age of the subjects, standard scores could not be computed and the resultant profile of abilities is irrespective of age. By merging some small groups where no meaningful clinical distinctions had been found, nine subgroups were formed which largely concurred with clinical intuitions while based on objective assessment criteria. These nine groups are described below and summarised in Table 2.XXVII.

Group 1. Speech. (Mainly speech problems; N 19, 16 boys and three girls). This group had minor comprehension and minor expressive language problems but severe speech production difficulties.

> 'Frank came to Dawn House when he was 9.0. His father had died two years earlier, leaving Frank's mother and the family to manage their small farm. Only when Frank's continuing lack of intelligibility and failure to begin to read or write began to change his originally cheerful and positive personality into a withdrawn and self-deprecating one, was his mother able to accept the need for special schooling. At entry to Dawn House he was found to have average verbal and non-verbal intelligence and good comprehension of language. He had many minor problems with expressive syntax but could formulate complex sentences and express ideas fluently, in spite of a considerable word-finding problem. He had a major difficulty with speech phonology and he was a non-reader. Tongue movements were poor and his speech sound system was extemely limited, he could not sequence two consonants at an adequate rate and his vowels were abnormal. The speech therapist commented that in spite of some dyspraxic elements in his speech, with daily therapy the prognosis was good.'

Group 2. Speech Plus. (Still mainly speech but more handicapping language problems; N 23, 20 boys, three girls.) Speech was equally severely impaired in this group but additionally expressive language was moderately impaired. Comprehension was either minimally or moderately impaired.

> 'George was a small baby (2175g) born by caesarean section. All his milestones were late. He had frequent catarrhal colds as an infant and a slight squint. His previous school commented on his distractibility which interfered with his learning, and his frequent retreat into a world of his own. George's speech difficulties which rendered him unintelligible when he came to Dawn House aged 7.6, were compounded by a minor palatal insufficiency which gave his speech a nasal tone. Tongue movements were accurate but slow. All articulatory movements were weak, with poor muscle tone. Some vowel

47

sounds were distorted and he made both immature and atypical speech errors. His comprehension of language was within low average range and was less of a day-to-day problem than his distractibility. Expressively George was functioning about a year below his age in vocabulary, content and syntax. He had made a start with reading and had some phonic skills. Writing and drawing were affected by poor motor control.'

Group 3. Classic. (Expressive language problems; N 46, 36 boys, 10 girls.) This group comprises children with the most traditionally described language impairment. Expressive language is severely impaired, speech production is also generally severely impaired, but may be moderately impaired. Comprehension impairments are minor or moderate.

'Alice was a timid and tearful six-year-old whose problems had become central to the life of her warm and loving parents. Language assessment showed her comprehension to be about 18 months behind her age, but functionally Alice only understood what was happening concretely in the here and now. Conceptual development was very limited. Her auditory memory was short and her persistence not good. Her expressive language was mainly at a single-word level, but occasionally she could relate two words. Although she would produce a string of words there was no grammatical structure to the string ('Mummy Daddy Richard look go choo-choo'). Expressively she had not attained the level of a normal two-year-old. Her articulation of speech was at a similar developmental level. Her phonological system was very immature but not atypical. Because her utterances were so short and related to context, it was normally possible to understand what she was trying to say.'

Group 4. Semantic. (Comprehension problems; N 30, 22 boys, eight girls.) This is a group of children whose problems with the meaning of language are at the lower edge of their disability profile. Comprehension may be severely or moderately impaired. Either expressive language or speech or both are superior to comprehension.

'The problems of Warren took staff at Dawn House a while to understand. A quiet, serious and thoughtful boy he produced no words until he was over four years old, the latest of a series of delayed developmental milestones which included walking at 16 months. His considerate and helpful behaviour at entry to Dawn House was hard to reconcile with reports of his early negative behaviour, aggression and tantrums. Unusually for language-impaired children, he was particularly good at both drawing and dancing, and was a leader in his social group. Some of his problems became apparent at his assessment for a place at Dawn House, aged nine, when he described 'train' as 'a long word' confusing the characteristics of concept and label. He had a non-verbal IQ of 126, his highest scores being in the least verbal aspects of the test. Assessment at entry found only minor immaturities of speech articulation and more severe, if subtle, problems of language, with comprehension scores being worse than expressive scores. He produced a lot of spoken language but could confuse his listener with his failure to relate elements semantically. The therapist commented on his "semantic problems, failure to grasp the whole situation, inappropriate replies and failure to understand the therapist's comments." Once admitted to school, his precise and logical thinking were noted alongside basic conceptual gaps and confusions, unexpected irrelevancies and occasional panic. He was reading about nine months behind age level, his writing was vivid and imaginative though rather muddled; he had an ability to learn and a good store of general knowledge.'

Group 5. Residual. (N 10, all boys) and *Group 6. Moderate.* (N 13, all boys.) In the relative terminology employed here (no children admitted to Dawn House could truly be said to have minor or moderate disabilities) these are children without severe impairment in any area of spoken language. Although their profiles measured at entry to Dawn House are similar, those in Group 5 have previously attended special language schools or language units, and represent the results of up to four years of intensive help. The early profiles of such children, still in need of intensive help in spite of such early advantage, would surely have been in one of the more severe categories. Group 6 includes those children accepted with severe problems of written language accompanying lesser oral language problems. All children in Groups 5 and 6 have impairments in each oral language category no worse than moderate.

'Andy transferred to Dawn House after two years at a similar school with a younger ceiling age. He was a plump and rather babyish eight-year-old with a lot of warmth and zest for life. At entry to his previous school he had been found to have age-appropriate passive vocabulary, but some difficulty in the comprehension of complex sentences which did not affect his ability to understand and respond in the classroom. At that time his articulation was approaching normal but his expressive language was very immature, being three or four years below chronological age. He could not read or write. When he came to Dawn House, aged 8.8, the pattern of difficulties was similar. His skills of speech discrimination and auditory short-term memory were below average and may have contributed to his continuing errors in understanding syntax. He still made grammatical errors and omissions and was inclined to ramble, but could express quite complicated ideas. The only remaining articulatory problems were a confusion of /r/ and /w/, and retention of somewhat immature forms such as "chimbley". Reading and spelling were major problems. Although Andy had made a start, he was functioning at a low level, two years below age. He is included in the *Residual* subgroup.'

'Wesley is included in the *Moderate* subgroup. He entered Dawn House as a day pupil just before his sixth birthday. He seemed a little confused at first but soon became sociable and friendly, showing an appreciation of verbal humour which is uncommon among SLI children. He had no problems with speech discrimination, but scored poorly on a test of basic concepts, at about the 5th centile. He could follow instructions and answer straightforward questions, but had increasing difficulties as questions became open-ended and abstract. Expressively also his subject matter was restricted to the current context, and lacked specificity, he used "empty" terms such as "it", "do", "thingy" rather than specific ones. Although sentence structure was very immature, there were positive indicators of a good potential outcome, such as his use of colloquial language and contracted verbs ("that's the doctor", "I'd got it") both unexpected in SLI children.'

Group 7. No Language. (N 6, five boys and one girl.) These children, who were graded severely impaired in all linguistic areas, were without any capability of speech or oral language production at school entry other than a few speech sounds. Five of the six were unable to understand speech unless aided by gesture, sign language or lip-reading.

'Gemma was not progressing at the school for the deaf she attended until, after two years attendance when she was six years old, she was put into a class where Paget Gorman Signed Speech was used as a teaching medium. She then began to make good progress, and this led to the discovery that her hearing acuity was quite normal, and that she was one of a rare group of children with the Landau-Kleffner syndrome. This meant that although Gemma heard sounds, she was not able to discriminate them as meaningful speech. When she transferred to Dawn House, aged 8.4, she used no spontaneous speech. She could vocalise and attempt to imitate words, but these were not recognisable. She had some ability to recognise individual spoken words, and could point to pictures and objects. When Paget Gorman Signing was used her understanding was at a 4.0-year level, and she could produce signed language at a 2.6-year level. She was making good progress with reading and her reading age was only six months behind her chronological age. Gemma was never daunted by her difficulties, she enjoyed people and communication and brought an expectation of success and enjoyment to all activities.'

Group 8. Young Severe Unclassified. (N 6, four boys and two girls.) These children, who were under seven years of age when assessed and who were severely impaired in all three areas measured, had abilities too low to be graded: although unlike the children in Group 7, they all had some capability of understanding and using language. Since there is a developmental aspect to almost all language skills it did not seem possible to assign group membership to these very young children on the basis of this initial very low grading. Nor is there a typical child to use as an illustration, as their eventual patterns of disability, and therefore subgroups, differed.

Group 9. Severe. (N 3, all boys.) This comprises three children who were over the age of seven at school entry and who fell into the lowest grade in each linguistic area, but who unlike the children in Group 7, were able to demonstrate some basic language knowledge .

> 'One of the most disabled children ever to attend Dawn House was Arthur. He came at the age of 7.10, a thin rather nervous little boy, who smiled readily and only ever seemed completely happy and secure when receiving the attention of an adult. He was the youngest of three children of a widowed mother, and there had been many family problems. Arthur himself was a sickly infant and had some visual problems for which he wore glasses. He had no hearing problem although this had been queried when he was younger, and his non-verbal IQ was in the normal range. At his previous school, he was described as immature and dependent with poor co-ordination. At the selection interview for Dawn House he produced a mixture of grunts, mime and single words. His attention was fleeting and he made a lot of speech discrimination errors. He could not repeat two digits or point consistently to two objects sequentially. At the first assessment after admission as a pupil, he was found to have comprehension skills at a four- to six-year level and expressive skills between two and five years, with language structure being the poorest and vocabulary the best of his skills. He could produce a wide range of speech sounds, and some single words were clear but attempts to combine words led to a breakdown of his phonological system. He was a non-reader.'

APPENDIX 2.A

Criteria for assigning staff evaluations to functional comprehension abilities. Examples of assignments based on reports from teachers and care staff during first year at Dawn House

Good
'No problems', 'understands well', 'good', 'very good', 'follows easily'

Qualified
'Understanding variable', 'better with written language', 'difficulty with long sentences', '—— with complex language', '—— in groups', 'poor when he's tired', 'switches off if it's noisy'

Tangential
'Misses the most important point', 'goes off at a tangent', 'responds to peripheral information, not central theme'

Poor
'Poor', 'very poor', 'major problem', 'everything has to be explained very simply', 'often misses the point', 'can't cope with spoken instructions'

APPENDIX 2.B

Criteria for including subjects in LARSP stages of clause and phrase level

Clause Stage I to V and Phrase Stage I to IV
A minimum of five utterances and at least two different structures

Phrase Stage V
Three utterances

Stage VI
A minimum of five utterances using at least two different structures, or three utterances using three different structures. Positive as well as negative features must be present

Stage VII
Five utterances using a minimum of two structures or three utterances using three structures

Imitated LARSP
50 per cent of structures or more repeated correctly

APPENDIX 2.C

Phonological processes in Dawn House speech assessment
 1. Reduplication. Repetition of syllable, *e.g.* 'mama', [bibi] for 'biscuit'
 2. Final consonant deletion, *e.g.* [do] for 'dog'
 3. Neutralisation of vowels. Vowels replaced by a central neutral vowel [uh]
 4. Diphthong reduction. Diphthongs replaced by single vowel, *e.g.* [epen] for 'aeroplane'
 5. Glottalisation of final consonant. Final plosive replaced by glottal stop
 6. Consonant harmony. Two consonants within one syllable harmonised to one place of articulation, *e.g.* [doat] for 'goat', [koak] for 'coat'
 7. Stopping. Fricatives and affricates replaced by homorganic stops, *e.g.* [tam] for 'Sam'
 8. Palatalling of velars. Velar articulation moved forward to palate
 9. Fronting of velars. Velar articulation moved to alveolar ridge, *e.g.* [finda] for 'finger'
10. Weak syllable deletion. Omission of unstressed syllables, *e.g.* [efant] for 'elephant'
11. Confusion of liquids and glides. Any interchange of liquids /l/ /r/ and glides /w/ /y/, *e.g.* [gwuv] for 'glove', [lero] for 'yellow'
12. Context sensitive voicing. Voicing before vowels and devoicing word finally, *e.g.* [gat] for 'cat', [bik] for 'big'
13. Cluster reduction. Sequences of two consonants within one syllable reduced to one, *e.g.* [poon] for 'spoon'
14. Fronting of palato-alveolars, alveolars and dentals. Articulations of these sounds moved towards the front of the mouth, *e.g.* [fis] for 'fish'
15. Epenthesis. Inserting a vowel in consonant sequence, *e.g.* [galuv] for 'glove'
16. Metathesis. Transposing consonant sequence, *e.g.* [deks] for 'desk'
17. Idiosyncratic. Recurring patterns in any child's system not common in normal development, *e.g.* lateralisation of alveolar and palato-alveolar fricatives; glottalisation of initial fricatives, *e.g.* [hun] for 'sun', [hat] for 'fat'
18. Rule-free variability. Variations of pronunciation not consistent or rule bound, *e.g.* [my soon your foon] for 'my spoon, your spoon'

3
ANTECEDENT FACTORS

Children with a specific speech and language impairment comprise a selected sample of children with language disorders, and the aetiology of their impairments is still obscure. There is growing evidence that genetic influences may be at work (Robinson 1987, Tallal *et al.* 1989*a*). Adverse conditions before, during, immediately after birth and neonatally—some possibly related to brain damage or dysfunction—have been implicated causally in subsequent language learning problems (Stewart 1984, Low *et al.* 1985, Hadders-Algra *et al.* 1986). Environmental disadvantage co-occurring with threatening perinatal circumstances may both contribute to these and later exacerbate language-learning problems in a developmentally vulnerable child. Similarly environmental conditions may mitigate or worsen the problems of a child with an inherent propensity towards language disorder.

In this section we examine antecedent data of possible aetiological significance: family histories of language difficulty, prenatal and perinatal histories and later potentially damaging illnesses, and family and social background. Severe hearing loss, known to be associated with language difficulty, has been excluded by the school entry criteria. A question mark remains over the influence of minor degrees of loss and also of middle-ear infections. Each antecedent factor is explored separately. Children having a specific language impairment do not constitute a homogeneous group clinically. The language-test profiles on which our nine subgroups are based (see Chapter 2) take account of patterns of disability which are discernible to us in our many years of working with the children. It is possible that some of these subgroups are expressions of different conditions, each with a particular aetiology and outcome. The frequency with which each antecedent factor occurs in each subgroup is also examined. It is possible, even if single aetiological factors should emerge as significant, that a multiplicity of factors is operating more commonly (Robinson 1987).

The final part of the chapter examines interrelationships between antecedent factors, the effect of combinations of factors upon measures of language, and the distribution of absent, single and multiple factors in the language subgroups.

Family history of language problems
Family histories in a language-related learning disorder, dyslexia, have been the subject of investigation for many years. The common finding of a concentration of reading difficulty in certain families strongly suggests a genetic component in the aetiology of this disorder. But only relatively recently has similar enquiry been made of SLI children. Luchsinger (1970) referred to some interesting very early

investigations into the heredity of stuttering and speech disorders, and reported that 'heredity was recorded' in 35.5 per cent of 127 children whose retarded speech was associated with a variety of factors including deafness and mental handicap. Ingram (1959) drew attention to the familial background of children with a specific impairment when he commented on the high proportion of SLI children whose parents, grandparents, uncles and aunts had had a history of similar speech problems.

Recent estimates of the frequency of a positive history in the immediate family, parents and siblings, vary between about 30 to 40 per cent (Fundudis *et al.* 1979, Martin 1981, Robinson 1987). Tomblin (1989) reported an incidence of 51 per cent despite the stringency of his criterion for a positive history, namely treatment by a speech-language clinician. More commonly, a positive history is accepted on reports by a member of the family (usually the mother) of past or present speech and/or language problems. On the basis of broad criteria, Tallal *et al.* (1989*a*) found that 77 per cent of their carefully selected sample of 62 SLI children had at least one affected first-degree relative, classified as such if there was a history of problems with language, reading, writing or other learning disabilities or, in the case of parents only, if they had been kept back a year at school. Data from control groups of unselected children or those with a known absence of speech or language problems suggest that in the general population the incidence may range from 3 to 14 per cent (Fundudis *et al.* 1979, Bishop and Edmundson 1986, Neils and Aram 1986*a*, Tomblin 1989).

The strength of familial tendencies with implications for transmission has been explored by computing rates or ratios of impairment (Robinson 1987, Tallal *et al.* 1989*a*). Tallal *et al.* found that their sample of 62 SLI children had a total of 99 siblings of whom 37 were affected, giving a 37.4 per cent rate of sibling impairment. The comparable rate for a control group of 50 children was significantly lower at 19.3 per cent. Robinson (1987) reported that one in 5.2 of all the siblings of 75 SLI children had a history of speech delay. The ratios for SLI boys and girls varied, the highest being for brothers of SLI boys (1:3.9) and the lowest for sisters of SLI girls (1:11). The recognised excess of boys among SLI children was to a lesser degree mirrored in the ratio of boys to girls among their siblings, the ratio of brothers to sisters being significantly higher (1.5:1) than that in the normal population (1.06:1). Similar findings are reported by Tallal *et al.* (1989*a*), whose SLI sample had almost twice as many male as female siblings.

Although the mechanism of transmission is not known, there is growing evidence of a genetic component in some language disorders, particularly those for which there is no obvious aetiological or associated factor such as deafness, overt brain damage or mental disability.

In this chapter we examine the incidence of speech and language problems in the immediate and extended families of our whole sample. We also ask what effect, if any, family histories may have on different measures of speech and language. This SLI sample is not homogeneous linguistically. Nine groups are identified on the

TABLE 3.I

Positive family history of speech or language problems
in the immediate family

	Positive history		Total N
	N	%	
Girls	9	33.3	27
Boys	55	42.6	129
No significant gender difference			
One relative	39	25.0	
Two relatives	13	8.3	
Three relatives	11	7.0	
Four relatives	1	0.7	
All	64	41.0	156

basis of different levels of impairment on measures of comprehension, production of language and speech (see p. 60). If these are separate conditions with different aetiologies, we would expect them to exhibit variations in relative frequencies of positive family histories.

The relevant data, and those relating to the perinatal history and the family environment (see below), were obtained by the school's social worker, who liaised between home and school. Her first pre-admission visit was arranged to enable both parents to be present. Questions were asked about problems of speech, language, reading or spelling difficulties among the child's relatives and about the relationship of affected members to the child.

Family history in Dawn House children
THE WHOLE SAMPLE
A positive history was recorded for direct relatives who were reported (usually by the child's mother) to have a history of language delay, language disorder or speech problems including stuttering. We also noted difficulties with written language, reading and spelling, but it was not always clear whether these were associated with or separate from oral language problems. Relatives for whom a reading difficulty only was reported are not included in any analysis unless stated. Just over half of the total number of children, 53.8 per cent, had at least one relative with a history of speech or language problems. This percentage is reduced to 41 per cent when only parents and siblings are considered. A positive history was recorded within the nuclear family for a slightly higher but non-significant proportion of boys (55 out of 129) than girls (nine out of 27). Twenty-five children had two or more affected relatives (Table 3.I).

These findings are comparable to those obtained by Fundudis *et al.* (1979) and Martin (1981), but higher than Robinson's incidence of 28 per cent for the nuclear family (1987).

If we include parents and siblings who had experienced difficulties with written

TABLE 3.II

**History of language problems in siblings, grouped by gender of
Dawn House children and gender of their siblings**

Dawn House subjects	Siblings		
	Total N	Affected N	Ratio
Boys (119)			
brothers	101	32	1 in 3.2
sisters	121	11	1 in 11.0
Girls (26)			
brothers	30	7	1 in 4.3
sisters	25	1	1 in 25.0
Boys and girls (145)	277	51	1 in 5.4
brothers	131	39	1 in 3.4
sisters	146	12	1 in 12.2

language, reading or spelling, but not oral language, a further 13 families are added raising the percentage of our SLI children with a positive history in the nuclear family to 49.

Parents. Thirty-four children had one affected parent, and in a further five cases both parents had a history of language problems, making a total of 39 (25 per cent) with a positive parental history, a proportion similar to that reported by Ingram (1959) who found that 24 per cent of 75 language-disabled children had a similar parental background. In our study, affected fathers were slightly more numerous than mothers (25 against 19). Tallal *et al.* (1989*b*) reported a similar trend, as did Tomblin (1989) when he accepted reports of impairment as evidence of a positive history instead of a history of treatment by a speech therapist.

Siblings. Of our 156 children, 11 had no siblings. The remaining 145 had 277 full siblings, half or adoptee siblings being excluded. Among them are slightly fewer brothers, 131 (47.3 per cent), than sisters, 146 (52.7 per cent). In this respect, our findings differ from those of Robinson (1987) who noted a significantly high 1.5:1 ratio of brothers to sisters, and from Tallal *et al.* (1989*b*) who also reported an excess of brothers to sisters among the siblings of their SLI sample. Of the 277 siblings in our sample, 51 had speech and/or language problems, producing a sibling ratio of 1:5.4. This is almost identical to that of 1:5.2 reported by Robinson (1987). Table 3.II shows the number and percentage of affected brothers and sisters of our male and female subjects separately.

The incidence of language problems is appreciably higher among brothers of both our male and female SLI children than among their sisters. Our findings strongly resemble Robinson's, who quotes his findings from another sample of SLI children, and who refers to a study by Sonksen (1979), all of which produce similar results. Their ratios range from 1:3.4 to 1:4.4 for brothers. Our findings are 1:3.4. While the proportions of affected sisters show slightly greater variation, there is agreement that the incidence is much less, 1:7 and 1:11 (Robinson 1987) and 1:15 (Sonksen 1979) than for brothers. Again our findings, 1:12.2, are similar.

Taken together these findings strongly suggest that there is a one in five chance of a sibling of the SLI child being similarly affected and that brothers are two or three times at greater risk than sisters.

The similarity of results from several studies, including this one, supports the existence of a genetic factor. It could be argued that the presence of a history of familial language problems may operate through the environment thus created, not through genes. This argument is weakened when the reported difficulties have ocurred in the early years of adult relatives and have disappeared before the SLI child's birth. Affected siblings may conceivably act as models for younger brothers and sisters: but it is difficult to imagine that the deviant patterns of language described here could be produced by a child whose language would otherwise develop normally, and who has been exposed to normal language from all but one of his social contacts within and outside the family. Unfortunately our sibling data were not recorded in a manner which enables us to determine whether affected siblings were older or younger than our subjects. But we can say that 46 subjects were either only children or the first child in a family, with no possibility of being affected by elder siblings.

Family history and language measures
Did the performance on the language measures of children with a positive family history of language problems differ from those with no known history?

Children with and without a positive family history, scored as 0 or 1, in the extended family were compared on the language and speech measures listed on page 36.

The means and standard deviations of each of the nine measures of speech and language, and the distribution of LARSP stages for children with and without a positive family history, are given in Table 3.III. Differences between the two groups are insignificant, with two exceptions. Both relate to gaps between test and chronological ages, large gaps reflecting greater degrees of retardation. Children with a positive family history were on average 21 months below age on the test of general comprehension (RDLS), compared with 30 months for those with no known history (Mann-Whitney U test, z−2.604, p<0.01). However, they functioned at similar levels on the more formal tests of comprehension, vocabulary and grammar. Likewise the mean gap was significantly smaller (Mann-Whitney U test, z−2.523, p=0.011) for the children with a positive family history when retelling a story immediately after hearing it (Bus Story). But again on the more formal aspects of language production, vocabulary, syntax, and morphology there were no differences between the groups. Nor were differences found between mean EAT raw scores, an index of the development of a child's speech sound system, and mean EAT atypical scores, a measure of deviant as opposed to immature sounds.

For reading, two analyses for family history were made. For the first, as for all other language measures, a positive history was based on reports of language problems which may or may not have included reading. For the second, we added

TABLE 3.III

Language measures at entry by a familial history of language problems

Language measures	N	Family history	
		Present mean (SD)	None known mean (SD)
Comprehension			
Vocabulary	148	84.3 (12.1)	85.2 (14.5)
Grammar	100	−0.8 (1.2)	−0.9 (1.2)
General~	97	21.3 (14.9)	30.4 (17.9)**
Language production			
Vocabulary~	135	23.1 (14.9)	26.4 (16.9)
Structure (see below)			
Morphology	97	21.9 (10.5)	19.0 (10.6)
Content~	80	36.7 (18.4)	47.3 (15.9)**
Speech			
Maturity	152	29.1 (17.5)	27.6 (18.7)
Deviance~	151	15.5 (13.5)	17.3 (15.0)
Written language			
Reading age	144	78.2 (10.9)	79.9 (12.7)
Structure	145	N	N
Stage III−		20	9
Stage IV		16	18
Stage V		17	22
Stage VI+		24	19

~ Lower score = better performance
**$p<0.01$ (Mann-Whitney U test)

relatives reported to have a reading difficulty but no language problem. This caused a slight rise in the number of children with a positive family history and a slight fall in those with no known history, but the results of both analyses were almost identical. The reading ages quoted are derived from the former in keeping with the other analyses (Table 3.III).

It is not clear why there are differences between children with and without a known family history of language problems. The effect is to produce differing language profiles with greater discrepancy between general communicative competence, revealed by the general comprehension (RDLS) and story-retelling (Bus Story) tests, and formal linguistic skills among those with a positive family history. Families with a positive history may have a greater understanding of the language-disabled child's frustrations and be more sympathetic to a child's conversational efforts. This in turn may encourage persistence when communicating, resulting in greater ease and better general communicative skills. If this is so, such attitudes do not appear to have an effect on the more formal aspects of syntax, morphology and vocabulary which are so poor in both groups.

Family history and language subgroups
Different patterns of language impairment were recognisable clinically as we

TABLE 3.IV

Language subgroups by family history of language problems

Language subgroup	Total N	Family history	
		present	none known
Speech	19	9	10
Speech Plus	23	12	11
Classic	46	29	17
Semantic	30	16	14
Residual	10	8	2
Moderate	13	6	7
No Language	6	0	6*
Young Unclassified	6	3	3
Severe	3	1	2
Total	156	84	72

*p<0.02
Binomial test, P=0.46, two-tailed

worked with the children. We have attempted to identify these objectively by using language test result profiles as described in Chapter 2. It is possible that all or some of these subgroups represent different conditions, in which case one could expect to find differences in aetiology in the antecedent factors considered here. Our findings on positive family histories are close to those of other studies, pointing to a genetic basis for the impairments of at least some children. The clustering, or absence, of family histories in one or more subgroups would suggest that different aetiological factors may be associated with different subgroups (Table 3.IV).

The nine language subgroups are:
1. Speech (19)—children with mainly severe speech difficulties
2. Speech Plus (23)—children with severe speech and moderate language problems
3. Classic (46)—children with severe problems in language production and minor or moderate comprehension problems
4. Semantic (30)—children with mainly severe or moderate comprehension problems
5. Residual (10)—children with continuing moderate oral or severe written language difficulties after attending a special language school or unit
6. Moderate (13)—children with severe written and minor or moderate oral language problems
7. No Language (6)—children severely impaired in all linguistic areas
8. Young Severe Unclassified (6)—children severely impaired in all areas and unclassifiable
9. Severe (3)—older children in the lowest grade in each linguistic area.

In six of these groups (Speech, Speech Plus, Semantic, Moderate, Unclassified and Severe) there are almost equal numbers of children with and without a positive family history, the distribution expected from the total numbers of children with and without a positive family history. In the small group of six No Language children, none has a positive history, the probability of this being less than 2 per cent (binomial test, P = 0.46, family history negative). In the opposite direction the Classic and Residual groups reveal a raised incidence of positive family histories. The children were classified on the basis of information elicited on entry to Dawn House School but our knowledge of the previous history of children in the Residual group, many of whom came to us from another I CAN school, would place several in our Classic language group. In respect of family histories, the Residual group bears some similarity to the Classic group.

Although a very small group, the finding of a negative history for all in the No Language group may not be a chance one. They constitute that minority among SLI children sometimes described as aphasic or with a receptive language disorder whose histories suggest brain damage perinatally or in early childhood, a question pursued in the following section.

Summary
Our finding in respect of reports of language problems in the families of our pupils closely resembled those of other studies recently carried out in this country. Within their immediate family, 41 per cent of the children had at least one parent and/or at least one sibling with a positive history. Of their full siblings, one in five had a language problem. Brothers of our subjects were two or three times more likely than sisters to be affected. When direct relatives in the extended family are included, 53.8 per cent have a positive history of language problems.

No significant differences were found between those with and without family history, on a range of tests which explored specific language skills, the comprehension of vocabulary and grammar, expressive vocabulary, sentence structure, morphology and reading. Both groups demonstrated equally severe problems. Nor was any difference found in speech, both developmental and deviant. However on two tests of general communicative ability—one of comprehension, the other involving retelling a story—children with a positive history were retarded to a significantly *lesser* degree. Those with a positive family history present a more uneven linguistic profile than those without. They perform most poorly on the formal rule-based aspects, grammar and sentence structure, and on tests of vocabulary which involve the recognition and retention of verbal labels.

Positive and negative family histories are fairly evenly distributed in six of the language subgroups. Of the remaining three, family histories were remarkable for their absence in one group, the No Language. In two groups, the Classic (characterised by expressive language disorders) and the Residual, positive histories were found more frequently than in the remainder, but not significantly so.

Our findings support the existence of a genetic factor in the aetiology of some language impairments. This is absent in the No Language group and raised in the Classic and Residual groups.

Perinatal history and early illness
The child with a specific speech and language disorder is, by definition, one for

whom overt abnormalities of the central nervous system have been excluded. Nevertheless, many who work closely with SLI children believe that most disorders of language function are the result of neurological dysfunction affecting the transmission of information from ear to brain, within the brain itself or from brain to organs of articulation (Rapin and Wilson 1978). In the absence of overt neurological abnormality, the possibility has been considered that some learning and language difficulties may stem from minimal brain injury or dysfunction. Prenatal and perinatal events such as low birthweight and short gestation, known to be associated with increased perinatal mortality and cerebral damage, have been implicated as factors which might lead to minimal injury and consequently adversely affect development as an effect of a 'continuum of reproductive casualty' in the survivors of these hazards (Pasamanick and Knobloch 1960). When there are no obvious neurological abnormalities, it cannot be assumed that injury has been sustained however minimal. All we can say is that the risk of damage is increased. This applies also to diseases such as meningitis, encephalitis and other events in early life which threaten neurological integrity and may adversely affect later neuropsychological development including speech and language skills.

Perinatal history—background
Of the events surrounding pregnancy and birth, low birthweight and short gestation are the most frequently implicated precursors of disability. In their follow-up of the national sample examined for the 1958 Perinatal Mortality Survey (Butler and Alberman 1969), Davie *et al.* (1972) demonstrated a persisting relationship between length of gestation and educational subnormality, visuomotor function and clumsiness, after allowance was made for social class and birth order. The prevalence of educational backwardness was raised at both extremes of the gestation period, before 37 weeks and after 42 weeks, especially the former. The mitigating effect of social conditions was demonstrated when educational backwardness was related to birthweight for gestation. The prevalence of educational backwardness in small for gestational age (<10th centile), large for gestational age (>90th centile) and optimal (10th to 90th centile) children was examined in both the least and most socially privileged groups. Children born before 37 weeks were excluded. Among the least privileged—the fifth-born of fathers in manual occupations—there were 2½ times as many educationally backward children among the small for gestational age as among children between the 10th and 90th centiles. A similar proportion was found between small for gestational age and optimal groups among the most privileged: the first-born of fathers in non-manual occupations. The mitigating social effect was evident in the different prevalence rates between the underprivileged small for gestational age (nearly 17 per cent) and the most privileged (1.5 per cent).

From the same national sample, a subgroup of 215 children with marked speech defects but normal hearing was selected. The information available did not permit distinctions between dysarthrias and specific language disorders and the

62

sample included all levels of intellectual ability. Premature birth (<37 weeks) was the only significant perinatal feature to emerge when this sample was compared with the rest of the national sample. No differences were found in birthweight, maternal age, history of haemorrhage during pregnancy, prolonged labour, fetal distress or abnormal delivery (Sheridan 1973).

In the 1970 British Births Survey, children with speech problems were identified at five years (Paterson and Golding 1986). No distinction was made between speech and language difficulties, and features such as deafness, cleft palate, cerebral palsy and mental handicap were not excluded. Socio-economic background of the study group did not differ from the rest of the population. Children of low birthweight, <2500g, were at greater risk of persisting speech problems, but this association disappeared when other factors were taken into account: sex of the child, number of children in the household and maternal smoking habits. Although low birthweight is more prevalent among the lower socio-economic groups, it has been shown in all three British cohort studies (1946, 1958 and 1970) that the primary associations are not with socio-economic class but with other factors such as maternal smoking habits, maternal height and age of mother (Golding and Butler 1986a).

There are few studies which examine the effects of perinatal events on specific speech and language disorders, when gross mental and/or physical disability and sensory loss are excluded. After such exclusions had been applied, a study of 243 low-birthweight children revealed significantly lower levels in a wide range of speech and language skills compared with those obtained from a control group of full birthweight children at four years. At 6½, differences were also found in short-term auditory memory and verbal IQ (Washington et al. 1986).

Some prospective studies have looked at the outcome of various neonatal factors, again excluding major disability. In a small group of nine neonatally at-risk children, six were found to be experiencing receptive, expressive, grammatical or phonological deficits compared with only two out of 20 normal full term children without neonatal cerebral symptoms and of similar social background (Jensen et al. 1988). In a much larger sample of neonatally at-risk children in Finland, examination at nine years permitted the consideration of background factors such as prenatal and perinatal events, socio-economic and familial factors. Cerebral depression and smallness for gestational age were risk factors for poor psychol-inguistic ability, but low social class was a very important predictor. Adverse prenatal and neonatal factors, along with a positive family history of 'developmen-tal disturbance' and low social class, were associated with poor scholastic achievement. The authors commented on the multifactorial nature of the aetiology of developmental disorders and the importance of the background pathology of the neonatal conditions (Lindahl et al. 1988).

The abnormal outcome of a neonatal neurological examination was the basis for the selection of 76 children by Hadders-Algra et al. (1986). Excluding children with severe neurological impairment at six years, 17 per cent of their study group were found to have speech/language problems, compared with 5 per cent of a control group of neonatally normal children. The difference was not significant.

There are few reports of the perinatal history of children selected for their speech and language disorders. An early American study (Pasamanick *et al.* 1956) located over 400 white children who did not have cerebral palsy or mental deficiency but who were receiving speech therapy, largely because of defective articulation or stuttering. Compared with a matched control group of similar socio-economic status, no differences were found in hospital records of pregnancy, delivery, preterm birth, abnormal neonatal conditions and previous reproductive casualty. However, the speech-disordered were significantly more likely to be the third- or later-born children.

One hundred and two children in the Newcastle Child Development Study, who had failed to string together three words at the age of 36 months, became the subjects of a detailed study of speech and language retardation (Fundudis *et al.* 1979). They were compared with a control group matched for sex, age and postal district. Among the 102 speech-retarded children were 18 classified as 'pathologically deviant' (PD) because of severe psychological, mental or physical abnormalities. The remaining 84 were termed 'Residual Speech Retarded' (RSR). The mean gestational ages of both the PD and RSR groups were significantly lower than that of the control group. There was also a significant difference in birthweight, but only when the total speech-retarded sample was compared with controls: a comparison which also revealed a significantly longer second stage of labour. A perinatal risk index was computed by giving an equal weighting to each of 10 extreme perinatal obstetric experiences, which included toxaemia of pregnancy, complications of delivery and fetal distress. No significant differences were found between the three groups.

The results of national surveys show that events surrounding birth, particularly low birthweight and short gestation, are associated with mental, physical and educational disability. It is also clear that social conditions are influential in exacerbating or mitigating their effects. The long-term effects on specific speech and language disorders are still open to question, but there is evidence that at least some disorders may be associated with perinatal events.

In this study, we examine the incidence of prenatal, perinatal and neonatal problems in the whole sample and in the language subgroups, and consider the possible effect on different measures of speech and language. We also look at the relationship with neurological illnesses occurring in early life.

Dawn House children
The prenatal, perinatal and neonatal information on Dawn House children comes from maternal responses to a list of questions put by the school's social worker on her pre-admission visit to the home. Maternal reports of perinatal events may suffer from unreliability of recall and lack of knowledge about the exact significance of events. With any group of disabled children there is the danger that a

mother may over-report, perhaps in an attempt to explain her child's disorder. To overcome some of these difficulties, a list of questions was drawn up. For example mothers were asked specifically whether they had suffered from rubella, high blood pressure or toxaemia, and at what period during pregnancy these had occurred. An opportunity was also given for them to relate any event they regarded as abnormal.

The accuracy of the information must vary. Mothers are likely to have spoken honestly about their health during pregnancy, but the severity of any reported conditions like high blood pressure or toxaemia is unknown. Possibly not all adverse events were reported. Schwartz (1988) commented that some mothers were unaware of the significance of mid-term bleeding and had not reported it. Greater reliability can be placed on some features such as length of gestation, birthweight and whether the newborn had been placed in a special care unit. Golding and Butler (1986a) found that mother's recall of birthweight corresponded closely to that recorded at birth, but that it tended to be the baby's lowest weight during the first few days after birth rather than the actual birthweight.

Most mothers at some point could not remember the detail requested. Where an indication was given that there had been no problems, the response was recorded as negative or falling within the normal range. Only six children lived in a household which did not include the natural mother, but two of these lived with the father. No information was available in four cases.

PRENATAL AND PERINATAL HISTORY

Pregnancy. Nineteen of the mothers had been young, less than 20 years old, and three had been 40 or above when their children were born. Two mothers had had rubella, one during the last trimester. Eight had been toxaemic and an additional 12 had had a raised blood pressure but no toxaemia. Two mothers stated that they had experienced a threatened miscarriage. Altogether 24 mothers (15.8 per cent) reported one or more pregnancy risk factors, including maternal age >40, rubella during the first trimester, and a history of toxaemia or high blood pressure.

Birth. Mothers were asked about the length of labour, divided into first and second stages, but few were able to give such information. The duration of labour reported relates to first and second stages combined. For the majority, 82.2 per cent, this was thought to be between two and 24 hours. It was precipitate, less than two hours in all, for 10 children (6.5 per cent) and long, more than 24 hours, for 17 (11.2 per cent). Eleven (7.2 per cent) were caesarian births, more than 2½ times the 2.7 per cent reported nationally (Butler and Bonham 1963). A further eight (5.3 per cent), about twice the national average, were breech deliveries. The mothers of 14 boys (10.1 per cent) reported that delivery was assisted by forceps. Two of 156 births (1.3 per cent) resulted from a twin pregnancy, an average proportion. One or more risk factors (twin birth, precipitate or long labour, caesarian or breech delivery or the use of forceps during delivery) was recorded for 47 children (30.9 per cent).

Gestation. Maternal recall or knowledge of the precise number of weeks of

TABLE 3.V
Birthweight of Dawn House children compared with the 1970 cohort (Butler and Golding 1986)

Birthweight	Children %	
	1970 cohort (N 12,755)	Dawn House sample (N 152)
<2500g	6.9	12.5
≥2500g	93.7	87.5
Total	100.0	100.0

Chi-square 7.188, df 1, p<0.01

TABLE 3.VI
Birthweight and social class

Birthweight	Social class	
	Non-manual	Manual
≤2500g	4	15
>2500g	34	98

Chi-square 0.195, df 1, NS

gestation varied. On the assumption that mothers are likely to know and recall both a preterm delivery and one that occurred well past the expected date of delivery, a response of 'normal' or 'no problems' has been recorded as occurring between 37 and 42 weeks. Twelve children (7.9 per cent) were born after a gestation period of less than 37 weeks. Seven (4.6 per cent) were postmature babies born after more than 42 weeks. Preterm and post-term babies were slightly more common in this sample than nationally.

Birthweight. The birthweight of most children (87.5 per cent) exceeded 2500g. Of the 19 children with a birthweight below this, four (2.6 per cent) weighed less than 1500g. Compared with a national birthweight distribution (1970 cohort) reported by Golding and Butler (1986*a*), who also based their figures on maternal reports, this sample contains a significantly greater proportion of low-birthweight children (Table 3.V). Low birthweight has been associated with low socio-economic status. It will be seen in the following section that the Dawn House sample includes a greater proportion of children from the manual social groups than was found in a national sample. Within our sample, however, low birthweight was no more associated with low social class than were children of birthweight ≥2500g (Table 3.VI).

While very low birthweight is associated with perinatal risk, it is not as important as birthweight which is low for gestational age. Small-for-gestational-age babies were identified by reference to the norms for weight and gestational age given by Babson *et al.* (1970). Taking the 10th and 90th centiles as cut-off points, 22 children (14.5 per cent) were small for gestational age and four (2.6 per cent) large for gestational age.

TABLE 3.VII
Perinatal risk factors

	Score
Rubella during pregnancy	1
Toxaemia of pregnancy	1
High blood pressure—no reported toxaemia	1
Mother aged 40 or over	1
Twin	1
Precipitate labour—<2 hrs	1
Long labour—>24 hrs	1
Caesarian birth	1
Breech presentation	1
Forceps assisted delivery	1
Birthweight <1500g (not small for gestational age)	1
Small for gestational age—<10th centile	1
Large for gestational age—>90th centile	1
Late to breathe	1
Admission to special care unit	2
Convulsion(s) during the first 4 weeks	1

Maximum score 12

Neonatal. Mothers were asked about the condition of the baby immediately after birth and during the first four weeks. No problems were reported for 63 per cent. Breathing was delayed in 13, by more than 10 minutes in four cases. Three had had convulsions. Twenty-nine babies had been admitted to a special care unit for some period of time. Children were regarded as at risk neonatally if one or more of the following were reported: birthweight <1500g, birthweight for gestation below the 10th or above the 90th centile, late to breathe spontaneously, convulsions or admission to a special care unit. A history of one or more of these conditions was given for 54 children (35.5 per cent).

Problems with sucking, swallowing or milk dribbling through the nose were reported for 28 babies during the first weeks. If the eight with structural oral abnormalities are excluded, 13 of the remaining 20 had a perinatal risk rating (described below) of more than 1. In 11 cases the risk related to the neonatal period and possibly reflected a neurological abnormality.

PERINATAL RISK RATING

While some single perinatal factors carry a high risk for later development, the presence of more than one risk factor is thought to increase the risk potential (Hadders-Algra *et al.* 1986). In some studies which have considered the relation between perinatal events and later development, a perinatal risk rating has been constructed by summing the number of adverse factors. The factors included and the criteria for inclusion vary, much influenced by the method and detail of data collection, the professional background of the data recorder, and the prospective or retrospective nature of a study.

Ratings are usually based on information relating to pregnancy, birth and the

TABLE 3.VIII

Distribution of perinatal risk scores

Score	N	%
0	62	40.8
1	43	28.3
2	17	11.2
≥3	30	19.7
Total	152	100

TABLE 3.IX

Measures of language and speech by perinatal history

Language measures		Perinatal history	
	N	No problem mean (SD)	Some problem mean (SD)
Comprehension			
Vocabulary	143	85.7 (11.7)	84.2 (14.3)
Grammar	97	0.88 (1.3)	0.83 (1.0)
General~	94	23.7 (16.6)	25.9 (17.2)
Language production			
Vocabulary~	132	25.6 (16.4)	23.5 (15.9)
Structure (see below)	141		
Morphology	94	21.2 (11.1)	20.3 (10.6)
Content~	78	42.6 (21.9)	40.8 (15.9)
Speech			
Maturity	148	28.9 (18.8)	27.7 (17.7)
Deviance~	147	17.2 (15.2)	16.2 (13.6)
Written language			
Reading age	140	78.1 (10.5)	79.9 (12.6)
Structure (LARSP)		N	N
Stage III−		13	16
Stage IV		15	18
Stage V		15	22
Stage VI+		16	26

~Lower score = better performance
No significant differences

neonatal period (Mellor 1977, Bishop and Butterworth 1980, Schwartz 1988). In selecting factors for a perinatal risk rating, we have been guided particularly by Bishop's Birth Risk Rating and Mellor's list of adverse perinatal factors. Our information is more limited than theirs. Since it is based on maternal histories, it cannot be compared with Mellor's carefully recorded hospital data. With one exception, each of the factors listed in Table 3.VII has been given an equal score of 1 as degrees of severity are unknown (*e.g.* in toxaemia or failure to breathe immediately after birth). Admission to special care unit after birth has been weighted with a score of 2, since this would have followed a decision by medical personnel on their judgement of the baby's condition. On this basis the maximum score is 12, but none was higher than 7.

TABLE 3.X

Perinatal risk scores in language subgroups

Language subgroup		Perinatal risk score			
	N	0	1	2	≥3
Speech	19	5	8	2	4
Speech Plus	22	10	5		7
Classic	46	23	8	10	5
Semantic	30	12	10	3	5
Residual	10	3	2	1	4
Moderate	11	5	4		2
No Language	6	2	1		3
Young Unclassified	6	2	4		
Severe	2		1	1	
Total	152	62	43	17	30

PERINATAL RISK RATING IN THE WHOLE SAMPLE

Table 3.VIII gives the distribution of risk ratings for the 152 children for whom data were obtained. No adverse factor had been reported in less than half of the children (41 per cent). Only one was recorded for a further 43 (28 per cent). Almost a fifth of the children had three or more adverse pointers in their perinatal histories. The birth-risk scores described by Bishop and Butterworth (1980) are based on a much larger number of pointers and our results are not strictly comparable. However, in their unselected sample of 169 eight-year-old children, a history of no problem was obtained in 45 per cent and one problem in 23 per cent, figures not dissimilar to those obtained here.

PERINATAL PROBLEMS AND MEASURES OF LANGUAGE

Measures of comprehension (vocabulary, grammar and general comprehension), the production of language (vocabulary, structure, morphology and content) and speech (maturity and deviance) were analysed for the effect of perinatal risk. Children with a perinatal risk score of 0 (no problems) were compared with those with a score of 1 or more. No significant differences were found in any field of speech or language. Nor was any trend discernible which might have been suggestive of the adverse effects of increasing perinatal risk on one or more speech or language skill (Table 3.IX).

PERINATAL PROBLEMS IN THE LANGUAGE SUBGROUPS

Are perinatal problems distributed proportionately evenly among the speech and language subgroups? If not, this would suggest possible aetiological differences, with some types of impairment being related to perinatal risk factors.

We have already noted the absence of a positive family history of language problems in our No Language group. Would perinatal problems be found more frequently in this group?

The distribution of perinatal risk scores in each of the language subgroups is described in Table 3.X. There is a suggestion that scores of 3 or more are most frequent among the No Language. Because of small numbers, scores of 1 or more were combined and expected frequencies of no perinatal problem and some problem were calculated in the four largest subgroups—Speech, Speech Plus, Classic and Semantic—the remaining groups being too small for the calculation of chi-square. Only the Speech and Classic groups appeared to depart from expected frequencies, the Speech group containing more children with problems and the Classic fewer, but the differences did not reach a level of statistical significance.

Summary
No perinatal problems were reported in 41 per cent of this sample, and only one problem was recorded in a further 28 per cent. The similarity between our findings and those of Bishop and Butterworth (1980), for unselected normal children, suggests that our findings are not exceptional.

Some features occur more frequently than those found nationally. Caesarian births were 2½ times more common and breech deliveries twice as common as those reported for the 1958 cohort (Butler and Bonham 1963). Almost twice as many SLI children were of low birthweight, <2500g, as were found in the 1970 cohort, p<0.01, (Golding and Butler 1986a).

14.5 per cent of our pupils were small for gestational age, compared with 10 per cent in the standardisation population. There was only a fraction of large-for-gestational-age infants. 2.6 per cent against an expected 10 per cent. This sample includes a greater number of children who had been tiny infants. This may be partly due to a bias towards the lower social classes, but within our sample no association between social class and birthweight was found.

No association was found between a range of language measures and perinatal risk. Levels of comprehension, language production and speech did not vary with perinatal risk. Nor were perinatal risk factors found significantly more or less frequently among the language subgroups.

Early neurologically threatening illnesses
Other early events such as meningitis and encephalitis might feasibly result in long-term neurological dysfunction with an associated SLI.

As part of the developmental history, mothers were asked about the health of their children from infancy until school entry. They were asked whether the children had suffered from meningitis, encephalitis, epilepsy and convulsions, in addition to common childhood diseases like mumps, measles and chicken pox, and when these had occurred.

Twenty-four children (15 per cent) had had one or more of the following: meningitis, encephalitis, epilepsy or convulsions (Table 3.XI). We have no control group with which to compare this incidence, but Bishop (1980a) had found that 5.9 per cent of 170 unselected children had a history of convulsions, meningitis or head injury.

70

TABLE 3.XI

Neurologically threatening conditions (not mutually exclusive)

	N
Meningitis	2
Encephalitis	2
Epilepsy	3
Convulsions including febrile	21
Total	28
Number of children with one or more	24

TABLE 3.XII

Children in language groups with adverse neurological history

Language subgroup	Total N	Adverse neurological history N
Speech	19	1*
Speech Plus	23	6***
Classic	46	6*
Semantic	30	6
Residual	10	1
Moderate	13	0
No Language	6	3*
Young Unclassified	6	0
Severe	3	1
Total	156	24

*Each asterisk represents one child with supra-bulbar palsy (known cases only)

NEUROLOGICALLY THREATENING CONDITIONS IN THE LANGUAGE SUBGROUPS

The distribution of threatening conditions among the nine language subgroups is detailed in Table 3.XII. The medical reports forwarded to the school by the referring education authority sometimes included reference to supra-bulbar palsy. Unfortunately information received varied greatly and we could be sure of such a diagnosis only when this was confirmed by the school's honorary paediatric neurologist (Chapter 5). Of the six children known to be palsied, four were already included among those with an adverse neurological history.

Children with an adverse history do not appear to be similarly distributed between the language subgroups. Numbers are very small, and it would be clinically meaningless to combine language subgroups to increase cell numbers and compute a chi-square value. Binomial tests were carried out on each subgroup, the expected P proportion, 0.15, based on the frequency of an adverse history in the whole sample. The subgroup with the proportionately largest number of children with an adverse history are the No Language, three out of six, while the Speech,

TABLE 3.XIII

Combined perinatal and neurologically threatening conditions in the language subgroups

Language subgroup	N	A* N	B* N
Speech	19	14	5
Speech Plus	22	11	11
Classic	46	36	10
Semantic	30	19	11
Residual	10	6	4
Moderate	11	9	2
No Language	6	1	5
Young Unclassified	6	6	0
Severe	2	2	0
Total	152	104	48

A* = perinatal score ≤2 and no adverse neurological condition
B* = perinatal score ≥3 and/or adverse neurological condition

Moderate and Young Unclassified groups are at the other extreme with none or one. In no group, however, did the observed proportion depart significantly from the expected.

Combined risk factor
Finally, we looked at the possible effect on the language subgroups of a risk factor which combined at-risk perinatal and later neurologically threatening conditions. The children were divided into two groups. On the assumption that the presence of several perinatal risk factors would increase the risk potential. Group A included those with two or fewer perinatal risk factors and no history of adverse neurological conditions (104 children). Group B included those with three or more perinatal risk factors and/or a neurologically threatening history (48 children). The numbers of Group A and Group B children within each language subgroup are shown in Table 3.XIII. The numbers in the two groups are distributed approximately 2:1. If there is no association between risk factors and language subgroups, one would expect to find roughly a 2:1 ratio of Group A to Group B in each subgroup.

The distribution of A and B children suggests that risk factors may be more common among the No Language (five out of six) and the Speech Plus (11 out of 22), and that they may be less common among the Classic (10 out of 46), the Moderate (two out of 11) and the Young Unclassified (none out of six). A chi-square test was carried out for the first four groups, Speech, Speech Plus, Classic and Semantic (chi-square 6.11, df 3, $p > 0.05$). Within these four groups, the Speech Plus and the Classic groups departed from the expected frequency. These differed significantly from each other, the Classic including fewer children with a history of risk factors, and the Speech Plus including a greater number (chi-square 4.323, df 1, p<0.05). Only one child in the No Language group fell into Group A. The proportions of Group A to B departed significantly from those expected (P=0.68 for A, p<0.03). Binomial tests for the remaining small groups gave no significant results. In two of these subgroups, the Speech Plus and the No Language, a history of neurologically threatening events is significantly frequent. It is less frequent among the Classic.

Summary
One or more postnatal neurologically threatening episodes had occurred in 24 children (15 per cent). Compared with the 5.9 per cent affected in Bishop's (1980*a*) normal sample on a slightly different scale, our findings suggest a higher incidence than might be expected from a normal population.

The distribution of adverse conditions between the language subgroups pointed to a greater frequency among the No Language.

Perinatal risk factors and a later adverse neurological history were combined. The No Language group, for whom no evidence of a positive familial history of language problems had been found, had a significantly high incidence of risk factors, suggesting that early traumatic events are at least partly responsible for the impairments of this small group. The Classic, among whom a positive family history was common, included fewer children with neurologically threatening episodes than the Speech Plus group.

Environment
Language develops with apparent ease for most children within their family home, with a primary care-giver (most often their mother) and possibly in the company of siblings. If children fail to learn to speak, one investigation must be into the possible inadequacy of this nurturing medium. In extreme cases of deprived environmental conditions, such as those suffered by the so-called wolf children, there is a clear and unsurprising result: a lack of linguistic input results in a speechless child. There is only weak evidence for abnormal language resulting from lesser degrees of deprivation, although there are some positive correlations between aspects of the environment (social class, presence of primary carer) and aspects of language (size of vocabulary, rate of language acquisition). Even when environmental deprivation of linguistic input has been so severe as to preclude language development, transfer of the deprived child into a physically and emotionally nurturing situation can enable language to develop late but normally (Skuse 1988). Schiff (1979) found that children of deaf mothers with poor speech caught up with language peers when given only 10 to 15 hours per week normal input. This evidence suggests that environmental conditions alone are not sufficient cause for language impairment, although they may interfere temporarily with normal language development.

Several demographic studies include some information about environmental factors and language, but in early studies the language data are scant. The

TABLE 3.XIV

Parental situation compared with 1970 cohort (Butler and Golding 1986)

Parental situation	Children (%)	
	1970 cohort (N 13,135)	Dawn House sample (N 156)
2 natural parents	90.2	80.8
2 parents (1 substitute)	4.6	5.8
1 natural parent	3.9	10.9*
Other	1.3	2.5
Total	100	100

*Chi-square 17.9, df 1, p<0.001

application of linguistics to the study of language pathology is relatively recent, only generally practised since the early 1970s. It is now recognised that many speech-production failures in children are essentially language problems operating at the phonological level, *i.e.* they are systemic breakdowns. Other speech-production difficulties, such as cleft palate speech and cerebral-palsied speech, may be classified as articulatory problems, caused by difficulty with the neuromuscular production of individual speech sounds. Previously these conditions were both described as defective speech, whether or not there were other linguistic problems with the structure and use of language (Morley 1965, Davie *et al.* 1972). It is certain that the children whom we would now categorise as specifically language-impaired were included in studies of speech-defective children, together with children with other types or lesser degrees of disability.

Environmental data for the Dawn House children are provided by the questionnaire filled in by the social worker and child's parents before school entry. There are questions on the number and relationship of parent figures, the subject's rank in the birth order of siblings, the age, health, ethnic group and social status of the parents, the language(s) used in the family, and parental awareness of the nature of the child's language difficulty.

Household composition

Family patterns change in a changing social system, and must be related to current norms. The children in this study were born between 1964 and 1981, and the household composition is that reported at the time of school entry, between 1974 and 1987. In Table 3.XIV subjects' parental situation is compared to that of the cohort of all children born in Britain during one week of 1970, at the time of their fifth birthdays in 1975 (Butler and Golding 1986).

There are more single-parent families in the Dawn House sample, 11 per cent as opposed to the 4 per cent reported in the Butler and Golding (1986) cohort, and this is highly significant (chi-square 17.9, df 1, p<0.001). Although Dawn House family composition was recorded when the children were a little older (mean age at entry 7.10), this is unlikely to affect the comparison seriously, as Popay *et al.* (1983)

TABLE 3.XV
Maternal age compared with the 1970 cohort (Butler and Golding 1986)

Maternal age at birth	Children (%)	
	1970 cohort (N 13,135)	Dawn House sample (N 131)
Under 20	8.6	14.5
20 to 34	83.0	77.8
35 or over	8.4	7.6
Total	100	100

No significant difference

reported only 6 per cent of single-parent families in all families having children below 16 years of age recorded in the 1981 census.

Presence of a stepfather or stepmother implies some degree of family disruption to which the child must adjust. A single parent suggests a degree of hardship, possibly economic, possibly in reduced parent-child contact, although these conditions do not always apply.

Parental age and health

Since language develops in social interaction, the effects of environmental disadvantage may impinge upon the child directly, or indirectly through their effects upon the primary care-giver. A mother who is ill, stressed, depressed, too busy with other children or unaware of her child's problem, may not be providing the same number or quality of communicative opportunities as a mother without these difficulties.

The children of sick parents are known to be disadvantaged in a number of ways (Rutter 1966), but we know of no study which explores this with regard to language development. A persistent health problem in either parent could affect the quality of the child-parent interaction, and thence the development of communicative skills in the child. Depression in the primary care-giver will plausibly lead to reduced or qualitatively different social interaction between care-giver and child. Although Morley (1965) found no correlation between defective articulation and maternal inability to cope, recent studies have found an association between maternal depression and impoverished language or poor attention skills in children (Cox *et al.* 1987, Breznitz and Friedman 1988). Fourteen mothers and 16 fathers in this study suffered from persistent health problems by their own report, and 31 mothers described themselves as depressed while the subject children were infants. The nature and severity of the health problems were not defined. In subsequent analysis, only those children with depressed mothers or with two chronically unwell parents will be counted as disadvantaged.

Parental age was examined. It is possible that older parents may have less energy and more children, and therefore less time to devote to the child. The problems faced by very young parents are different, but could include economic and socio-emotional disadvantage. There is some evidence that the babies of adolescent mothers are less responsive to social stimuli (Thompson *et al.* 1979). Butler and Golding (1986) found that several aspects of child health and behaviour in the first five years, including increased dysfluency of speech, were associated with teenage mothers. In a study which considered the effects of maternal age on verbal reasoning skills in 11-year-olds, Record *et al.* (1969) found that scores increased as mother's age at birth increased, children born to mothers under 20 years of age scoring lowest, and those born to mothers between 35 and 40 years scoring highest.

Table 3.XV compares maternal age in the Dawn House sample with the 1970 cohort. Although there is a raised incidence of young mothers in the Dawn House sample, this does not reach significance. In subsequent analyses, children of teenage mothers or with two parents over 40 when the child was born were considered to have a potential disadvantage.

Family size and birth order
The number of children in the family and the child's increasing birth rank have been negatively correlated with a range of attainments: physical, cognitive, social, educational and linguistic. Although there is usually a high correlation also with social class, family size and birth order have been found to have effects independent of social class and of each other (Belmont and Marolla 1973, Fogelman 1983). Children of lower birth rank and from smaller families generally have superior language development, which is reflected in measures of speech intelligibility (Davie *et al.* 1972, Butler and Golding 1986), verbal reasoning (Rutter and Madge 1976) and vocabulary (Douglas 1964). This could relate to the available amount of 'adult time per child' (Fogelman 1983), an argument that finds support in the Bristol study of normal language development, in which the two-year-olds who made the most accelerated language progress were those most often engaged conversationally in joint activities with an adult (Wells 1975).

If SLI has a distinct and separate aetiology from the delays in language development associated with environmental factors, one might expect to find no effect of family size or birth order on SLI. But if language impairment stems from some genetic predisposition, with a number of possible triggering factors, an underlying impairment might be exacerbated by environmental disadvantage.

Studies of other language-impaired populations seem to support the latter view. When Morley (1965) carried out the survey of speech development and disorders in 1000 children in Newcastle upon Tyne, interest focused on abnormal speech rather than language, but the most impaired group (44 children with unintelligible speech persisting until 4.9 years) also had language delay. Among this group, the low number of first-born children (nine) was significant at the 1 per cent level. In the later study of 3300 children born in Newcastle in 1961, first-born children were found to be advanced in their development of three-word sentences, compared with children produced by second to fourth pregnancies and by later pregnancies (Neligan and Prudham 1969*a*). Those children who could not string

TABLE 3.XVI

Family size of normal children (1970 cohort) at age 5 and Dawn House children at school entry (age 5 to 12, mean 7.10)

Family size	Children (%)	
	1970 cohort all families (N 13,121)	Dawn House sample (N 156)
1 child	10	7
2	49	38
3	25	30
4	10	15
5+	6	10
Total	100	100

1970 cohort and Dawn House children
Chi-square 14.5, df 4, p<0.01

three words together meaningfully at three years of age were the subjects of a further study when they were seven years of age (Fundudis *et al.* 1979). When children with pathological conditions were excluded there remained 84 'residual speech retardates', a specifically language-disordered group, who were matched for age, sex and postal area with a control group. The disordered group had more siblings and contained a significantly smaller number of first-born children than controls in the study. Butler *et al.* (1973) also found that children with markedly poor speech were more likely to be the younger children of large families. When children with learning difficulties were excluded, they found family position to be highly significant in a group of 120 speech-impaired seven-year-olds. In the 1970 cohort (Butler and Golding 1986), the term 'speech problems' referred to a large category of mixed aetiologies, and was not specific. Children with two or more siblings were twice as likely to appear in this group as children with no siblings. Richman *et al.* (1982) studied language delay in 705 London three-year-olds, and found that 45 per cent of those screened as language-delayed came from families of four or more children. Family size has also been associated with educational attainment and written language ability. Davie *et al.* (1972) found a marked advantage in reading attainment at age seven, for families of one or two, compared with families of five or more children.

The size of the families of the Dawn House sample at the time of their admission to school was compared with family size of the 1970 cohort, measured at a comparable time when the cohort children were five years of age (Table 3.XVI). The Dawn House children came from larger families and the difference was significant at the 1 per cent level. However the mean family size of the Dawn House sample (2.9) was smaller than the mean family size of four reported for the residual speech retardate group of Fundudis *et al.* (1979).

Table 3.XVII compares birth order among three disordered populations with the children in the 1970 cohort. Both Newcastle studies included a wider range of

TABLE 3.XVII

Birth order in normal and 3 speech/language-impaired populations

Birth rank	Percentage of children			
	1970 cohort all families (N 13,121)	Morley (1965) speech/language (N 44)	Fundudis et al. (1979) language (N 84)	Dawn House language (N 156)
1	38	20	19	30
2/3	51	57	61	55
4+	11	26	18	15

1970 cohort and Dawn House children
Chi-square 6.5, df 2, p<0.05

TABLE 3.XVIII

Ethnic origin and first languages of sample

Main family language	Ethnic group of parents					
	British	West Indian	Asian	Other European	Mixed	Total
English	143	7	0	0	4	154
Other	0	0	1	1	0	2
Total	143	7	1	1	4	156

TABLE 3.XIX

Parental and Dawn House perception of problems at school entry

	Parent-school concord		School only note problem		Parents only note problem	
	N	%	N	%	N	%
Comprehension (N 127)	98	77	24	19	5	4
Structure (N 97)	80	82	12	12	5	5
Articulation (N 116)	102	88	2	2	12	10

disability than the Dawn House sample: although Fundudis *et al.* (1979) excluded several pathological conditions from their residual speech-retarded group, they included children with WISC IQ of 65 or more. The more specifically language-impaired Dawn House children have a much higher proportion of low birth-rank children than the other disabled groups, but are just significantly different from the normal group.

Ethnic group and languages used in the home
We live in a multicultural society, and children from different ethnic backgrounds have differences of language vocabulary, form, pronunciation and use. These variations may result directly from the language environment in the home, and also indirectly from different child-rearing practices. These language differences may constitute a disadvantage when a member of the minority group is placed in a social or learning situation which is mediated in the linguistic style of the majority.

Wooster (1970) found that Jamaican children lost an initial advantage in language skills in their first year at school in the Midlands, compared to a group matched for social class. He suggested that competing language habits might make their language-learning task more difficult. There is also increased likelihood of language delay in children whose mother tongue is not English, or where a second language is used by some members of their family. Puckering and Rutter (1987), reviewing the literature on bilingualism, reported evidence that most children with good basic language abilities growing up in a bilingual environment will be a little slowed in their acquisition of each language, while children with poor potential for the first language will have marked difficulties if presented with two languages simultaneously.

Of the 156 children in this study, seven came from West Indian families, one from an Asian family where the main language was not English, and one from a mainland European family where the main language was not English. Four others had one non-English parent (Table 3.XVIII). Butler and Golding (1986) found an increased proportion of speech problems among West Indian children and children of other European groups compared with those whose parents were of British, Asian, or African origins. However, half the children of West Indian parents in that study were in large families of four or more children, also associated with an increased risk of speech problems. The family language of the 'other European' children was not recorded by Butler and Golding, so it is not possible to examine the effect of two languages on subsequent speech problems. We included data concerning non-British mothers, a mother tongue other than English, and the presence of another language in the home, in a scale of environmental disadvantage described on page 83.

Awareness of language problem
Communication can break down when one interlocutor is unaware of the language deficiences of the other. The social worker's questionnaire includes questions about the parental perception of the child's language difficulties. Parents are asked if the child has a problem with language comprehension, language structure (syntax), and pronunciation. Parental perceptions of the child's problems are compared with the results of standardised tests at school entry (Table 3.XIX).

The greatest disparity was found in awareness of comprehension problems, where 19 per cent of parents assumed normal comprehension in children who had measurable comprehension deficits. Parents also under-reported problems with language structure in 12 per cent of children. This tendency was reversed in reporting articulatory competence, however, with 10 per cent of parents reporting articulatory problems which were insignificant on standardised tests. Although generally there was a high degree of agreement between school and parental perception of the nature of children's language difficulties (between 77 and 88 per cent agreement) there was some tendency for parents to perceive language problems as affecting mainly speech, a common misconception with the general public. We felt that under- or over-expectation of a child's comprehension was potentially the most damaging to communication, and included a mismatched perception of comprehension abilities in the environmental disadvantage index described below.

Social class
Socio-economic groups in Britain have different language styles. This is almost a defining feature of class membership. Many controversies have centred around the proposal that one language style may be 'better' for communicating, or 'more successful' for learning than another. Our interest is with disordered language, not language which is in some way impoverished, but this division is not always easy to decide. There are three key questions:
1. Are social-class differences a significant factor in the aetiology of SLI?
2. If social class is significant, what are the specific effects on language?
3. If social class is significant, what is the mechanism of its effect?

Several studies have reported positive correlations between social class differences and language ability (Wooster 1970, Davie *et al*. 1972, Silva *et al*. 1982*b*) but others have failed to find any association (Butler and Golding 1986). Wells (1986) described social class as 'probably the most controversial of all the dimensions of variation of child language'. In his research into normally developing language in three-year-old Bristol children, he found no social-class differences either in the amount of language produced in varying contexts, or in the rate of language acquisition, or in the number of pragmatic functions the children could control. However he did find that the poorest and highest scores on a scale of language development were obtained by children in the lowest and highest social groups respectively. These scores were sufficient to produce a statistically significant class effect, although over-all there were larger differences within social groups than between groups.

Specific effects of social class have been reported for verbal comprehension (Wooster 1970, Silva and Fergusson 1980), vocabulary (Wooster 1970), explicitness (Bernstein 1965), verbal reasoning skills and reading ability (Davie *et al*. 1972, Fogelman 1983). Deficiencies in all of these linguistic abilities may be representative of language impairment, or be part of the continuum of normal language skills. Delayed language acquisition and poor speech intelligibility are more likely signifiers of pathological language development. Studies generally concur in finding no effect of social class on the age of language acquisition (Morley 1965, Neligan and Prudham 1969*a*, Wells 1986), but in Morley's study and in that of Davie *et al*. (1972) there is some link between social class and speech articulation. While finding no significant correlation between social class and intelligible speech as a whole, Morley (1965) found a highly significant association with social status in her most severely affected group, those whose severe articulatory defects persisted until age 4.9. Davie *et al*. (1972) found a trend for speech test scores to decrease from Social Class I to V. However, their speech test was somewhat superficial, and assessment

TABLE 3.XX

Social-class membership of 1970 cohort (Butler and Golding 1986) and Dawn House sample

Social class	Children (%)	
	1970 cohort (N 12,268)	Dawn House (N 151)
Non-manual	35.2	25.2
I	6.9	7.3
II	19.6	13.9
III NM	8.7	4.0
Manual	64.8	74.9
III M	46.7	47.7
IV	13.2	19.9
V	4.9	7.3
Total	100	100

Chi-square 13.1, df 5, $p<0.05$
Based on parental occupation using the classification of Office of Population Censuses and Surveys, 1970 and 1980. Unemployed and unknown excluded

also relied on the judgements of teachers and doctors, which could be contaminated by their own cultural norms and expectations (Fogelman 1983). Very little of significance has emerged from the study of social class within language-impaired populations. Fundudis *et al.* (1979) also considered the general effects of social class on non-specifically and specifically language-impaired groups in a population study. There was a tendency for both groups to come from lower Social groupings than the whole sample, but this only reached significance level in the globally impaired group. Two studies (of four-year-olds in Adelaide and of three-year-olds in Dundee), noted the same direction of effect: increased incidence of speech problems in lower social groups, which did not reach significance (Johnston 1980, Drillien and Drummond 1983).

The possible mechanism of a social-class effect is not easy to plot. It is difficult to distinguish the effects of social factors from those of genetic and other variables which have previously been associated with environment, such as antenatal care, family size and parental education (Puckering and Rutter 1987). There is some evidence associating better language abilities with the higher social classes, but no evidence that reduced language ability in lower social groups amounts to SLI. There is, however, an association between speech defect and lower social class in several of the studies cited above.

The social-class membership of the Dawn House sample was based on paternal occupation (classified according to the Office of Population Censuses and Surveys, 1980). If the father was absent, maternal occupation was used. Five children (3.2 per cent) had no employed parent. The social-class groups of the remainder are presented in Table 3.XX. In comparison with the normal 1970 cohort of Butler and Golding, there is an increase in the representation of manual occupations (Groups III manual, IV and V) which just reaches significance.

TABLE 3.XXI
Language measures and environmental factors

Language measures	Single	Teen	Old	Ill	Foreign	Family+	Fourth	Mismatch	SC
Comprehension									
Vocabulary					*				
Grammar					*				
General					*				
Language production									
Vocabulary									
Structure									
Morphology		*							
Content		*		*					
Speech									
Maturity									*
Deviance									*
Written language									
Reading age									*

*Mann-Whitney U-test $p<0.01$

Single = one-parent family. *Teen* = mother under 20 years when child born. *Old* = both parents aged 40+ at child's birth. *Ill* = both parents chronically ill or mother depressed during infancy of child. *Foreign* = non-British mother, English not first language or other language spoken at home. *Family+* = family of 4 or more children. *Fourth* = birth rank of 4 or greater. *Mismatch* = difference between home and school perception of child's understanding of language. *SC* = social class.

TABLE 3.XXII
Language measures and environmental disadvantage index (envrisk)

Language measures	Mean scores	
	0 or 1 envrisk	2+ envrisk
Comprehension		
Vocabulary	85.7	82.6
Grammar	−0.9	−0.8
General ~	22.1	28 *
Language production		
Vocabulary ~	22.7	26.6
Structure (see below)		**
Morphology	22.9	19.2*
Content ~	37.6	40.8
Speech		
Maturity	29	28.1
Deviance ~	16	16.9
Written language		
Reading age	80.1	77.3
Structure	N	N
Stage III−	15	5
Stage IV	16	8
Stage V	13	20
Stage VI+	20	18

~Lower score = better performance
*$p<0.05$ Mann-Whitney U test
**chi-square 7.9, df 3, $p<0.05$

Environmental factors and language measures

We considered the effects of a number of individual variables on the language measures. Results are presented in Table 3.XXI. Because of the large number of analyses, significance level was set at 0.01.

All three measures of language comprehension—vocabulary, grammar and general understanding— were significantly affected by the presence of non-British mothers or by use of a foreign language in the home. Since no expressive measures were affected by these factors, it seems probable that language learning was circumscribed but not impaired by these factors. The child in such a home is likely to have some additional comprehension of other language or dialect variation which is not tested in our array, possibly at the expense of standard English. This could lead to a delay in his or her comprehension of English. However, expressive communication is no more impaired than in other subjects in this sample. Another possible explanation is that whatever is being tapped by this variable specifically affects language comprehension. If the latter is true, and deviant rather than delayed comprehension is the result, problems with comprehension are likely to persist (see Chapter 7).

Subjects of very young mothers, aged less than 20 years at the birth, had significantly poorer performance in grammatical morphology. Teenage mothers, and also the presence of persistent ill-health in both parents or depression in the mother during the infancy of the subject, significantly affected the content of language measured by Bus Story. It may be that a high level of communicative interaction generally, as well as language content in this particular form—story telling—is more likely to occur in families with the advantages and energy of two care givers in good physical and mental health. We know from Wells (1986) that accelerated language development in normal children is associated with a high level of communicative interaction.

The effects of social class were limited to speech and reading, with immature and atypical speech and delay in starting to read being more likely in the children of manual workers.

An environmental scale of disadvantage, based on the research findings discussed above, was constructed. Factors with a large number of missing data were excluded from the composite scale which comprised the following items:

	Points
Single parent	1
Birth rank four or greater	1
Non-British mother	1
English not first language	1
Other language spoken at home	1
Social Class III manual	1
Social Class IV or V	2
Maximum possible score	7

TABLE 3.XXIII
Language subgroups and environmental disadvantage

Language subgroup	Environmental scale			
	N	0 or 1	2	3+
Speech	19	10	5	4
Speech Plus*	23	7	12	4
Classic*	46	36	8	2
Semantic	30	17	7	6
Residual	10	7	2	1
Moderate	13	5	5	3
No Language	6	3	2	1
Young Unclassified	6	4	1	1
Severe	3	1	1	1
Total	156			

*Chi-square 12.9, df 1, p = 0.0003

We looked at the effects of this composite scale on the language measures (Table 3.XXII). Generally the scores of children with some adverse environmental factor tend to be lower than those of children not so disadvantaged. Only on two tests does this not apply, both tests of language form: the understanding of grammar (TROG) and production of grammatical structures (LARSP). Only the latter is significantly different. On all other measures the environmentally disadvantaged children fare worse, significantly so on the general comprehension measure (Mann-Whitney U one-tailed, z-score −2.1, p<0.05) and grammatical morphology (Mann-Whitney U one-tailed, z-score −1.7, p<0.05).

Morphology, as assessed by the grammatic closure subtest of IPTA, measures small grammatical changes within words such as plural and possessive forms of nouns, comparative forms of adjectives and adverbs, and tense markers on verbs. To some extent these are the refinements of grammar, the niceties of 'correct' English which are sometimes associated with educational status. Morphological mistakes rarely impede communication in the broad sense, nor do they imply a limitation of structural language range. To some degree they may be considered as an index of language style, not necessarily a facet of language disorder.

The children who come from less advantaged homes are slightly slower to develop language comprehension and to produce correct English. They do not demonstrate the particular problems with form, which are basic in SLI, to any greater extent than others in this sample.

Environmental factors and language subgroups

The distribution of environmental scale scores in the language subgroups is shown in Table 3.XXIII. Inspection suggests a difference in environmental risk between the four largest subgroups (Fig. 3.1), and taking a risk score of 2 and above as a cut-off point, this difference is highly significant (chi-square 15.23, N 118, df 3, p<0.0016). In particular there are fewer children with environmental disadvantage

84

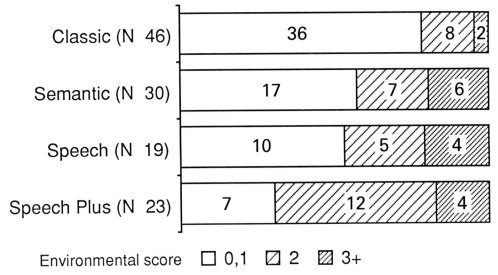

Fig. 3.1. Environmental problems in language subgroups.

in the Classic language subgroup and more in the Speech Plus subgroup which comprises children whose predominantly articulatory or phonological problems are accompanied by marked difficulties at other language levels. The table also suggests that members of the Residual and Young Unclassified groups—who may be past or future members of the Classic group—are not environmentally disadvantaged.

Summary
Compared with the normal population, Dawn House children have a raised incidence of single parents, big families, high birth-rank and parents who are manual workers. All of these factors have been associated with delayed language development in the general population, and also with more globally disabled groups (Fundudis *et al.* 1979). The few specific effects we found on language skills (social class with immature speech and reading, foreign influence at home with reduced comprehension of English, reduced parent-child interaction with impoverished language content) are the same as those quoted in essentially normal populations where they are described as language delay (Bernstein 1965, Wells 1986, Puckering and Rutter 1987).

Environmental disadvantage was most likely to be found in the mixed disability Speech Plus group, and least likely to accompany a Classic language impairment.

These results support the following views:
1. The effect of environmental disadvantage on the language skills of Dawn House children is similar to the effect on the normal population and other disabled groups;

comprehension and reading are delayed and grammatical correctness is reduced, but production of vocabulary and syntax are not specifically affected.

2. Environmental disadvantage may act synergistically with other predisposing factors to exacerbate the effects of language impairment.

3. Environmental disadvantage may be associated with language delay but it is not a significant cause of SLI.

Middle-ear problems and mild conductive hearing loss

Severe hearing impairment is a major cause of language disability, resulting in late, deviant and impoverished language skills. Investigators have therefore frequently considered the possible implication of mild to moderate hearing impairments, or temporary impairment at a critical stage of language acquisition, as a causative factor of SLI. A considerable body of research has produced very variant results concerning the relationship between middle-ear disease, hearing levels and language development, but a strong clinical belief persists that otitis media leading to mild to moderate conductive hearing loss is a significant factor in developmental language disorder.

In this section, we ask: (i) whether there is an association between middle-ear disease (otitis media) and language impairment, (ii) whether such an association, relates to failure to acquire language at a critical period, or to continuing hearing impairment, or to other factors, (iii) what the specific effects of such an association might be, and (iv) whether the effects are permanent or reversible.

Middle-ear disease

DESCRIPTION

Anything which impedes the transmission of sound from its source to the inner ear mechanism can cause a conductive hearing loss. This includes impacted ear wax, foreign bodies such as beads or cotton-wool, and malformations of the auditory tract such as a narrow external auditory meatus. However the commonest cause in children is middle-ear disease, also known as otitis media (Kerr 1984). In young children with their short Eustachian tubes, which are more horizontal than in adults, this is a common sequela of catarrhal colds and other upper respiratory-tract infections. Effusions which cannot drain away from the middle-ear through the blocked Eustachian tube build up and may become infected. The transmission of sound is impeded, with resulting conductive hearing loss. Otitis media exists in various forms: it can be acute or chronic, with or without effusion, and infected or sterile. Effusions can remain after infection has been cured, and can thicken to the consistency of mucus or glue. This condition may be treated surgically by inserting pin-sized ventilation tubes, called grommets, through an incision in the tympanum. Unrelieved middle-ear pressure can cause rupture of the tympanum, and in this case there will be a noticeable discharge of pus from the ear canal. Other possible symptoms are acute earache and impaired hearing. These various presenting symptoms must be taken into account if early history is based on parental reports (as in the present study). Otitis media can recur frequently; each occurrence may last for days or for several weeks and some episodes may go unnoticed. Concern has frequently been expressed about the potential damage of chronic intermittent conductive hearing loss to the developing child.

PREVALENCE

Quoted prevalence of middle-ear disease varies but it is accepted that the condition is very common in children. Teele *et al.* (1980) found that one third of children had experienced three or more episodes before the age of three, and Shah (1981) found evidence by otoscopic examination of previous otitis media in 35 per cent of the population of a London nursery. It has been estimated (Murphy 1976) that as many as 20 per cent of primary schoolchildren at any one time may be suffering from middle-ear related hearing loss.

Hearing loss
LEVEL OF HEARING LOSS ASSOCIATED WITH DISABILITY

The degree of hearing loss associated with otitis media is generally given as between 0 and 55dB (Furukawa 1988). While a hearing loss of 25dB and more has generally been accepted as a significant disability, many audiologists now suggest that this figure should be revised downwards. Skinner (1978) found that some elements of connected speech were inaudible with a hearing loss of 14dB. Quigley (1978) and Downs (1981) both argued that losses of around 15dB are disabling to the child who is still developing communicative skills (the condition in which all Dawn house children are admitted to school). Not only are Dawn House children still developing communication skills at school entry, but they are developing them with considerable difficulty. Rabbitt (1986) described an early experiment, in which a level of crackle introduced on to a telephone line at 15dB below signal strength did not affect accuracy of word repetition, but did affect the ability of subjects to remember the words they had heard, and to answer questions about the content of passages. Because of the extra degree of attention devoted to listening, processing availability may have been reduced to a level below that necessary to fix the words in memory and to decode the passages semantically. Compared with their unimpaired peers, children with language disorders need more processing time to decode at semantic, syntactic and phonological levels, as frequently none of these systems is complete at the time of school entry. A hearing loss of 15dB which used up some processing capacity could therefore be a significant disability. Haggard and Hughes (1990) suggested that children with a history of otitis have particular difficulty in perceiving speech against a background of noise or competing speech, and that this may be the reason for cognitive, linguistic or educational difficulties. It is sometimes claimed that the effects of early otitis media, on hearing, language and educational attainments are reversible (Bennett *et al.* 1980). But five years after otitis media ceased, the subjects of Dalzell and Owrid (1976) had a continuing hearing loss of around 15dB, although hearing acuity and linguistic skills had improved. In contrast with a control group, no child scored above average in any linguistic test.

Association between middle-ear disease and language

MECHANISM OF EFFECT

There are a number of possible ways, not necessarily causative, in which middle-ear disease might be associated with impaired language development. It could be associated with other physical or environmental factors which affect language independently. The National Child Development Study cohort of 1958 (Davie *et al.* 1972) found separate effects of social class on purulent ear discharge and on oral abilities, although no effect of social class on ear discharge was found in the 1970 cohort (Golding and Butler 1986*b*). Otitis media is an illness, which may be accompanied by fever, and can result in a listless, fretful or passive child who does not develop at an optimal rate. Both restlessness and passivity are characteristics which have been associated with otitis-prone children. Otitis can cause a temporary or permanent hearing loss, but hearing loss may co-occur with middle-ear problems and have quite different causes. This means that middle-ear disease and hearing loss may have separate and/or interactive effects on language, complicated by such factors as age of onset, severity and duration. Haggard and Hughes (1990) concluded that 'there are as yet no unequivocal data which would allow us to state with certainty whether hearing-loss effects or disease effects are more important'. Almost all language systems have been cited as vulnerable to otitis and/or reduced hearing acuity, either developmentally during the acquisition of language, or pragmatically in the communicative limitations of a child suffering current impairment.

PREVIOUS STUDIES

Investigations into the possible association between otitis media and language impairment have adopted two basic methods:
(1) prospective, longitudinal studies of language development and educational attainment in children suffering from early middle-ear problems, and
(2) retrospective studies, which have looked for a raised incidence of history of middle-ear problems in a currently language-impaired population.

Both have produced variable results. In the first group, Bax *et al.* (1983) followed up 870 children for five years and found a highly significant relationship between otitis media and language delay, as did Friel-Patti *et al.* (1982) who prospectively studied 35 infants in an 'at-risk' nursery. In a well controlled study by Roberts *et al.* (1986), however, there was no correlation between verbal deficits and prolonged periods of otitis.

A longitudinal study of children who had otitis media with effusion was carried out in Dunedin, New Zealand, by Chalmers *et al.* (1989). Deficits in language development and speech articulation, first identified at five years, persisted into the mid-childhood years, and were still present at 11 years of age.

Retrospective studies are similarly inconclusive. Gottlieb *et al.* (1979) found that children with auditory processing problems and poor school performance had a significantly raised incidence (45 per cent) of early otitis media, while Bishop and Edmundson (1986) found no significant difference in the number of episodes of ear infection experienced by language-impaired four-year-olds and controls.

The majority of papers seem to favour some sort of positive association, but the size of effect is often small (Fischler *et al.* 1985) or relatively short-lived (Bax *et al.* 1983). Paradise (1981), in a review of the major studies up to 1980, was dubious and indicated methodological flaws in the studies; but in a very extensive critical review of the field, Haggard and Hughes (1990) concluded that the case for developmental sequelae of otitis media is convincingly made, although liable to be overstated. While clinical opinions continue to polarise between Bishop and Edmundson's scepticism (1986) and Gordon's (1988) suggestion that all language impairment has its roots in inadequate auditory input, it seems worthwhile examining any available data.

SIGNIFICANCE OF DEVELOPMENTAL LEVEL FOR IMPAIRMENT

Children need accurate auditory input in order to derive and use language rules at phonological, syntactic and semantic levels. Prelingually profoundly deaf children do not naturally develop normal speech and language. Animal deprivation studies also suggest that lack of auditory stimulus at critical periods might lead to permanent perceptual abnormality, even though auditory acuity is later restored to an adequate level. The critical period for language development is extended, so that during the first six years there is an overlapping succession of critical periods for different language skills. Normal babies in their first month of life are able to differentiate between minimal pairs of speech sounds such as ba/da, and are already showing lateralisation to the left hemisphere for this activity, indicating that this is in some measure a prelinguistic categorisation (Entus 1977). By six months, infant babble is becoming language-specific, able to reproduce prosodic features of the input language (Laufer 1980, Crystal 1986). Towards the end of the first year of life, the infant begins to respond to words at the semantic rather than the acoustic level, and categorises them according to meaning. The evidence suggests that between this time and about four years of age, words are stored as gestalts and not phonologically analysed (Menyuk *et al.* 1986), but this does not impair categorical perception of words, and familiar words are well discriminated by three-year-olds (Barton 1976). During the same period, the child is learning many rules of grammar and testing production hypotheses (Crystal 1976). Vocabulary is increasing rapidly. Between four and six years of age, the ability to analyse words phonemically develops and a grapheme-phoneme correspondence can be learned as a preliminary to reading (Bradley and Bryant 1978). More complex grammatical structures are acquired, and internalised language can be used to reason and solve problems (Gaudena 1982). This ability continues to develop into adolescence.

In the child whose hearing is impaired at the relevant period, it is reasonable to assume that any of these processes can be interfered with, and that incapacity in one area may affect others. For example, the failure phonologically to categorise word-final /s/ /z/ and /d/ would prevent the development of the major morphological rules for nouns and verbs, and their associated semantic distinctions. Menyuk (1979) argued that an inconsistent hearing loss is particularly damaging to phonological development and to the interface of phonology and morphology.

Some studies have claimed that mild to moderate hearing loss may affect the development of semantics, syntax, phonology and verbal intelligence. Results are not consistent; this must reflect to some extent the very varied research designs.

SPECIFIC LINGUISTIC EFFECTS ASSOCIATED WITH MIDDLE-EAR DISEASE

Otitis is known to peak in the second six months of life (Sipila *et al.* 1987), when normally developing infants are internalising the phonological system. Therefore receptive and productive disorders of the phonological system are perhaps the most convincing evidence of the effect of early otitis media (Shriberg and Smith 1983). Paden *et al.* (1987) examined 40 preschool children with a positive otitis history and phonological impairment to determine which factors might predict persisting difficulty beyond three years of age. She found that early onset and late remission from otitis were among the most important variables. Shriberg and Smith (1983) used phonological analysis to pinpoint particular sound-change categories (affecting word-initial consonants and nasal consonants) which were associated with children with a positive middle-ear history. They concluded that these related to inconsistent auditory input. However Bishop and Edmundson (1986) were unable to replicate Shriberg and Smith's findings, or to find any significant differences in a range of phonological processes. Needleman (1977) found no effect of otitis history on measures of auditory discrimination, normally associated with phonological ability.

The effects on syntactic and semantic development of a positive middle-ear history are suggestive, but even less compelling than those at the phonological level. A broad range of language skills, including acquisition of words, verbal comprehension, vocabulary, linguistic concepts, grammar, reading and spelling, has been cited as being significantly associated with (i) a history of otitis (Lewis 1976, Zinkus and Gottlieb 1980, Sak and Ruben 1981, Friel-Patti *et al.* 1982), (ii) continuing otitis (Holm and Kunze 1969), or (iii) minor hearing impairment (Davis 1986). Several studies have also found associations with low verbal IQ (Gottlieb *et al.* 1979, Zinkus and Gottlieb 1980, Sak and Ruben 1981). However, Roberts *et al.* (1986) found no relationship between early otitis and any subsequent verbal or academic achievement, and Bishop and Edmundson (1986) failed to find any difference in the pattern of language impairment or rate of progress in their language-disordered groups, with and without an otitis history. Haggard and Hughes (1990) concluded that while there is sufficient evidence to accept linguistic sequelae of secretory otitis media, the effects are diverse and occur only in some children.

TABLE 3.XXIV
Reported middle-ear problems at entry (N 125)

	Onset before 2.0	Onset after 2.0 (or unknown)	Total (%)
Otitis media	7	29	36 (29)
Ear discharge	3	24	27 (22)
Recurrent earache	6	18	24 (19)
Myringotomies	2	18	20 (16)
Total with problem	14	42	56 (45)
Total no problem			69 (55)

Numbers in the first four categories are not exclusive

Dawn House Data
Middle-ear data are (i) retrospective, and (ii) current.

HISTORY OF MIDDLE-EAR PROBLEMS

We asked the parents of all new entrants to give information about early ear infections and hearing. Since the age of onset of otitis media is considered to be related to the extent of interference with language development (Hall and Hill 1986), data before and after two years of age were recorded separately (Table 3.XXIV). Parental accounts are not entirely reliable and may be vague; sometimes the primary carer was no longer available for questioning and no information could be obtained. Those mothers who were not able to remember dates, however, could often associate episodes of ear infection with a stage of development (such as the infant still being in a pram), or recalled infection as a recurrent problem throughout infancy associated with frequent colds. Otitis media was assumed to be present only if ear discharge or recurrrent earache was reported or if a doctor had treated the child for an ear condition or had performed a myringotomy. Single episodes of untreated earache may have been wrongly attributed to a fretful child, and were not included. Altogether the parents of 125 children were able to report.

The incidence of almost 45 per cent is high, and similar to that found by Gottlieb *et al.* (1979) in children with poor school performance. However Bishop and Edmundson (1986) suggested that incidence may be raised artificially because parents of children who are not developing language are more likely to report ear problems and to seek treatment. The language-disordered sample in their study did not have significantly more episodes or ear infection than their control group, but did have more referrals to ear, nose and throat (ENT) departments.

MIDDLE-EAR PROBLEMS WHILE PUPILS AT DAWN HOUSE

The prevalence of otitis media decreases with age, particularly after the age of seven (Klein 1983). The 1972 National Child Development Study found otoscopic evidence of past or present otitis in just over 8 per cent of seven-year-olds. Freeman and Parkins (1979) also used otological examination to assess middle-ear function in 50 learning-disabled 10-year-olds and 32 controls. The relative incidences of

TABLE 3.XXV

Ear problems in boarding pupils (age 5.7 to 13.5)

	Children N (%)	Occurrences
Referrals to health centre for ear problems	67 (51)	204
Removal of impacted wax	12 (9)	29
Removal of obstruction	3 (2)	3
Family doctor treatment for middle-ear infection	49 (37)	89
ENT referrals	10 (8)	10
Myringotomy + grommets	6 (5)	6
Total having middle-ear problem	51 (39)	
Total number of boarders	131 (100)	

TABLE 3.XXVI

Hearing loss in decibels at entry and finally

	Left ear mean (SD)	Right ear mean (SD)	Combined average mean (SD)
Entry N 119 (mean age = 8.0)	14 (10.8)	12 (8.9)	12.8 (8.1)
Final N 82 (mean age = 11.4)	12.6 (12)	8.4 (7.3)	10.1 (7.5)

TABLE 3.XXVII

Hearing loss greater than 15dB and 24dB at entry, by age

Age (N)		Under 15dB N (%)	15–24dB N (%)	Over 24dB N (%)
5.0–6.11	(39)	22 (56)	12 (31)	5 (13)
7.0–8.11	(47)	29 (62)	14 (30)	4 (8)
9 yrs or more	(33)	28 (85)	3 (9)	2 (6)
Total	(119)	79 (66)	29 (24)	11 (9)

TABLE 3.XXVIII

Hearing loss greater than 15dB and 24dB at discharge, by age

Age (N)		Under 15dB N (%)	15–24dB N (%)	Over 24dB N (%)
6.6–8.11	(9)	7 (8)	2 (2)	0
9 yrs or more	(73)	59 (71)	12 (15)	2 (2)
Total	(82)	66 (81)	14 (17)	2 (2)

TABLE 3.XXIX

Mean hearing loss at first and final assessment of children with and without otitis history

		Left ear mean (SD)	Right ear mean (SD)	Combined average mean (SD)
First				
Otitis media absent	(N 67)	12.5 (9.3)	11.3 (9.4)	12 (8.6)
Otitis media present	(N 52)	16 (12.3)	13 (8.3)	14 (7.4)
Final				
Otitis media absent	(N 46)	11.5 (9.8)	6.7 (4.9)	9.3 (7)
Otitis media present	(N 36)	14 (14.2)	10.5 (9)	11.1 (8.2)

reduced function were 20 per cent and 9.5 per cent. A high current incidence of middle-ear disease in Dawn House pupils would suggest the continuation of early problems, indicating the risk of continuing conductive hearing problems (Table 3.XXV). Full records of medication and clinical and hospital visits are kept for boarding pupils while they are resident in school, but this information is not always available for day pupils, so only the figures for boarders are presented.

Fifty-one of 131 pupils (39 per cent) had some diagnosed middle-ear problems while resident at Dawn House. Six had myringotomies performed. Twenty-eight had also reported early history of problems. No early information was available for 24 boarders, but five of these suffered bouts of otitis media while at Dawn House.

The available evidence suggests a raised incidence of early middle-ear disease in the Dawn House sample, with many problems continuing into school age. However, any such evidence in a language-disabled population has to be interpreted cautiously, as ear problems which might be ignored or treated lightly in an unimpaired child may be more likely to provoke investigation and treatment in a child with speech or language difficulty.

HEARING LEVELS IN DAWN HOUSE PUPILS

Each pupil has his or her hearing tested yearly by a speech therapist using a pure-tone audiometer in a specially designed, sound attenuated room. We give six-monthly tests to pupils with a history of middle-ear disease or hearing problems, mild hearing loss or poor response to sound. We also test after episodes of ear infection or staff reports of inattention to auditory input. Any child found to have a raised hearing threshold is referred to the school doctor for otoscopy and treatment if necessary. The mean pure-tone average hearing threshold for otologically normal five-year-olds has been measured at 7.6dB, based on levels at 0.5, 1 and 2kHz (Rahko and Karma 1989). Using their figures but including frequencies of 0.25 and 4kHz (as recommended for the formulation of mean hearing thresholds in the British Journal of Audiology 1976) the means for the normal children increase to 8.3dB in the right ear and 8.1dB in the left ear, with an over-all average of 8.2dB. Tables 3.XXVI to 3.XXVIII show the mean hearing levels of all Dawn House pupils who could be tested by audiometry at school entry and discharge, and

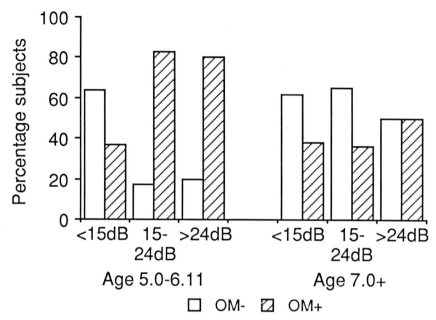

Fig. 3.2. Hearing loss and otitis media by age at first assessment.

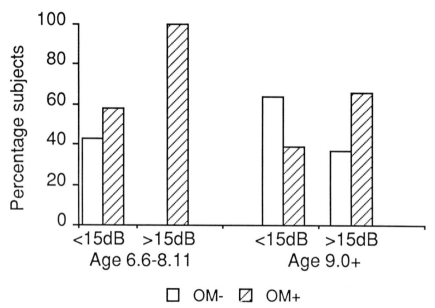

Fig. 3.3. Hearing loss and otitis media by age at final assessment.

numbers having mean losses greater than 15dB and 24dB. Children at the initial assessment who were not able to respond adequately to pure-tone testing for any reason have been excluded. Children with an air-bone gap of 15dB were referred for otoscopy and retested after any prescribed treatment. For such children the second assessment has been assumed to be more representative of their normal hearing acuity, and has been treated as the initial one.

Table 3.XXIX shows the mean hearing losses at first and final assessment for children with and without a history of otitis.

In Figures 3.2 and 3.3 the hearing thresholds have been divided at 15 and 25dB (levels which are suggested to produce disability). Taking 15dB as a cut-off point, chi-square was used to compare the two groups. Significantly more children with a positive otitis history had average hearing losses greater than 15dB at school entry (chi-square 3.86, df 1, $p<0.05$) and this was particularly true of the children under seven years of age (chi-square 6.48, df 1, $p<0.01$). This significance disappeared by the final hearing test. Age unrelated to time of testing was not significant. There was no difference between children with an onset before and after two years of age.

The evidence suggests that children with an early history of otitis media enter school with mildly impaired hearing, which is likely to exacerbate problems of poor attention and may contribute to language and learning problems. This is particularly true for children under the age of seven.

Early middle-ear problems, hearing level and language measures
A middle-ear risk scale was computed. Reported problems were scored and the points summed to form a scale of 0 to 8. Children with problems reported before the age of two years were considered to be more at risk of interference with language development. Points were awarded as follows:

Otitis media starting before age two	2
Otitis media starting after age two	1
Otitis media recurring 'frequently'	1
Effusion before age two	2
Effusion after age two	1
Effusion recurring 'frequently'	1
Myringotomy/grommets before two	2
Myringotomy/grommets after two	1

Our interest is in middle-ear problems as a possible cause or aggravating factor in language impairment, either as a debilitating condition, or indirectly through temporary hearing disability. The language abilities of children entering school were examined for any effect of early otitis using the middle-ear risk scale, and also for any effect of raised hearing thresholds (over 15dB) at school entry, using the language measures described on page 36. None of the results reached significance and the scores were in fact extremely close. Subjects were then grouped into four categories, otitis media present (a score of two and more on the risk scale), with

TABLE 3.XXX
Language measures, history of otitis, and hearing levels

Language measures			Means			
	Otitis history		Hearing loss		Otitis present/	Otitis absent/
	Present	Absent	dB15+	dB<15	dB15+	dB<15
Comprehension						
Vocabulary	86.4	82.6	83.8	85.2	85.6	83.4
Grammar	−0.97	−0.8	−1.1	−0.75	−1.4	−0.79
General~	23.4	26.3	26	24.3	20.9	23.6
Language production						
Vocabulary ~	22.3	26.3	24.7	24.4	21.9	25.7
Structure (see below)						
Morphology	21.9	20.6	19.2	22.2	21.2	22.5
Content~	34.5	41.6	32.7	41.7	28.6	42.3
Speech						
Maturity	28.7	29.9	29.4	29.1	30.5	30.4
Deviance ~	16	16.5	15.8	16.6	15.4	16.5
Written language						
Reading age	79.9	78.4	78	79.6	78.6	78.4
Structure	N	N	N	N	N	N
Stage III-	12	8	8	9	6	4
Stage IV	10	14	14	9	6	11
Stage V	11	24	25	10	4	18
Stage VI+	18	20	26	10	6	15

~Lower score = better performance
No significant differences

and without hearing thresholds above 15dB, and otitis media absent with the same hearing categories. Even between the extreme groups (otitis media present and hearing loss >15dB *vs* otitis media absent and hearing loss <15dB), there was no significant difference in language scores (Table 3.XXX). Since early middle-ear disease and minor hearing losses have been frequently cited as damaging to phonological development, we also looked at the effects of otitis on the phonological simplification processes being used by those children for whom data were available. Although we do not have data on the sound-change categories (processes) found significant by Shriberg and Smith (1983), processes affecting word endings might be expected to increase where hearing was less than adequate. In our data such processes are final consonant deletion and glottalisation of the final consonant. Neither of these processes, nor the total number of phonological simplification processes, was associated with otitis or hearing thresholds of 15dB or more (Table 3.XXXI).

Language subgroups and otitis media
Table 3.XXXII and Figure 3.4 show the distribution of children with early middle-ear problems in the subgroups of impairment. Analysis of the distribution of the four major groups confirms the lack of any significant association of subgroup with a history of otitis media.

TABLE 3.XXXI

Word final phonological simplification processes, a history of otitis media and mild conductive hearing loss

Processes	Otitis history		Hearing loss	
	Present	Absent	dB loss 15+	dB loss <15
Final consonant				
deletion present	10	11	7	14
absent	23	26	18	31
Glottalisation				
of final present	19	17	11	25
absent	14	20	14	20

No significant difference

TABLE 3.XXXII

Language subgroups and history of otitis media

Language subgroup	Otitis media	
	Absent	Present
Speech	8	8
Speech Plus	14	7
Classic	16	15
Semantic	16	10
Residual	4	4
Moderate	4	7
No Language	2	2
Young Unclassified	3	3
Severe	2	0
Total	69	56

No significant difference

Fig. 3.4. *(below).* Otitis history and language subgroups.

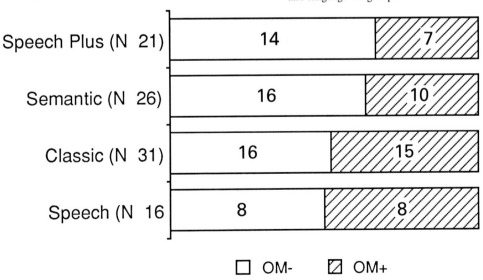

Speech Plus (N 21)   14   7

Semantic (N 26)   16   10

Classic (N 31)   16   15

Speech (N 16   8   8

□ OM-   ☑ OM+

Summary and discussion

Dawn House children were found to have a raised incidence of early middle-ear problems compared with a normal population, and early middle-ear problems were associated with reduced hearing acuity at school entry, particularly for children below seven years of age.

The disabilities associated in the literature with otitis media are all common at Dawn House. Children with SLI have delayed acquisition of speech and deficits at every linguistic level. It has frequently been suggested that mild hearing loss is a major or contributory cause of language problems, and that middle-ear disease is a sufficient cause of diminished hearing. It has also been suggested that the recurrent ill health of the otitis-prone child can cause a range of developmental problems.

Although the raised incidence suggests that otitis may have a causative role in SLI, we found no specific effects of early otitis or raised hearing threshold on any of a wide range of speech and language abilities. Scores were remarkably similar, even comparing children having a positive otitis history plus reduced hearing with children with no history plus better hearing. Most of the studies which have found positive effects have used non-disabled children as controls. An important difference here is the fact that the whole population suffers from severe language impairment. If SLI springs from diverse roots, all capable of producing severe impairment, our findings are understandable and similar deficits could be caused by otitis media in some children and have another root cause in others.

Our data are only retrospective, and based on retrospective parental reports rather than on otoscopic examination. It has not been possible to distinguish cases of secretory otitis media, thought to be most harmful, from non-secretory episodes. Nor has it been possible to measure the dimensions of severity and persistence which Haggard and Hughes (1990) indicated as major predictors of disability. However, as no hearing tests or assessments were undertaken when children were suffering from middle-ear problems or colds, we have excluded from our sample the presence of current otitis which has sometimes been claimed as a *sine qua non* of persisting language disability (Bennett *et al.* 1980). Rapin (1979) called for more sensitive assessment procedures to detect some of the subtle effects of minor hearing impairment. Clearer data and finer language tests may be necessary to provide conclusive answers. We must regard both middle-ear disease and minor hearing impairment as potential hazards and continue to make every effort to avoid them, but there is no clear evidence from these data that otitis media is an important cause or an exacerbatory factor in SLI.

Interaction of antecedent factors

The role of possible antecedents may be considered according to two models of the aetiology of language impairment. The first of these stresses the multi-causal nature of SLI (Rapin and Wilson 1978, Rapin 1982). Genetic, traumatic, social or physical events may be independently responsible for a similar cluster of language symptoms in this model: in which case, each of the possible antecedents would be

TABLE 3.XXXIII

Children with a positive family history, with and without environmental disadvantage, and language measures

Language measures	Mean scores	
	Family history, no envrisk	Family history with envrisk
Comprehension		
Vocabulary	85.9	81.7
Grammar	−0.9	−0.8
General ~	17.9	27.2*
Language production		
Vocabulary~	21.8	27.1
Structure (see below)		
Morphology	23.8	20.1
Content~	32.9	37.6
Speech		
Maturity	29.5	29.5
Deviance~	16	14.2
Written language		
Reading age	79.6	77.1
Structure	N	N
Stage III−	12	4
Stage IV	10	2
Stage V	6	11
Stage V+	13	8

~ Lower score = better performance
*Mann-Whitney U test, z −2, p<0.05

dissociated from the others. The second model is a synergistic one in which children with a predisposition to language impairment have overt occurrence of symptoms only in the event of a further triggering factor. Genetic, perinatal, environmental and physical factors might be expected to co-occur and have a cumulative effect.

Association between antecedents

Chi-squares were used to examine the association between the following potential antecedents: (i) family history of language problems in the extended family, (ii) neurisk: perinatal risk score of 3 or more and/or neurological risk, (iii) environmental disadvantage index of 2 or more, and (iv) otitis positive history (2 or more on the middle-ear risk scale). The only significant associations involved the environmental index. Environmental disadvantage was associated with a negative family history of language problems (chi-square 3.9, N 156, p<0.05) and with negative history of otitis (chi-square 5.3, N 125, p<0.05).

Environment and family history are therefore significantly dissociated, and if they have aetiological significance they must be assumed to act independently. The same dissociation is found between environment and otitis history: the likelihood of one diminishes in the presence of the other. But environmental risk and neurisk were positively associated, so perinatal risk or neurologically threatening conditions were more common in adverse environmental circumstances (chi-square 5.5, N 152, p<0.05).

TABLE 3.XXXIV

Language subgroups and number of possible antecedent factors

Language subgroup	Antecedents		
	None	One	More than one
Speech	2	6	8
Speech Plus	1	3	16*
Classic	5*	13*	13
Semantic	0	14	12
Residual	0	3	5
Moderate	2	4	4
No Language	1	2	1
Young Unclassified	0	4	2
Severe	0	1	1
Total	11	50	62

*Chi-square of 4 largest groups 12.6, N 93, df 6, p<0.05

Antecedents and language measures

So far in this chapter we have considered the effects of individual antecedent factors on the battery of language measures. It has been suggested that even if SLI can be attributed to a discrete cause, additional hazards such as frequent middle-ear illness or adverse psychosocial situations might be expected to shape the nature and outcome of the language impairment (Rutter 1987). We therefore examined the language measures when the additional hazards of otitis and environmental disadvantage occurred in children with a positive family history, and in children with increased perinatal/neurological risks. We also examined the language measures relative to the number of adverse antecedent factors present: none, one, or two or more.

The aggregation of possible antecedent factors had no effect on the language measures. Children with two or more possible aetiological factors performed in much the same way as those with a single suggestive aetiology. But there was a tendency for children with a positive family history and adverse environmental conditions to achieve poorer scores than those with positive history not environmentally disabled (Table 3.XXXIII). There was a significantly worse performance in the general comprehension measure (Mann-Whitney U test, z −2,p<0.05) by the group with family history and environmental disadvantage, but this assessment was also affected by environment alone. These data do not support a theory of cumulative antecedents increasing the severity of language problems.

Antecedents and subgroups

Finally for 123 subjects for whom data on all possible antecedents were available, we looked at the numbers and combination of antecedents present in relation to the language subgroups (Table 3.XXXIV). Over 90 per cent had some suggestive aetiology, and 50 per cent of the sample had more than one possible antecedent factor. In the four largest subgroups (Speech, Speech Plus, Classic and Semantic)

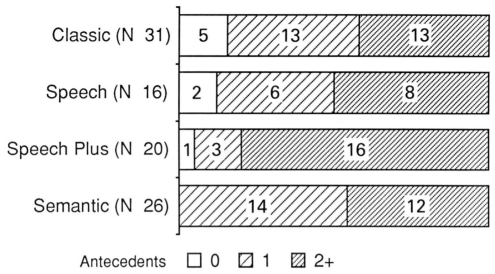

Antecedents □ 0 ▨ 1 ▨ 2+

Fig. 3.5. Language subgroups and number of antecedents (chi-square 12.6, df 6, p<0.05).

TABLE 3.XXXV

Constituents of combined antecedent factors by language subgroup

Language subgroup (N 123)	Antecedents (occurring singly, with others)			
	Positive family history	Neurisk	Envrisk	Otitis media present
Speech (16)	8 (2,6)	5 (1,4)	7 (2,5)	5 (1,4)
Speech Plus (20)	11 (0,11)	11 (0,11)*	14 (2,12)**	6 (1,5)
Classic (31)	22 (10,12)	5 (0,5)	6 (2,4)	10 (1,9)
Semantic (26)	15 (5,10)	8 (3,5)	10 (4,6)	7 (2,5)
Residual (8)	6 (2,4)	4 (0,4)	3 (1,2)	2 (0,2)
Moderate (10)	5 (2,3)	2 (0,2)	5 (2,3)	2 (0,2)
No Language (4)	0	3 (2,1)	1 (0,1)	0
Young Unclassified (6)	3 (1,2)	2 (0,2)	2 (1,1)	3 (2,1)
Severe (2)	1 (0,1)	1 (0,1)	2 (1,1)	0

Numbers with combined antecedents are not exclusive
* p<0.05
**p<0.01

there was a significantly different distribution of antecedent factors (Fig. 3.5). The Classic group included more subjects than expected with just one antecedent, or without any, while the Speech Plus subgroup had more subjects than expected with two or more antecedents.

When we broke down the constituents of antecedent combination by language group (Table 3.XXXV) we found that children showing the symptoms of a Classic language disorder were likely to have some genetic factors, and that the very severely handicapped No Language group had a traumatic history. There was also a positive family history in six of the eight children in the Residual group, possibly deriving from an earlier Classic impairment, although numbers were too small for analysis. The 20 children in the Speech Plus group, in which multiple antecedent factors are most likely to occur, had a significant number of combinations which included neurisk (chi-square 8.5, df 3, p<0.05) and environmental risk (chi-square 13, df 3, p<0.01). Seventeen of 20 children had one or both of these antecedents.

What is the evidence that these antecedents are causes of SLI?
Parents of any disabled child need to find a cause for their child's problems. An explanation—something to blame—can help family adjustment, but may lead to fairly normal events being exaggerated. The reports of antecedent factors present in 91 per cent of our subjects must be viewed in this context.

A positive family history significantly increases the risk of a child, particularly a boy, developing SLI. Such an impairment is most likely to be of the predominantly expressive, classic type where language *form* is particularly impaired. Environmental disadvantage may exacerbate this problem to some degree, but mild conductive hearing loss is not a significant additional hazard for the SLI child with positive family history.

The aetiological significance of an adverse perinatal or neurological history is not proven. Although some individual risk factors had a higher than expected incidence (caesarian and breech deliveries, small-for-gestational-age babies), no association was found between particular language functions and perinatal risk, on its own or combined with other antecedents. There was suggestive evidence that children with a perinatal problem and/or postnatal neurological problem (neurisk) were found more often in the No Language and the Speech Plus groups. In the Speech Plus group neurisk always occurred in combination with other antecedents. As expected (Davie *et al.* 1972) there was a positive correlation between perinatal and environmental disadvantage (rho 0.24, N 152, p<0.002), but we have no evidence that the combination of these factors increased the likelihood or severity of the impairment.

Our inability described earlier to find any evidence of aetiological significance in a history of otitis media, extends to an examination of the presence of otitis media in combination with other possible antecedents. No increased impairment on any of the language measures or increased membership of any language subgroup was found. The slightly odd finding that children with otitis media are more likely to be environmentally advantaged may have a social explanation. Bishop and Edmundson (1986) found a high ENT referral rate among language-impaired children relative to bouts of earache, compared with normal controls, and inferred that this was due to parental anxiety about the failure of language development. Our environmental disadvantage scale indexes large families, minority cultures, single parents and lower socio-economic groups. Such families may be expected by reason of other stresses to be less attentive to language delay, less likely to seek an explanation in ear problems, or less likely to report and remember incidents.

The analysis of environmental factors produced rather different results from the analysis of the other three antecedents under consideration. Environmental risk was associated with each of the other factors, positively with neurisk and negatively with the presence of otitis media and a positive family history. We have suggested (see p. 85) that the linguistic effects of environmental disadvantage may not be deviant but fall within a normal range of language behaviour. If this is true then the linguistic effects of environmental disadvantage in the SLI child would be superimposed onto the deviant language behaviour and exacerbate a problem stemming from a different root. Our Speech Plus group may provide an example of how this could occur. This somewhat heterogeneous group, in which severe speech disability is accompanied by a considerable degree of mixed language problems, could be the product of mixed aetiology. Sixteen out of 20 children have multiple antecedents. Neurisk (11 occurrences) and environmental disadvantage (14 occurrences) figure largely in these combinations of antecedents. It is possible that within this subgroup, a child might present with a cluster of symptoms derived from different aetiologies: with motor speech problems perhaps resulting from neurological trauma and any associated language problems made worse by problems in the environment.

Out data give weak support to a heterogeneous causal model of SLI. All four putative antecedent factors—genetic links, perinatal or neurological trauma, environmental disadvantage and early middle-ear problems—have a high separate occurrence rate among Dawn House pupils, and there are certainly other possible aetiologies for which we have no data. The most convincing association found in this sample is between SLI and family history of language problems. There is little evidence to support a synergistic causal model. In spite of the fact that more than one antecedent factor is present in half of the subjects, there is no decrease in language achievement with the increasing number of antecedents. Of the four possible antecedents considered, only environmental causes interact with all the others, and may be the triggering factor that pushes into impairment a child who is already at risk.

103

4
DEVELOPMENTAL FACTORS

First words and phrases

Normal development

The production of meaningful words by a child depends upon the development and co-ordination of cognitive, perceptual, and neuromotor skills and on an emotionally adequate nurturing environment. Lenneberg (1976) considered that meaningful speech originated only when the brain achieved a particular level of neurological maturity. Piaget (1926) stressed the necessary basis of mental representations before speech could develop. In the last 20 years psycholinguists have been more concerned with analysing the complex mechanism of language development at the different linguistic levels of semantics, syntax and phonology, and with cataloguing the variety of rates and styles with which normal children attain these skills. No longer is passive imitation thought to underlie first words; instead the infant is deemed actively and creatively to form conceptual and phonological hypotheses which must map together in order for words to be produced. Many first 'words' are in fact holophrases, such as 'allgone' or 'gimme', which are the distillates of phrases. Real phrase and clause use begins when the child is able to use simple permutations of concepts—'car gone', 'Simon car'. Many of the descriptions of speech and language acquisition in the literature are based on parental reports. These vary from the detailed diaries of parent–linguists to the more common responses to questions put at varying periods after the event. There is however a fair measure of agreement between observation and recall, and between professional and parental judgements. The general course of events is summarised here (based on Morley 1965, Davie *et al*. 1972, Crystal 1976, Elliott 1981, Fletcher and Garman 1986).

BABBLING

The non-linguistic vocalisations between birth and six months merge into a period of babble, usually between the ages of six and nine months, in which sounds and intonation patterns echo the language heard by the child, and meanings, such as anger, satisfaction or requesting, may be consistently associated with sequences of sounds or pitch movements. From nine to 12 months babbling sounds more and more speech-like, and an occasional real word may be incorporated into the stream of jargon.

FIRST WORDS

The first meaningful single words are usually produced at about one year of age. In a demographic study of Newcastle children (Morley 1965), 73 per cent of the sample had some words at 12 months of age, although acquisition age ranged from six months to 30 months, with a mean of 12 months. Only 2 per cent were two years or more when their first words were produced. Around 50 words are expected at 18 months, and 200 words by two years.

PHRASES

Between 18 months and two years of age, children acquire the ability to relate two concepts linguistically in their first phrases. As with word production there is considerable variation in the age at which this occurs and in the topics selected. Forty per cent of Morley's normal sample were joining words by 18 months and 89 per cent had some word combinations in use by the age of two years. Acquisition age for word combination ranged from 10 to 41 months, with a mean of 19 months. A relationship has been noted between the number of individual words in a child's vocabulary and the ability to combine words into phrases. Commonly an infant acquires 10 to 15 words fairly slowly, and then gains vocabulary much more rapidly until about 50 words can be used. At about this stage, the child begins to put some of these words together (Peters 1979).

Some studies find a gender difference in the rate of language acquisition. Where there is a difference it is in the direction of earlier acquisition by girls. Morley (1965) found girls to be on average a month ahead of boys in developing both words and phrases. However, a more recent study suggests that any such differences are as likely to be environmentally as biologically caused (Wells 1986).

Abnormal development

Delayed language acquisition is symptomatic of a wide variety of developmental disorders. About half of the non-communicating three-year-olds referred to paediatricians have sensory, neurological or intellectual deficiencies; those with no such underlying problem may have a specific language impairment (Mellor 1980). Several ages have been proposed as cut-off points beyond which non-development of language indicates pathology, but in the present state of knowledge these ages must be somewhat arbitrary, and it is not always made clear what constitutes non-development. Morley (1965) looked at a group of 162 children in a study of 1000 Newcastle families, who had 'defective articulation or delayed development of speech'. The average age for the first use of words for this group was 15 months, four months later than her normal sample, with the ages for first use of phrases being 24 months and 18 months respectively. In the same study, a small group of 44 children with longer-lasting 'severe defects of articulation' had very similar acquisition mean ages, 15 months for words and 25 months for phrases. These relatively small delays could indicate a wide spread of language ability with some minor handicaps in Morley's speech defective group. Allen and Rapin (1980) suggested the likelihood of pathology in any child not communicating at three, and considered that the delayed onset of 'communicative language' beyond the age of four years indicates a *severe* developmental language disorder. Communicative

105

language in this context seems to mean use of phrases and/or sentences and a range of communication functions such as *demanding* and *referring to others*. Fundudis *et al.* (1979) classified speakers as retarded if they were at or below the third centile of a normal population study. Such children were not able to string together three or more words at 36 months. In a large recent study, Teris Schery (1985) examined data from 718 Los Angeles children diagnosed as having severe and specific language problems. The mean age of first words for these children was 21 months, and 38 months for two-word combinations. It seems that there is a wide variation in acquisition age for abnormal as well as for normal language-learners.

Rutter (1987) drew attention to the variation that can exist within normal development, but recommended investigation of all those infants not using words by 24 months or phrases by 33 months. He stressed the need to examine patterns as well as rates of development, and (unusually among modern writers) attached some diagnostic importance to late or reduced babble.

If delayed language acquisition is a good predictor of future language problems, does the extent of the delay relate in a linear way to the severity of the eventual impairment? The minimal difference between acquisition age in Morley's more and less severe groups can probably be attributed to the presence of some children in her study with speech (phonological) problems only. Allen and Rapin (1980) found that the most severely disabled children among 22 they studied longitudinally were those acquiring communicative language at or after four years. In her longitudinal study, Schery (1985) incorporated age of first words and phrases in a language history cluster of 11 variables which also included attention and crying in infancy, hearing, current use of gesture, imitation, comprehension, use of language and articulation. This cluster of variables was a significant predictor of the degree of impairment in children when they entered the programme, with age of first words being one of the stronger predictive variables. However, the language history cluster was non-significant in predicting the amount of progress which the children made. Fischel *et al.* (1989) used vocabulary size as a gauge of acquisition age in a prospective study of 26 two-year-olds with expressive language problems. They were able to predict improvement over five months with 81 per cent accuracy, and concluded that two-year-olds using less than eight words were least likely to make progress. There is general agreement in these studies that the degree of retardation in acquiring language correlates with the severity of subsequent impairment.

Dawn House data
Because eager parents may **discern 'mama'** in early babble and wrongly attribute meaning to it, parents were **asked in the** pre-entry questionnaire at what age a child could use four or five single words, and the ages at which the child began to join words together and to speak clearly and intelligibly. Questions were also put about the presence and quality of babble. Because the parents of only 10 children considered that they had achieved intelligible speech by school entry, this variable

TABLE 4.I
Babbling by gender

Babble	Boys	Girls	Total
Normal	48	15	63
Scant	37	5	42
Absent	30	5	35
Total	115	25	140

No significant difference

TABLE 4.II
Age of acquisition of words, by gender

Age (mths)	Boys	Girls	Total (%)
Under 12	3	0	3 (2)
12-17	10	5	15 (10)
18-23	5	2	7 (5)
24-35	26	11	37 (25)
36-47	40	4	44 (30)
48-59	26	2	28 (19)
60 and over	10	2	12 (8)
Total	120	26	146 (100)

No significant difference

TABLE 4.III
Age of acquisition of phrases, by gender

Age (mths)	Boys	Girls	Total (%)
Under 24	1	2	3 (2)
24-35	6	1	7 (5)
36-47	29	5	34 (25)
48-59	35	7	42 (31)
60-71	22	8	30 (22)
72 and over	17	2	19 (14)
Total	110	25	135 (100)

No significant difference

has not been entered into any analysis. Parents who could not remember exact ages of language milestones, and who had no baby record book to which to refer, could often recall events before or after which words and phrases first appeared. These data were collected and have been amalgamated into acquisition age bands. (Tables 4.I to 4.III). One hundred and forty parents had recall of the baby babbling—normally, scantily or not at all. Word acquisition data are available for 146 subjects, and phrase acquisition data for 135. No differences were found between boys and girls regarding the presence of babble in babyhood or the age of acquiring words or phrases.

There is a predictable correlation between word and phrase acquisition age (Spearman's rho = 0.6, N 131, p<0.0001). There are no acquisition data of any sort for six subjects. For the other 150 a language acquisition band has been assigned based on whatever word or phrase data are available. Since the recollections of the reporting parents generally related to birthdays (*e.g.* 'no words before he was four years old'), these have been used as cut-off points. Where word and phrase data are both available and indicate different bands, phrase data have been used.

LANGUAGE ACQUISITION BANDS

1. *Normal or mildly retarded.* Phrases before 48 months and/or words before 36 months. There are 36 children in this category.
2. *Moderately retarded.* Phrases between 48 and 59 months and/or words between 36 and 47 months. This group comprises 58 children.

107

TABLE 4.IV

Mean acquisition ages in months for 3 impaired groups

		Morley (1965)		Schery (1985)		Dawn House	
		N	Age	N	Age	N	Age
	Boys	103	14.5	520	20.8	62	39.4
Word	Girls	59	15.2	198	22.8	15	32.5
	All	162	14.9	718	21.3	77	38.1
	Boys	102	24.7	520	38.3	57	53.8
Phrase	Girls	57	25.5	198	35.7	10	48.5
	All	159	25.2	718	37.6	67	53

Range of acquisition ages at Dawn House: words 8-72 mths, phrases 18-96 mths.
Only subjects with exact acquisition ages included

TABLE 4.V

Acquisition age by babbling

Acquisition delay	Babble normal	Babble scant or absent
Mild	21	13
Moderate	23	28
Severe	17	34
Total	61	75

Chi-square 6.6, df 2, $p < 0.05$

3. *Severely retarded.* Phrases at 60 months or over, and/or words at 48 months or over. Fifty-six children fall into this group.

The degree of retardation in Dawn House pupils is considerable, even compared with other pathological groups. Our least retarded group contains children who are in fact extremely retarded by comparison with normal development. Mean acquisition ages could only be calculated for children whose parents gave exact ages. These are compared with Morley's speech-defective and Schery's language-impaired samples in Table 4.IV. Maternal report is not always accurate, particularly after a gap of years as in this case, and it is possible that anxiety leads to some overestimation of the delay in a language-disabled child. Nevertheless our knowledge of the very low language levels of these children at school entry lends credence to the parents' reports.

The age of language acquisition was compared for infants with normal or reduced babble (Table 4.V). Those infants in whom babble was scant or absent were more likely to be delayed in language acquisition.

LANGUAGE ACQUISITION AND ANTECEDENTS

Chi-square tests were used to examine any relationship between acquisition age and family history of language problems, perinatal or neurological risk, environmental disadvantage or early middle-ear disease. No significant associations were found.

TABLE 4.VI

Language measures at school entry: severely retarded language acquisition band compared with combined mild and moderate delay groups

Language measures	Mean scores		
	Mild delay	Moderate delay	Severe delay
Comprehension			
Vocabulary	84	85.5	83.3
Grammar	−1.3	−0.7	−0.8
General~	20.1	23.3	29.8**
Langage production			
Vocabulary~	21.7	22.1	28.5*
Structure (see below)			
Morphology	22.9	21.5	17.7*
Content~	40.5	38.9	44.3**
Speech			
Maturity	32.7	27.3	28
Deviance~	13.5	15.6	17.7
Written language			
Reading age	78.4	79.3	78
Structure (LARSP)	N	N	N
Stage III−	5	10	13
Stage IV	4	13	15
Stage V	9	16	13
Stage VI+	14	17	11

~ Lower score = better performance
Mann-Whitney U test (one-tailed)
*p<0.05, **p<0.01

LANGUAGE ACQUISITION AGE AND LANGUAGE MEASURES AT SCHOOL ENTRY

There has been considerable discussion in the literature as to whether SLI children have delayed language development which follows the normal pattern but develops more slowly, or whether they are more properly described as having deviant language which is essentially different from normally developing language (Liles and Watt 1984). Several authors (Menyuk 1964, Leonard 1972, Crystal 1987) have promoted the view that deviance relates to a qualitative rather than quantitative language difference, demonstrated by an imbalance of development within and across language areas. We therefore analysed the effect of acquisition age on the language measures to see if children with the greatest delay in beginning to speak were still the most severely impaired at school entry, and if so, whether this was a general delay across all language skills.

Results are presented in Table 4.VI. There was little difference in scores between those children whose acquisition age we have called mildly retarded and those we have classified as moderately retarded, but some differences emerged between the moderately retarded group (phrases at 48 to 60 months, words at 36 to 48 months) and the severely retarded group (phrases after 60 months, words after 48 months). The Mann-Whitney U test was used to examine the significance of differences between the severely retarded group and the other two groups combined.

109

TABLE 4.VII
Language subgroups and language acquisition

| Language subgroup (N) | Delay | | |
	Mild	Moderate	Severe
Speech (18)	6	9	3*
Speech Plus (22)	4	11	7
Classic (44)	5	17	22*
Semantic (30)	10	10	10
Residual (10)	2	5	3
Moderate (12)	6	3	3
No Language (5)	1	0	4
Young Unclassified (6)	1	3	2
Severe (3)	1	0	2
Total (150)	36	58	56

*p<0.05

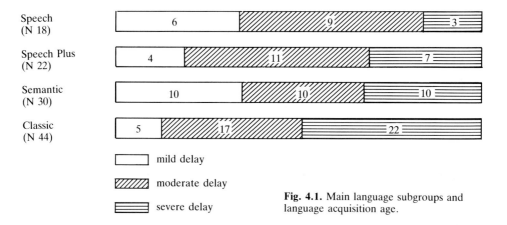

Speech (N 18)   6   9   3

Speech Plus (N 22)   4   11   7

Semantic (N 30)   10   10   10

Classic (N 44)   5   17   22

☐ mild delay

▨ moderate delay

☰ severe delay

Fig. 4.1. Main language subgroups and language acquisition age.

Children who had been slowest beginning to speak were performing least well in language skills when they entered school, but this was not evenly distributed across the language areas. Specifically they were most severely retarded in general understanding of language, and in expressive vocabulary, morphology and content. Language structure measured by LARSP level also related to acquisition age, although just failing to reach a level of significance (Kruskal-Wallis one-way ANOVA, p = 0.056). There was no significant difference between acquisition bands in development of passive vocabulary, understanding of grammar, or phonological development.

ACQUISITION AGE AND LANGUAGE SUBGROUPS

In order to examine the pattern of language impairments associated with delayed acquisition, we looked at subgroup membership (Table 4.VII).

Children in the No Language group were naturally found in the latest acquisition band, since by definition they have not acquired any language at the time of school entry. The one child in this group who appeared in the mildly retarded acquisition band was a boy with Landau-Kleffner syndrome who was reported to be using words and phrases before language ceased to develop and then disappeared at the age of 18 months. The other subgroups which had more members in the very severely delayed band than in the moderate or mild delay groups, were the Classic group, and the numerically tiny Severe group. Figure 4.1 shows the proportion of late, very late and extremely late speakers in the four large subgroups. Subjects with mild or moderate delay were more often found in the Speech subgroup, and subjects with the greatest delay were more likely to be members of the Classic subgroup (chi-square 7.34, df 2, p = 0.02).

Discussion of language acquisition delay
Children with such severe language problems that they require special education and intensive speech therapy have considerable delay in language acquisition. Those with the greatest acquisition delay are the most impaired in later years. This impairment is not a flat lag in all language domains, but tends to assume the balance we have called Classic. We found a probability that children with onset of speech after four years of age would eventually show the symptoms of a classic language impairment with marked difficulties of language production: vocabulary, form and content. Our data here concur with those of Allen and Rapin (1980), which also implicated onset after four years as an indication of severe disorder. The group least likely to have been severely retarded comprised children with predominantly articulatory or phonological difficulties.

Two paths are thought to lead to the development of words in the infant, the cognitive-conceptual path whereby meaning is established, and the phonological-articulatory path whereby the appropriate speech sounds are selected, programmed in sequence and produced. When these two paths map on to each other the child begins to use words (Carey 1978). Most language-impaired children have difficulties in both the conceptual and phonological domains, which could lead to delay in the use of words and phrases, reflecting in the first case a more language-biased, and in the second case a more speech-biased, aetiology. Almost all the children in this study were considerably delayed speakers, but those who exhibited principally speech problems came from the least severely delayed group, while the most severely delayed children later displayed the symptoms of a classic language impairment with problems of vocabulary, form and content.

The development of phrases does not rely on entirely the same abilities as the development of words. The use of phrases requires additional cognitive operations in order for two conceptual ideas to be related creatively. Children with cognitive-conceptual impairment might be expected to experience particular problems at this stage. Although there was a high correlation between word and phrase acquisition in Dawn House subjects, some children either narrowed or widened the gap between these milestones. Twelve children narrowed the gap slightly:

111

i.e. they moved from severe word delay to moderate phrase delay, or from moderate word delay to mild phrase delay. Half of these children became members of the Speech or Speech Plus subgroups, although this association was not significant. Nine children increased the gap and moved from mild word delay (before three years) to severe phrase delay (after five years), seeming to find the relationship of ideas in two-word combinations a particularly difficult hurdle. One of these was a child in the No Language group, whose language development deteriorated after single words had been established, and another was in the Speech Plus group. The remaining seven were members of the Classic group for whom linguistic expression of semantic and grammatical relationships remained a central problem, and this association was significant at the 1 per cent level (chi-square 9.13, df 1, p<0.01).

Summary

SLI is associated with considerable delay in the production of words and phrases; the extent of the delay relates to later language abilities.

Babies who did not produce normal babbling were among the slowest to develop words and phrases.

Infants developing words after four years, or phrases after five years, are likely to have a language impairment characterised by some difficulties in comprehension and speech, but with their major difficulty in language production. A lag of two years between word and phrase development is a particularly good predictor of such a language profile.

Language delay associated with articulatory and phonological problems is less extreme and less persistent than acquisition delay associated with language impairment in semantics and syntax.

These findings could have some diagnostic significance in planning future provision for non-speaking children.

Oromotor problems in infancy

Some pupils are admitted to Dawn House with physical or neurological pathology. These include pupils with cleft palate and pupils with supra-bulbar palsy who have additional language handicaps. Although language can develop normally, or even exceptionally well, in the absence of speech productive capability (*e.g.* in the case of Christy Nolan, poet and author), some language deficit frequently accompanies the lack of intelligible speech. Some children with overt pathology affecting articulation suffer from an additional language impairment, and the relationship between their speech and language difficulties is not always clear (Rapin and Allen 1983). These children can be admitted to Dawn House and would be expected to have a history of early oromotor difficulties affecting feeding.

A more tenuous connection between early oromotor problems and Dawn House children may be hypothesised in children with general motor difficulties. Many SLI children without overt pathology of any musculature are considered to be

TABLE 4.VIII
Early oromotor problems in 139 Dawn House pupils

Problems	N*	(%)
Dribbling milk through nose	6	(4)
Sucking	17	(12)
Swallowing	10	(7)
Chewing late	14	(10)
Chewing before 5 yrs	33	(24)
Chewing after 5 yrs	17	(12)
Drooling before 5 yrs	24	(17)
Drooling after 5 yrs	15	(11)

*Numbers not mutually exclusive

clumsy children with poorly developed fine and/or gross motor co-ordination (see Chapter 5). In the language-impaired population, general clumsiness has been associated with dyspraxia of speech (Gubbay 1975). There is no consensus on a definition of dyspraxia of speech, or even on the term used to describe the condition. As Tempest (1986) pointed out, the two commonest words in the opening paragraphs of papers on dyspraxia are 'controversial' and 'confusion', and in the 1980s the term 'dyspraxia' in child language disorders was increasingly used in a non-specific sense to refer to unremitting functional speech problems. However, in the specific sense of an impaired ability to produce voluntary sequential movements of the oral musculature for speech, there is some evidence of an associated history of feeding problems: notably regurgitation of milk, and late and lazy chewing (Eisenson 1984). Therefore an association may exist between early oromotor problems and speech problems, either articulatory or phonological. We collected data on feeding and other oromotor problems in the Dawn House children, and examined the data for answers to the following questions: (i) are early oromotor difficulties associated with any of the antecedent factors which are being considered, (ii) are specific oromotor problems particularly associated with later language or speech difficulties, and (iii) are particular subgroups of language disorder subsequent to early oromotor problems?

Dawn House data
During the social worker's pre-admission visit, parents were asked if their child had experienced any difficulties in the neonatal period with sucking or swallowing or regurgitating milk through the nose; at what age s/he had started to chew; if there were any problems with chewing; and whether there had been any drooling at any age (Table 4.VIII). As a measure of persistence of difficulties, data have been entered separately for occurrence before and after five years of age.

Six children dribbled milk through the nose as infants; of these, two had palatal clefts and one was later diagnosed as having supra-bulbar palsy. The other three had no overt neurological problems. Sucking and swallowing problems also occur at the early stages of the baby feeding at the breast or the bottle. We

TABLE 4.IX

Severity of oromotor problems, measured by risk scale

Oromotor risk scale	N children
0	82
1	24
2	17
3	7
4	7
5	2
Total	139

considered that the terms *sucking* and *swallowing* may have been used interchangeably by mothers to describe infant feeding problems at this stage. This view is supported by the fact that only two subjects were described as having both sucking and swallowing difficulties; usually only one or the other was reported. For the purpose of analysis, we combined sucking and swallowing problems and dribbling milk through the nose into one variable 'early feeding problems', which affected a total of 28 children. Difficulties with chewing and drooling were noted a little later, and may indicate at least delayed neuromuscular development. Chewing problems or drooling, persisting beyond five years of age, could indicate long-term oromotor difficulty and therefore difficulty with speech. Thirty-three children had chewing problems, and in 17 cases these problems continued after the age of five. Twenty-four children drooled, and 14 of these still had a drooling problem after the age of five, although this was sometimes of a minor nature. An oromotor risk scale was constructed with a range from 0 to 5 as follows:

Early feeding problems	1
Chewing problems	1
Chewing problems after age five	1
Drooling	1
Drooling after age five	1

The frequency of oromotor risk scores is shown in Table 4.IX.

OROMOTOR PROBLEMS AND ANTECEDENT FACTORS

Oromotor risk scores of 0, 1, and 2 or more were examined in relation to the antecedent factors discussed in Chapter 3. An expected positive association was found between the combined perinatal-neurological risk scale (neurisk) and oromotor problems (chi-square 7.6, df 2, $p = 0.02$). There was a smaller positive association between oromotor problems and a history of otitis (chi-square 6.1, df 2, $p = 0.047$). Family history of language problems and oromotor problems showed some dissociation, but this did not reach a level of significance (chi-square 4.96, df 2, $p = 0.08$). There was no association between oromotor problems and environmental disadvantage, or the age of language acquisition.

TABLE 4.X

Language measures and severe oromotor impairment

Language measures	Mean scores	
	0-2 problems	3 or more problems
Comprehension		
Vocabulary	84	85.7
Grammar	−0.9	−0.4
General~	23.7	27.4
Language production		
Vocabulary~	23.9	26.9
Structure (see below)		
Morphology	21.3	14.1
Content~	41.8	35
Speech		
Maturity	30.5	15.4**
Deviance~	14.8	26.9**
Written language		
Reading age	78.9	81.4
Structure	N	N
Stage III−	22	2
Stage IV	27	4
Stage V	30	4
Stage VI+	37	4

~ Lower score = better performance
**$p<0.01$

OROMOTOR PROBLEMS AND THE LANGUAGE MEASURES

Delayed development of good oromuscular function leads to late development of articulatory skills, which in turn could delay expressive abilities of language. Persisting problems of the oral musculature would also result in persisting articulatory abnormalities. Therefore we looked at the effect of oromotor problems on the full range of language, as well as speech, abilities. Only the two speech measures—maturity and deviance—were significantly affected, and this assumed significance only when a severe level of oromotor impairment (three points on the risk scale) was taken as a cut-off point. Drooling before or after five years of age, and chewing problems persisting after the age of five, were highlighted when we analysed the particular problems experienced by children with significantly slower and more deviant speech development. No other language measures were significantly affected by any oromotor difficulties. Mean scores for the language measures in children with and without severe oromotor problems are presented in Table 4.X.

SUBGROUPS AND OROMOTOR PROBLEMS

Tables 4.XI to 4.XIII show the subsequent subgroup membership of children with early oromotor difficulties. Figure 4.1 shows the proportion of oromotor problems in the four larger language subgroups. We found no significant associations between early oromotor problems and type of language impairment.

TABLE 4.XI

Language impairment subgroups of 28 children with early sucking or swallowing problems, or who dribbled milk through the nose

Language subgroup (N)	Overt pathology*	Other	Total
Speech (18)	1	3	4
Speech Plus (20)	3	2	5
Classic (41)	2	6	8
Semantic (28)	0	4	4
Residual (9)	0	2	2
Moderate (11)	1	1	2
No Language (4)	0	0	0
Young Unclassified (6)	0	2	2
Severe (2)	0	1	1
Total	7	21	28

*Includes cleft palate, cerebral palsy and supra-bulbar palsy

TABLE 4.XII

Language impairment subgroups and chewing problems before and after 5 years in children with and without overt pathology

Language subgroup (N)	Pathological* (continues after 5 yrs)		Other (continues after 5 yrs)		Total
Speech (18)	1	(1)	1	(1)	2
Speech Plus (20)	4	(3)	3	(1)	7
Classic (41)	1	(1)	11	(3)	12
Semantic (28)	0		4	(1)	4
Residual (9)	0		2	(1)	2
Moderate (11)	0		1	(1)	1
No Language (4)	2	(1)	1	(1)	3
Young Unclassified (6)	0		2	(2)	2
Severe (2)	0		0		0
Total	8	(6)	25	(11)	33

*Includes cleft palate, cerebral palsy, and supra-bulbar palsy

TABLE 4.XIII

Language impairment subgroups and drooling problems before and after 5 years in children with and without overt pathology

Language subgroup (N)	Pathological* (continues after 5 yrs)		Other (continues after 5 yrs)		Total
Speech (18)	1	(1)	3	(2)	4
Speech Plus (20)	5	(2)	0		5
Classic (41)	1	(1)	5	(2)	6
Semantic (28)	0		3	(2)	3
Residual (9)	0		2	(2)	2
Moderate (11)	0		2	(1)	2
No Language (4)	2	(2)	0		2
Young Unclassified (6)	0		0		0
Severe (2)	0		0		0
Total	9	(6)	15	(9)	24

*Includes cleft palate, supra-bulbar palsy, and cerebral palsy

Summary

Over one third of families with available data on early oromotor development (57 out of 139) reported some early problems. This could reflect the slow neurological development which has been associated with SLI. It is also possible that the figures are inflated by over-reporting. We have noted that parents of language-impaired children often begin by seeking an explanation for the impairment in some failure of the articulators.

Oromotor problems were found more frequently in children with some perinatal or neurological history, and were also associated with early middle-ear disease, but the effects of such traumatic events were very restricted. A variety of early feeding difficulties had no measureable effect on language and speech attainments at school entry. Only the more severe and remarkable problems of drooling, and chewing difficulties which persisted beyond five years of age, were significantly associated with later communication problems—and then specifically with speech articulation measures. Somewhat surprisingly, children with oromotor problems were not significantly more likely to be classified in the Speech or Speech Plus subgroups at school entry. To some extent this reflects the school admission policy of accepting children with predominantly language problems and varying degrees of speech articulation disability, but not children with speech articulation problems and no other language disability. The evidence suggests that among this selected population, speech disabilities are dissociated from problems at other linguistic levels, and that the type and degree of language impairment is independent of the degree of speech difficulty.

Some SLI children have early oromotor problems. These are not a cause of the language impairment, but severe oromotor problems such as drooling, and problems which persist after five years of age, are associated with speech articulation defects.

Walking

With few exceptions, the children in this study were very late in achieving the developmental milestones of talking, using single words and stringing words into phrases. Were they similarly slow to achieve the motor milestone of walking unaided? A low but highly significant correlation was found by Neligan and Prudham (1969*b*) between the ages of walking unaided and using sentences (three words strung together to make some sort of sense). Were these two milestones associated with each other in this sample of SLI children?

In their study of children with language delay, the age of walking was used by Fundudis *et al.* (1979) to differentiate between children with a specific language retardation (having delayed language but walking early), and those generally retarded (both language and walking being delayed). Using the age of walking as a distinguishing factor was later justified by the low levels of the latter on a wide range of cognitive (including IQ), and linguistic measures. Would age of walking in this sample be related to levels of performance on our range of language measures and IQ?

TABLE 4.XIV

Age of walking unaided, by gender

Age of walking (mths)	Boys N	Girls N	Total N	%
Before 12	17	2	19	13
12-14	36	11	47	31
15-17	27	7	34	22
18-21	25	5	30	20
22 or later	19	2	21	14
Total	124	27	151	100
Median age (mths)	16	15		15.5
Mean age (mths)	16.3	15.8		16.2
(SD)	(4.9)	(4.5)		(4.8)

Median and mean ages are based on exact ages given for 122 children, 97 boys and 25 girls
No significant gender difference

We compared our findings with the norms reported by Neligan and Prudham (1969a) in the Newcastle Survey of Child Development, which concerned all children born in Newcastle in 1961. Norms were based on contemporaneous data recorded by health visitors from information supplied by the mother. Commonly information about developmental milestones is obtained retrospectively. The authors again asked mothers about the age of walking around the time of school entry, thus providing retrospective as well as contemporaneous data. Norms were described in terms of median ages and centiles, the latter presented in the reverse of the usual order. Thus the age of 14.2 months, which falls at the 75th centile, indicates that 25 per cent of children were *not* walking at that age. Bax (1987) noted that in reporting milestones retrospectively, mothers 'tended to improve upon nature', a tendency also found by Neligan and Prudham (1969a) when they compared contemporaneous with retrospective ages of walking.

Dawn House children
Information about the age at which the children walked unaided was supplied for 151 children. An actual age was given in 122 cases, and forms the basis of the medians, means and standard deviations. Statements which indicated walking before or after a certain age have been incorporated along with exact ages into walking age bands (Table 4.XIV).

No significant difference was found between the ages given for boys and girls (Mann-Whitney u test, z −0.446), the combined median being 15.5 months. This may be compared with the Newcastle combined gender median of 13.1 months (retrospective), no gender difference emerging from that survey.

On the Newcastle norms, the 97th centile fell at 18.4 months, indicating that only 3 per cent of children did not walk by that age. In our sample, 34 per cent of the children did not walk until 18 months or later. At the other end of the scale, 25

118

TABLE 4.XV

Age of walking and language acquisition

| Language acquisition | Walking | | | |
| | by 17 mths | | 18 mths or later | |
	N	%	N	%
Words before 36 mths or phrases before 48 mths	25	25.8	11	22.5
Words 36-47 mths or phrases 48-59 mths	36	37.1	20	40.8
Words 48 mths or after, or phrases 60 mths or after	36	37.1	18	36.7
Total	97	100	49	100

Chi-square 0.263, df 2, NS
Correlation coefficient (Spearman rho) 0.05 between ages of walking and use of phrases for 55 children for whom exact ages were available for both variables

per cent of the normal population walked by 12 months, compared with our 13 per cent.

This picture of delay in walking is in keeping with other studies of speech- and languaged-impaired children. In her report of the 215 children found to have marked speech defects in the National Child Development Study of over 15,000 children, Sheridan (1973) noted that 16 per cent were not walking by 18 months, compared with 4 per cent of controls, while Robinson (1987) reported that 22 per cent of 82 SLI children were similarly delayed. In a study of 718 language-disordered children, Schery (1985) found the mean age of walking to be 14.9 months, also later than average—although lower than our mean of 16.2 months.

On all indices—median, mean and distribution of age groups—this sample includes a very much greater proportion of late walkers than would be expected from a normal population. If, as Neligan and Prudham (1969a) found, mothers tended to underestimate in retrospect, then the delays may have been greater than those here reported.

AGE OF WALKING AND ANTECEDENT FACTORS
The age of walking (in three age bands—by 15 months, between 15 and 17 months, and 18 months or later) was examined for the effect of the antecedent factors: a positive family history of language problems, a history of perinatal difficulty alone and combined with neurologically threatening events, adverse environmental conditions, and middle-ear infections. No association was found between any of these antecedent factors and the age of walking, nor was there any trend even suggestive of any antecedent effect.

IS AGE OF WALKING RELATED TO AGE OF LANGUAGE ACQUISITION? (Table 4.XV)
Neligan and Prudham (1969a) recorded significant correlations between the ages of walking and using sentences: r 0.16 for boys and 0.14 for girls. In this study, for the

55 boys and girls for whom a specific age for both walking and using phrases had been given, a correlation coefficient of 0.05 (Spearman rho) indicates a virtual absence of association between these two developmental milestones. Early walkers (walking before 12 months) were compared with very late walkers (walking after 21 months) for the age at which phrases began to be used. No child was using phrases before 36 months in either group. The very late use of phrases (after 60 months) was slightly more frequent among the very late walkers (nine out of 18, compared with six out of 19 of the early walkers) but the difference between them was not significant (chi-square 1.19, df 1). The lack of association was further borne out by the distribution of language acquisition age bands in children walking before 18 months, and those walking at or later than 18 months.

Within this sample of children with a severe SLI, only three of whom had begun to use phrases before two years, the age at which they began to walk independently bore no relationship to the age at which they began to acquire language. Compared with normal children, both language and walking were seriously delayed in almost all. Despite this, it would have been wrong to conclude in early childhood that these children were generally retarded.

AGE OF WALKING AND IQ

Fundudis *et al.* (1979) used age of walking to subdivide their sample of 84 Residual Speech Retarded children. Those walking early were described as having a specific delay, and the late walkers as generally delayed. Examination of the children at seven and eight years indicated that the former experienced a form of 'developmental dysphasia'. The latter displayed greater retardation on a range of language measures and the mean non-verbal IQ was significantly lower, resulting in a picture of general rather than specific retardation.

The language impairments of our sample are specific in terms of their non-verbal abilities, our criteria for selection demanding that each child functioned within or above the average range on an individually administered test of non-verbal intelligence, usually the WISC-R Performance Scale. Nonetheless it is possible that the very late walkers had a lower IQ than than those who walked earlier.

The 90th centile on the Newcastle norms falls at 15.8 months, the basis for the cut-off point of 16 months used by Fundudis *et al.* (1979). We employed a similar cut-off point for this analysis. There are 126 children with data on walking and a non-verbal IQ. (The tests of intelligence, their administration and results are presented in Chapter 5. The mean IQ for the 77 children walking by 16 months is 99, compared with a mean of 97 for 49 children walking after 16 months—both with a standard deviation of 10. (Mann-Whitney U test, $z - 0.827$, NS). There is no evidence that the children who are late in walking are duller at school entry than those who walk earlier.

AGE OF WALKING AND LANGUAGE MEASURES

Was the age of walking, particularly late walking, associated with the severity of language deficit on entry to the school?

TABLE 4.XVI

TABLE 4.XVI
Language measures and age of walking

| Language measures | N | Age of walking | | | | | |
| | | by 15 mths | | 15-17 mths | | 18 mths or later | |
		Mean	(SD)	Mean	(SD)	Mean	(SD)
Comprehension							
Vocabulary	144	84	(14)	84	(11)	84	(12)
Grammar	98	−1	(1)	−1	(1)	−1	(1)
General~	95	25	(18)	23	(15)	27	(16)
Language production							
Vocabulary~	132	24	(16)	20	(15)	29	(16)
Structure (see below)	140						
Morphology	95	23	(11)	20	(9)	18	(11)
Content~	78	38	(16)	41	(21)	45	(20)
Speech							
Maturity	147	29	(18)	27	(20)	29	(17)
Deviance~	146	15	(13)	20	(17)	16	(14)
Written language							
Reading age	141	78 mths	(11)	78 mths	(14)	81 mths	(11)
Structure		N		N		N	
Stage III−		14		7		6	
Stage IV		13		8		12	
Stage V		16		6		16	
Stage VI +		18		10		14	
Total	140	61		31		48	

~ Lower score = better performance
No significant differences

An examination of the scores on each of the comprehension, language production, speech and written language measures, for three walking age bands (by 15 months, between 15 and 17 months, and 18 months or later) produced no significant result (Kruskal-Wallis ANOVA for the nine tests with interval scores and chi-square for sentence structure). We also compared very late walkers (22 months or later) with those who walked very early (before 12 months) on each language test. Again, on no language measure did the difference between these two groups (Mann-Whitney U test) reach a level approaching significance.

There is no evidence that late walkers are more severely retarded at school entry on our array of language measures than those who walk relatively earlier (Table 4.XVI).

AGE OF WALKING AND LANGUAGE SUBGROUPS

The distribution of the three walking age bands in each of the nine language subgroups is detailed in Table 4.XVII. Inspection of the distribution suggested some possible differences. About half of the children in each of the Speech, Semantic, Moderate and No Language subgroups were walking before 15 months. On the other hand, late walkers (18 months or later) appeared to be slightly more

TABLE 4.XVII
Language subgroups and age of walking

Language subgroup (N)	Age of walking		
	by 15 mths	15-17 mths	18 mths or later
	N	N	N
Speech (19)	10	4	5
Speech Plus (22)	8	4	10
Classic (43)	16	13	14
Semantic (30)	15	6	9
Residual (10)	3	4	3
Moderate (12)	7	0	5
No Language (6)	3	1	2
Young Unclassified (6)	3	2	1
Severe (3)	1	0	2
Total (151)	66	34	51

numerous among the Speech Plus. Cell numbers are too small for the calculation of an over-all chi-square, but on the null hypothesis of no association between walking and subgroup membership, expected frequencies were calculated. These were very similar to those observed. The chi-square value for the first four major subgroups, (3.589, df 6) falls far short of significance. There is no evidence of an association between the age of walking and language subgroup membership.

Summary
Only 44 per cent of the children in this sample were walking unaided by 15 months. One third were not walking by 18 months more than 10 times the number to be expected from norms described by Neligan and Prudham (1969*a*).

Age of walking was not related to age of language acquisition. Each of these milestones appears to develop independently in this sample of SLI children.

Children who walked late, after 16 months (the cut-off point used by Fundidis *et al.* 1979), were not duller than those who walked earlier. The mean non-verbal IQS for late and earlier walkers were 97 and 99 respectively.

At school entry, age of walking was not related to the degree of language deficit on our range of comprehension, language production, speech and reading measures. Nor was any association found between walking and language subgroup membership.

No associations were found between walking age and a family history of language problems, perinatal or neurologically threatening events, environmental disadvantage or middle-ear disease.

Although not directly related to any of the linguistic variables examined, walking at a later than average age remains a common feature among our specifically language-impaired children. They present exceptions to the general retardation so often associated with marked delay in both walking and talking.

Bladder and bowel control
Early control of bladder and bowel is related primarily to physiological maturation,

with boys usually achieving control later than girls (Davie *et al.* 1972, Essen and Peckham 1976, Richman *et al.* 1982, Golding and Tissier 1986). Persistent day-wetting after the age of three years, and persistent bed-wetting after four years, were regarded as abnormal by Ellis and Mitchell (1968). Nonetheless both day- and night-wetting and soiling are not uncommon among young children. For example, in a one-in-four sample of 705 three-year-olds in a London borough, day-wetting (at least once a week) occurred in 16.9 per cent, bed-wetting (at least three times a week) in 37.4 per cent, and soiling (at least once a week) in 12.8 per cent—boys wetting and soiling significantly more frequently than girls (Richman *et al.* 1982).

Several explanations for delayed control have been postulated (Essen and Peckham 1976). Commonly found gender differences point towards physiological reasons, but not exclusively. Regular wetting and soiling are common in behavioural disturbances, even at the early age of three years (Richman *et al.* 1982). Among five- to seven-year-old children, Paterson and Golding (1986) found that wetting and soiling, one of a number of behaviour problems, were 50 per cent more likely to occur among children with speech disorders than among those without such problems.

While developmental delay may be one factor underlying both language impairment and incontinence, it is also possible that by five years, this and other behaviour problems follow from the great frustration experienced by most SLI children (see Chapter 5).

Dawn House children
In this study, information about the acquisition of bladder and bowel control had been collected mainly from mothers. Children were recorded as dry or not, and clean or not, by the age of three years. Just before the children entered school, parents were again asked about wetting and soiling. Information had not been collected systematically for the school's first entrants, with the result that numbers vary, with a maximum of 142 for the three-year and 149 for school-entry data. These were examined for their similarity or otherwise to survey findings with the expectation of higher rates of wetting and soiling among our SLI sample than have been found in population samples of comparably aged children.

Comparisons were made with findings from the follow-up studies of the second and third national surveys of all births in England, Scotland and Wales, the 1958 and 1970 cohorts (Davie *et al.* 1972, Butler and Golding 1986). The main source of normative data for the children at three years was the one-in-four sample of all three-year-olds in the London Borough of Waltham Forest (Richman *et al.* 1982. Such comparisons can be no more than suggestive, partly because of the differences in criteria for different behaviours, partly because of the slightly different ages to which information relates, and partly because our SLI sample includes only 27 girls, the ratio of boys to girls being almost five to one.

Most of our pupils were found to be late in walking, and if late bladder

TABLE 4.XVIII

Bladder and bowel control by 3 years, by gender

	Boys N	Girls N	Total N	%
Dry by day	85	19	104	75
Not dry	28	6	34	25
Total			138	
Dry by night	70	14	84	59
Not dry	47	11	58	41
Total			142	
Clean by day	81	19	100	76
Not clean	27	5	32	24
Total			132	
Clean by night	78	19	97	73
Not clean	30	5	35	27
Total			132	

No significant gender differences

and/or bowel control by three years is largely an expression of developmental delay, one would expect a positive association with walking.

Low social class has consistently been linked to bed-wetting in particular, and we look at social class and its relation to bladder and bowel control.

WETTING AND SOILING AT THREE YEARS

Table 4.XVIII shows early day and night bladder and bowel control at the age of three years. The occasional accident was ignored when determining whether children were dry or clean. The significant gender differences noted in surveys (Davie *et al.* 1972, Richman *et al.* 1982, Butler and Golding 1986) were absent in our sample. Values of chi-square for each with every other category of control ranged from 0.000 to 0.195 (df 1), indicating almost identical rates of control or lack of it for boys and girls.

Twenty-five per cent of our boys and girls combined were not dry by day, and 41 per cent were bed-wetting, compared with 16.9 per cent and 37.4 per cent for day- and night-wetting at the same age in the Waltham Forest study. While the incidence for SLI boys was 25 per cent for day- and 40 per cent for night-wetting, comparable to that found in the survey (namely 22.5 and 44.7 per cent respectively) day-wetting among our small number of girls was twice as common.

Soiling occurred in 24 per cent by day and 27 per cent at night, compared with a soiling rate of 12.8 per cent in the Waltham Forest survey. This last percentage conceals a gender difference of 17.8 per cent for boys and 8 per cent for girls. While soiling among the SLI boys was about 1½ times more common, the rate for girls was about three times higher.

TABLE 4.XIX

Bladder and bowel control at 3 years by age of walking

	Age of walking	
	by 17 mths N	18 mths or later N
Dry by day	73	29
Not dry	16	18*
Dry by night	56	26
Not dry	34	24
Clean by day	70	29
Not clean	16	16
Clean by night	67	29
Not clean	19	16

*Chi-square 5.733, df 1, $p<0.02$

BLADDER AND BOWEL CONTROL AND AGE OF WALKING

Are early wetting and soiling aspects of developmental delay? If late bladder and bowel control are related to neurophysiological delay, one might expect control after three years to occur more frequently among children whose motor milestone of walking unaided was also late.

Chi-square tests were used to find associations between age of walking (by or after 18 months) and bladder and bowel control. Late walkers had a consistently higher incidence of day- and night-wetting and soiling. The value of chi-square reached a significant level on day bladder control (Table 4.XIX) and fell just short of significance on day bowel control (chi-square 3.726, df 1, $p<0.054$).

BLADDER AND BOWEL CONTROL AND SOCIAL CLASS

An association between wetting and soiling and social class has been found in both the 1958 and 1970 cohort studies of children beyond the age of three years. This may be due to different family pressures, attitudes, and ages at which toilet-training was started (Golding and Tissier 1986). We looked at the distribution of children who had and had not attained bladder and bowel control by three years in the non-manual (Social Class I, II and III non-manual) and manual (III manual, IV and V). There was a consistent trend in the association between control and social class, but not in the direction expected from national surveys. Fewer children from the non-manual classes had control, compared with children from the manual classes, the strength of the association reaching a significant level for dry by day (Table 4.XX) and just failing to reach significance for clean by day (chi-square 3.596, df 1, $p>0.05$). Perhaps instead of exerting greater pressure, as has been suggested, the non-manual classes tend to be less exacting of children who are already demonstrating delay in reaching the developmental milestones for talking.

The relationship between walking, wetting and soiling, and social class, suggests that developmental delay and perhaps reduced expectation among the non-manual classes influences the achievement of early bladder and bowel control

TABLE 4.XX

Bladder and bowel control at 3 years, by social class
(excluding unemployed and unknown)

	Non-manual (I-III NM) N	Manual (III M-V) N
Dry by day	20	80
Not dry	14	19*
Dry by night	18	64
Not dry	17	38
Clean by day	20	77
Not clean	12	18
Clean by night	21	73
Not clean	11	22

*Chi-square 5.42, df 1, p<0.02

in this SLI sample. If developmental delay is an important factor, one might expect the children to achieve satisfactory control at a later age.

BED-WETTING AND SOILING AT THREE YEARS AND ON ENTRY TO SCHOOL

Because our information relates to only two points in time, it cannot be assumed that there had been no periods of continence between two reports of incontinence or that there had been no wetting or soiling between reports of early and late control. Nevertheless, late bladder control can be assumed in a child who was bed-wetting at three years but dry on entry to school, while bed-wetting and soiling at three years and at school entry suggests a persistent problem. Because of the range of entry ages in our sample, and the different ages at which information was collected in the surveys, any comparison with other studies can be no more than weakly suggestive.

Bed-wetting. Information at three years and at school entry was available for 142 children, 117 boys and 25 girls. Eighty-five children (60 per cent) were reported to be dry at three years and at entry to school. No child reported to be dry at night by three years was bed-wetting on entry to school. A further 44 children, 37 boys and seven girls (31 per cent) not dry at three years were reported to be dry on entry to school, suggesting that these may have been later than usual in attaining bladder control. Thirteen children, nine boys and four girls (9 per cent), were bed-wetters and had also been so at three years. Eleven of these were between five and seven years, 14 per cent of 79 children in that age group, a percentage which may be compared with the 11 per cent of children in the 1958 cohort reported to wet between five and seven years (Davie *et al.* 1972). It is more difficult to find a comparable figure for the two remaining bed-wetters, 3 per cent of 63 children aged eight years or over. Richman *et al.* (1982) found that 4 per cent of eight-year-olds

126

TABLE 4.XXI
Bed-wetting and soiling at 3 years and at school entry

	Boys N	Girls N	Total N	Total %
Dry at 3 yrs and at entry	71	14	85	59.9
Bed-wets at 3 yrs but not at entry	37	7	44	31
Bed-wets at 3 yrs and at entry	9	4	13	9.1
Total	117	25	142	100
Clean at 3 yrs and at entry	79	18	97	75.8
Soils at 3 yrs but not at entry	22	4	26	20.3
Soils at 3 yrs and at entry	3	1	4	3.1
Clean at 3 yrs but soils at entry	1		1	0.8
Total	105	23	128	100

were enuretic, while a prevalence rate of 4.8 per cent is reported for the 1958 cohort at 11 years.

Soiling. We had information about 128 children, 105 boys and 23 girls, at both points in time. Ninety-seven children, 79 boys and 18 girls (76 per cent), had been clean both at three years and at school entry. A further 22 boys and four girls (20 per cent) had soiled at three years but not on entry to school, suggesting bowel control after three years. Five children (3.9 per cent) were encopretic at entry, four occasionally and one frequently. Four had soiled at three years, suggestive of a persisting problem, while a fifth was reported to have been clean previously. Three were aged between five and seven years, 4 per cent of the 72 in that age group, compared with just over 1 per cent for the 1958 cohort. Two children (aged eight and nine), comprise just over 3 per cent of the 64 children aged eight years or over (Table 4.XXI). Richman *et al.* (1982) reported a higher rate of soiling (4 per cent) at eight years.

Bed-wetting at entry occurred only among children who were not dry at three years. The diminishing proportion of enuretics, when entrants are grouped by age (under eight years and eight years or over), reaches a point where the percentage corresponds quite closely to normal prevalence rates. The incidence for encopresis follows the same general pattern. Our incidence seems high by comparison with 1958 cohort rates, but not with the Waltham Forest survey.

Summary and discussion

At the age of three years, rates of wetting and soiling appear to be higher than expected from a survey sample.

Gender differences favouring girls have been consistently reported in national studies. No differences were found between boys and girls in this study. In effect this means that wetting and soiling were more common than expected among the girls.

An association between late walking and wetting and soiling suggests that neurophysiological delay is at least one contributory factor to late control.

Social class was linked to wetting and soiling, but not in the direction expected from national surveys. In this study the non-manual classes were associated with late wetting and soiling.

By the time the children entered school, rates of bed-wetting were comparable to those reported in national surveys. Encopresis diminished at a similar rate, but comparisons are inconclusive because of differences in survey findings.

The over-all picture from the three-year and school-entry data suggests that our SLI children tend to be late in achieving bladder and bowel control, but that ultimately bed-wetting (though perhaps not soiling) is not more common than in a normal population. We have suggested that developmental delay may be one factor, but the strong association between wetting and soiling as early as three years with behaviour disturbance (Richman *et al.* 1982) suggests that this may be an additional factor. Paterson and Golding (1986) found a higher rate of severe behaviour problems including wetting and soiling among five-year-olds with speech disorders. The high level of frustration experienced by children who wish to communicate but do not have the means to do so is discussed in Chapter 5. Both developmental delay and frustration could contribute to wetting and soiling at three years.

By the time of school entry, rates (particularly of bed-wetting) are not higher than might be expected. Paterson and Golding (1986) reported that only one in 23 of their speech-disordered five-year-olds had seen a speech therapist. All our SLI children had had speech therapy before school entry. Although this may not have been sufficient to meet their individual needs, the problems of the children had been or were being identified, and attempts were being made to remediate. School-entry data were collected after children had been accepted as pupils, usually to the great relief of parents. Both the pre-entry speech therapy and the acceptance of a place in the school may well ameliorate frustration and anxiety in both children and parents with a positive effect on behaviour, including toileting.

5
CORRELATES OF LANGUAGE IMPAIRMENT

The brief history of the study of SLI contains recurrent themes, derived originally from clinical observations and developed by research, of abilities and behaviours which also often veer from normality in children whose language is impaired.

Even when research seems to deny any firm basis for association with SLI, as has occured with auditory processing and with laterality, these themes recur as new observations and hypotheses are made.

Following the theories of minimal cerebral dysfunction which were current in the 1950s and 1960s, there have been suggestions that a non-damaged but different organisation of the brain may exist in SLI children. This has increased interest in neurological investigation, in the hope that new technology will in time provide some answers to old questions. One brain 'difference', the disparity between verbal and non-verbal ability, has long been used as one defining factor in specific impairment.

1. Auditory perception and processing abilities

Auditory processing is the term most often used to describe the post-cochlear categorisation, organisation, and interpretation of input speech, based on the listener's prior experience and innate species-specific capacity (Eisenson 1984). Lehiste (1972) proposed two processing levels, a primary level of 'listening in the speech mode' which is acoustic and phonetic, and a secondary linguistic level which is phonological and syntactic. Processing at these two levels is concurrent. While this division corresponds to some extent to the distance travelled along the neural pathway from the cochlea to the temporal lobe, and can be useful in teasing out and investigating auditory processing problems, it is unreal inasmuch as linguistic analysis is implicated from an early stage of speech perception. Luria (1966) wrote that 'the process of remembering is a direct continuation of the process of perception', and top-down processing (using semantic and syntactic knowledge to compute probabilities) interacts in a complex manner with the bottom-up processing of individual sounds into meaningful units (Marslen-Wilson and Welsh 1978). The complex interactive nature of this procedure probably accounts for some of the inconsistent results of the research into auditory processing problems. The auditory abilities most often selected for these studies have been speech perception and auditory verbal memory, although some researchers have looked for a composite auditory factor, and others have discussed 'auditory processing problems' without defining precisely what these are (Zinkus and Gottlieb 1980). In this chapter we consider speech perception and then auditory short-term memory in Dawn House pupils in the light of current theories.

A. Speech perception

Auditory discrimination was an early focus of interest for those working in the field of language impairment. Abnormal-sounding speech is a salient feature, and was the area of disordered child language which attracted most interest in the first half of this century. When children with speech problems were found to have normal intelligence and hearing acuity, and no overt neuromotor difficulties, questions were posed about their ability to perceive speech normally, and some of the earliest assessment measures used by speech therapists were tests of speech discrimination (Travis and Rasmus 1931, Templin 1943, Wepman 1958). At first speech perceptual problems were examined only in relation to disordered speech production, but the contemporaneous development of the fields of applied linguistics and acoustic technology led to investigations into the role of auditory discrimination difficulties at other linguistic levels.

The nature and development of speech discrimination

Speech consists acoustically of an unsegmented flow of sound, and motorially of continuous, variable, overlapping movements. The partitioning of the stream of sound into words and phonemes is a psycholinguistic act performed by the listener. Even the relatively mechanical aspects of sound analysis in terms of intensity and frequency, which are carried out at low levels of the auditory system, are influenced by the selective attention of the listener, who is 'listening in the speech mode'. Beyond this level all decoding becomes voluntary and interactive.

Selective attention serves to distinguish the chosen stimulus from a background of related distracting stimuli. It is only applied to stimuli which are recognised by the listener as relevant, and it is sharpened by perceptual expectancies. We do not pay much attention to completely unknown tongues which we have no chance of understanding, a fact which may have relevance to the poor attention to verbal input of the SLI child. Auditory material enters a brief echoic memory which lasts a second or two; the information then fades unless further processing takes place. The size of the unit that is processed is not fixed. Neisser (1967) suggests that it may vary according to the listener's need to detect sounds, words or meaning, but it will depend upon a knowledge of the appropriate phonetic, phonological, syntactic or semantic rules. Processing time is reduced by the dynamic interaction of all these levels and the continuous online computation of probabilities, so that a mispronounced word may be 'heard' correctly by the listener incorporating semantic expectancy into the decoding task. We make sense of what we hear, and become faster and more efficient listeners by doing so. It has been calculated from response times that the minimum perceptual unit in general conversational use is probably the word, and sometimes the syllable.

Young children are thought to perceive both words and individual speech sounds differently from adults. At first they perceive words as gestalts, not strings of sounds, with the sound quality of individual phonemes attached to the whole word (Waterson 1971, Ferguson and Farwell 1975, Menyuk *et al.* 1986). Important developments take place around the age of six, as the child begins to perceive words as consisting of sequences of sounds. This ability to separate words into their constituent phonemes is normally developed when children show a heightened awareness of phonological units associated with learning to read (Ervin-Tripp 1973). It is not yet established whether segmentation abilities precede and contribute to the development of reading, or derive from it, but it is most probably a reciprocal process (Morais *et al.* 1987, Ellis and Large 1988). From this stage onwards many aspects of language development (*e.g.* vocabulary development and memorising) are affected by the use of phonological coding.

The apparently arbitrary division of speech into units which contrast with each other, and can therefore build into words which have distinct meanings, varies in different languages. An example of this is the way languages distinguish between 'voiced' and 'voiceless' sounds. Voiceless sounds are not actually produced without any vibration of the vocal cords, but are classified as voiceless because voicing begins much later during the articulation of p, f, k and s, for example, than it does during the articulation of their 'voiced' equivalents, b, v, g and z. Most languages, including English, distinguish voiced from voiceless sounds using a voice onset lag which is innately discernible by babies. A minority of languages however, use different voice onset lags to distinguish pairs, or have developed three voicing categories.

The ability to recognise and categorise individual, *language specific* phonemes develops during infancy, and is not adult-like for some considerable time. It develops from the ability, found in babies as young as six weeks, to categorise some features of sounds which will later be incorporated into language (Morse 1979). This is a prelinguistic acoustic-phonetic categorisation. True linguistic categorisation begins towards the end of the first year, when together with context, facial expression, body language and prosody, it contributes to the development of comprehension. As infants gradually acquire the ability to categorise sounds phonemically, they may utilise or change the prelinguistic phonetic categories they have established, to produce the phonemic boundaries particular to their mother tongue (Simon and Fourcin 1978).

At first, infants use different perceptual features from adults to differentiate phonemes (Macken and Barton 1980), and only gradually do they begin to apply adult criteria.

In spite of these differing perceptual techniques, even young children under three years of age are able to distinguish pairs of words which differ by only one distinctive feature (such as 'fan' and 'van') without being aided by context (Barton 1978).

Auditory processing and specific language impairment
Many studies have compared language-impaired children with controls in auditory perceptual tasks. The suggestion is that some sort of perceptual impairment is fundamental to the language disability, although the nature of the relationship is

131

generally not made explicit. These studies have often tried to define the nature of the auditory perceptual defect, using synthetic or synthetically altered speech-like sounds in order to eliminate irrelevant features. Some early studies using tests of musical ability found that speech-impaired children had poor discrimination of pitch direction (Sommers *et al.* 1961) and minimal pitch differences (Mange 1960). Auditory processing of language necessarily incorporates a temporal and sequential element, and many experimenters have explored this aspect. Studies have investigated the inter-sound interval necessary to perceive separate rather than fused tones (Lowe and Campbell 1965, Haggerty and Stamm 1978), the ability to perceive sound differences (Rosenthal 1970, Tallal and Piercy 1973), and the ability to detect sequences having different variant features (Lowe and Campbell 1965; Rosenthal 1970; Tallal and Piercy 1973, 1978; Tallal *et al.* 1980). There have been some conflicting results from the first two areas studied but very consistent findings regarding the third type of perceptual judgement. There is now overwhelming evidence, mainly from the work of Tallal and her colleagues, that many language-impaired children are unable to process auditory sequences involving rapid frequency change, but the implications are not fully worked out. Some claim that slow processing speeds in SLI children may be a root cause of their problem.

Speech discrimination in language-impaired children: theoretical approaches
Probably the most commonly cited theory proposes that impaired auditory perception is symptomatic of some form of cerebral dysfunction or innate 'perceptual difference' (Eisenson 1984), and is a sufficient cause for language disability. The assumption here is that a child cannot decode verbal input because s/he cannot categorise it, and that s/he cannot reproduce something until s/he first perceives it accurately (Wepman 1960, Benton 1964, Powers 1971.) The strong form of this theory seems to predict that all SLI stems from perceptual inadequacy: in which case all SLI children would have auditory perceptual deficiencies, and those with the greatest perceptual impairment would have the most severe language impairment.

Several writers have discussed the involvement of impaired auditory memory in discrimination problems (McReynolds 1966, Weiner 1967). Both short-term and long-term memory have been invoked in connection with perceptual ability. Rosenthal (1972) argued that limited short-term storage underlay difficulties in processing the speech signal, but the finding that words were discriminated more accurately than non-words (Barton 1978), implicated semantic processing and long-term memory. If poor auditory memory is a significant cause of discrimination problems, one would expect the two to be strongly correlated.

Locke (1969) also thought that an adequate memory store was a prerequisite for the development of phonological categorisation. In the last two decades, resulting partly from the work in adult psychoneurolinguistics, there has been considerable interest in children's ability to develop phonological coding, as fundamental to how they perceive words, store them in memory, access vocabulary, speak, read and spell. The implication of these theories is that there is an interactive network of language-related problems, rooted in an inability to make efficient use of phonological code. If inefficient phonological coding is responsible for poor discrimination, the effect should disappear when the material to be discriminated is non-verbal and so cannot be phonologically coded. Phonological coding and memory are discussed further in the second section of this chapter.

The motor theory of speech perception (Liberman *et al.* 1967, 1985) has had considerable influence on theories of speech perception in the language- and speech-impaired population. In its simplest form, the motor theory states that perception of speech is achieved through an innate biological linkage to the phonetic gestures necessary to produce those sounds. One corollary of this may be that, since the speechless or speech-impaired child has inaccurate or non-existent phonetic gestures, perception cannot develop normally, and that speech discrimination difficulties mirror the production difficulties. Investigations into the relationship between perception and production have been manifold and inconclusive but the main findings can be summarised as follows:

1. Many children with phonological disorders do have reduced scores on tests of auditory discrimination (Wepman 1960, Marquardt and Saxman 1972).

2. Children with normally developing speech also sometimes score poorly on discrimination tests (Powers 1971, McReynolds *et al.* 1975).

3. Children can discriminate sounds which they cannot produce, and produce sounds which are not native to their language—sounds they have not perceived (Smith 1973). Some children make more discriminatory errors of speech sounds in which they also make production errors (Locke and Goldstein 1971, Powers 1971, Monnin and Huntingdon 1974).

4. However, the association between misperceived and misproduced speech sounds is found only in some children (Edwards 1974, Eilers and Oller 1976) or in some sound categories (Prins 1963, Schissel 1980).

5. Speech sound discrimination is a skill that continues to develop until the ninth year (Wepman 1960).

6. The association between discrimination and production errors is stronger in young children (Weiner 1967, Morgan 1984).

7. Improved discrimination may be subsequent to improved articulation and not *vice versa* (Prins 1963). This comes from the motor theory of speech perception, which implies that impaired perception is secondary to impaired articulation and that the worse the speech output, the worse discrimination is likely to be. In the motor theory, there is a strong relationship between the sounds which are misproduced and the sounds which are misperceived.

Another view is that auditory perceptual difficulties and language difficulties are not causally related but co-occur, both resulting from some diffuse brain dysfunction (Ludlow 1980). According to this theory, an increased level of impaired perception could be expected in SLI, but with no aetiological or correlational significance.

The failure to produce firm evidence of a causal relationship between auditory factors and language impairment caused Rees (1973) to argue that attempts to link auditory imperception to language impairment should be abandoned. However, the complexity of the processes involved, and the difficulty of disentangling theories which have overlapping predictions, suggest the need for caution. New investigatory techniques and increasingly complex models of language processing have kept the issues very much alive, and clinical acceptance of the importance of auditory perception in language impairment remains widespread.

It is not the intention of this study to solve the theoretical issues discussed above but to cast some light on the following questions:

1. How universal are discrimination problems in language-impaired children?

2. Does variability in discrimination ability account for a substantial amount of the variance in severity of language impairment?

3. Where discrimination difficulties are found, is this an enduring deficit or a temporary delay?

4. What is the relationship between auditory discrimination of words and auditory discrimination of non-verbal stimuli?

5. Are auditory discrimination difficulties associated with any antecedent factor?

6. Is discrimination associated with one particular language skill rather than another?

7. Are some subgroups of language impairment more likely to have discrimination problems than others?

Dawn House data

TESTS

Speech sound discrimination is assessed at least once a year in one of three ways.

Those children who understand the task, have a concept of 'same' and 'different' (although not necessarily knowing the labels), and have sufficient attention span are tested with the Wepman Test of Auditory Discrimination (1958) sometimes over several days if there are moderate attention problems. This test consists of 40 pairs of short words; 10 are identical and 30 vary by one phoneme, which may be the first or final consonant or the medial vowel. These word pairs are spoken in a level intonation by the tester whose lip movements are not visible to the testee. The child responds 'same' or 'different' (or 'yes'/'no', or with a nod or shake of the head).

Dawn House pupils who are not able to participate in the Wepman test may be assessed using the Picture Pointing Test (Renfrew 1972). In this test, children are shown coloured pictures of 38 items of vocabulary in four blocks of similar sounding words (*e.g.* 'sheep', 'sweep', 'sweet', 'sheet') and, after a vocabulary check, asked to point to the pictures as the examiner names them ('show me the ———'). Although the test format is simple and the use of pictures is an aid to attention, the vocabulary is often too difficult for language-impaired children ('cape', 'tar'). Rather than teach the vocabulary first as Renfrew suggests, the speech and language therapists at Dawn House may use only a subset of words for some children.

A third assessment possibility, used with younger and more disabled children, is a set of toys having similar sounding labels which are in the child's vocabulary (plane/plate, cars/cards). The child is asked to perform various activities with these toys, and discrimination errors noted*.

The Wepman test was standardised on children aged five to eight. At the upper end, performance reaches a ceiling so that rating scales for eight-year-olds apply to children aged eight and above. Raw scores are converted into five rating scales, 2,1,0,−1,−2. Ratings of 0,1 and 2 indicate average abillity or above, as found in 65 per cent of the standardisation sample. A rating of −1 (found in 20 per cent of Wepman's normal sample) indicates below average ability, and a rating of −2 (found in 15 per cent) indicates inadequacy and predicts learning problems (Wepman 1960).

Renfrew tried out her assessment with 300 normally developing five-year-olds. She found that on a page of nine to 11 items, the children made an average of one error. She suggested that there was a discrimination problem in any child aged five and above, making two or more errors. In this study, any child having a total of three or more errors in the Picture Pointing Test, or three errors in the discrimination of toys, was categorised as having a non-standardised discrimination problem.

NON-VERBAL DISCRIMINATION

A separate assessment has been developed at Dawn House which we call the Test of Prosodic Perception (Haynes and Tempest 1984). This was originally developed when it was noted that about 20 per cent of the school population had some abnormal production of prosody, possibly relating to perceptual difficulties. The test comprises four sections, discrimination of (i) loudness, (ii) pitch, (iii) length and (iv) rhythm. The sounds to be discriminated are generated by a pure-tone audiometer and musical instruments, and recorded on tape. In the first and third section the children are asked to indicate whether 10 pairs of sounds, varying only in loudness or length, are same or different. In the second section they listen for any pitch change in 10 series of four notes played on a recorder, and in the fourth section they respond to a change in each of four rhythmic patterns played on a piano.

When the test was devised, the results of Dawn House pupils were compared with 40 normal controls. We found significantly poorer performance in distinguishing length, pitch and rhythmic patterns in our SLI sample. There was suggestive evidence that pitch and length discrimination might be delayed, with nine-year-old

---

*This has now developed into the Dawn House discrimination assessment in which confusable items are introduced in a natural way into a format of play activities. This was not available at the time of the study.

135

<table>

TABLE 5.I		
Wepman speech discrimination ratings at school entry		
Ratings	*N*	*%*
+1 (above average)	3	3
0 (average)	11	13
−1 (below average)	13	15
−2 (inadequate)	60	69
Total	87	100

</table>

Mean age 8.6 yrs with a standard deviation of 16 mths

TABLE 5.II		
Non-standard measure of speech discrimination at school entry		
Evaluation	*N*	*%*
No problem	26	46
Problem	31	54
Total	57	100

Mean age 6.11 yrs with a standard deviation of 11 mths

Dawn House pupils performing similarly to normal six-year-olds, whereas perception of rhythm was deviant and did not relate to age (see also Lea 1980). No association was found between perception on this test and production of prosody in speech.

In the current study, 85 subjects have been assessed on the Test of Prosodic Perception.

RESULTS

The results have been considered in the light of the questions posed above.

1. *Discrimination problems in the language-impaired population.* Tables 5.I and 5.II show the results of Wepman test and non-standardised assessment at school entry. The percentage of children rated at initial assessment as inadequate (rating −2) on the Wepman test is 69 per cent (mean age 8.6, with a standard deviation of 16 months). On non-standardised assessment, 54 per cent of children have a problem. Given that the visually aided non-standard task is probably easier, these percentages are very similar. Combining these figures, 91 out of 144 children (62 per cent) have a discrimination problem at school entry, compared with Wepman's norms of 15 per cent having a rating of −2.

As a group, the SLI children attending Dawn House have extremely poor discrimination skills, but this is not universal. Fourteen (16 per cent) of the 87 children who were able to respond to the Wepman test scored at the average, above average or highly developed skill level. Although poor discrimination skills are general in the SLI population, our data undermine Eisenson's extreme position (1984) that discrimination deficits underlie language handicaps.

2. *Variance in discrimination and the severity of language disorder.* No over-all single measure of severity of SLI has been computed, since the profile of language disability varies from child to child, but chi-squares have been used to measure the effect of adequate or inadequate speech discrimination in the three broad areas of comprehension, language production and speech, using the categories of severe, moderate and mild disability in each of these areas (see Chapter 2). In all language areas there were more children than expected with discrimination difficulties in the

TABLE 5.III		
Wepman speech discrimin-		
ation ratings at interim test		
Ratings	*N*	*%*
+2	1	2
+1	1	2
0	10	19
−1	8	15
−2	33	62
Total	53	100

Mean age 9.8 yrs with a standard deviation of 13 mths

TABLE 5.IV		
Wepman speech discrimin-		
ation ratings at final test		
Ratings	*N*	*%*
+2	1	1
+1	6	6
0	39	40
−1	17	18
−2	34	35
Total	97	100

Mean age 10.11 yrs with a standard deviation of 19 mths

most severe category, but only in the area of comprehension did this reach significance level (chi-square 7.96, df 2, $p<0.02$).

3. *Persistence or transience of discrimination difficulties.* Tables 5.III and 5.IV show the Wepman ratings at the interim test, *i.e.* two years after entry for children staying at least four years at Dawn House, and at the final test. At the interim test there is little change; nearly all pupils can now undertake the standard Wepman test, and 62 per cent of these are in the inadequate category. The mean age at interim testing is 9.8 years, with a standard deviation of 13 months. By the final assessment (mean age 10.11 years, with a standard deviation of 19 months) there has been some improvement, but one third of the children are still categorised as inadequate. The poor performance at interim testing may reflect the greater problems of pupils who require intensive help for over four years. Only pupils who remained at Dawn House for four years or more had interim data recorded. The mean length of stay of the 97 pupils for whom final figures are available is 3½ years.

Auditory discrimination normally improves with age (Wepman 1960). Although Wepman indicated a levelling out in the ninth year, it has frequently been suggested that language-impaired children may have a general neurodevelopmental lag (Bishop and Edmundson 1987*b*), in which case it might be expected that they would take longer to reach test ceiling and would continue to increase raw scores beyond the age of nine years. Using the Kruskal-Wallis one-way analysis of variance (ANOVA), the scores of children aged between seven and nine were compared with scores of children aged nine or more at entry, interim and final test times. Mean raw scores for each age and test time are shown in Table 5.V; age of the group does not affect the discrimination score which is similar for seven- and nine-year-olds at a similar point in their school careers. However when we looked at the change in Wepman raw scores in individual children at initial, interim and final tests, we found that the improvement that takes place with subjects during their stay at school was highly significant (Friedman two-way ANOVA, N 28, df 2, $p<0.0001$). Since only 28 children were tested in all three test times, Wilcoxon

137

TABLE 5.V

Mean Wepman auditory discrimination raw scores, by age and test time.

	7.0–8.11			9 yrs and over		
	N	mean	(SD)	N	mean	(SD)
Entry	42	21	(5.2)	38	22.9	(4.1)
Interim	10	23.1	(4.5)	40	23.5	(3.9)
Final	12	25.8	(2.9)	74	25.3	(2.3)

Differences in scores with age non-significant

Differences in scores by test-time, Wilcoxon Signed Ranks test:
  entry–interim, N 63, p<0.001
  interim–final, N 36, p<0.01
  entry–final, N 65, p<0.001

TABLE 5.VI

Changes in Wepman rating over time

Change (N 44)				No change (N 44)			
Improve		Deteriorate		Stay adequate		Stay poor	
N	%	N	%	N	%	N	%
38	43	6	7	18	20	26	30

Lowest rating −2, counted as poor. All other categories grouped as adequate

Signed Ranks tests were used to compare individual scores between test times 1 and 2 (N 63), test times 2 and 3 (N 36) and test times 1 and 3 (N 65). All differences in scores were highly significant (p<0.001, p<0.01 and p<0.001 respectively).

Table 5.VI presents the patterns of change or otherwise in Wepman rating categories for the 88 children tested on at least two occasions. For children tested three times, the first and third ratings have been used to measure change. The lowest rank of −2 is classified as poor and all other ratings have been counted rather generously as adequate. The table charts any changes in either direction between these two categories for individual pupils. Although there was a significant over-all improvement in raw test scores during the period spent at Dawn House, a large number of pupils remained in the lowest rating category. Forty per cent of the 64 children who were graded −2 on their first assessment with the Wepman test (at test time 1 or 2) remained in that category. A further 7 per cent of the 88 children moved down to that category in their final assessment, and only 43 per cent moved up into rating −1 and above.

At first these results seem rather contradictory; improvement measured by raw score is highly significant, but relatively few children become average or even adequate in Wepman's terms. One explanation is that the therapy and teaching at

TABLE 5.VII
Prosodic perception problems by age at or soon after school entry

Age band	N	Pitch	Problems Length	Rhythm	Any problem
5.0–7.11	13	7	11	8	13
8.0–9.11	50	21	30	19	38
10 yrs and over	22	8	10	6	13
Total	85	36	51	33	44

Mean age 9.5 yrs with a standard deviation of 16 mths

Dawn House, both of which involve a great deal of work on phonological categorisation, push the children to maximise their discriminatory skills, but that this realised potential remains low. A second possibility is the one predicted by the motor theory of speech perception, that improved discrimination is secondary to speech-production improvement. Whichever reason accounts for the significant raw score improvement, discrimination ability remains poor relative to the normal population, and with so many children retaining inadequate levels, speech discrimination must be considered an enduring problem for most SLI children.

4. *Verbal and non-verbal discrimination.* The data on the test of perception of prosodic features, which are essentially non-linguistic although not without linguistic relevance, are not longitudinal (Table 5.VII). Success on eight or more of 10 discriminable pairs, or three of the four rhythm patterns, was accepted as adequate. The therapists who originally administered the test to normal and impaired children formed a clinical impression that subjects failing in the first part (loudness) often did so for reasons of poor attention, and as this could falsify their over-all results, children failing this section are excluded.

Previous studies have found an association between difficulties in non-linguistic discrimination (*e.g.* pitch) and articulation problems (Mange 1960, Sommers *et al.* 1961). We were interested in whether linguistic and non-linguistic discrimination might be associated, suggesting that they could both derive from the same sensory-acoustic substratum: in which case any association between speech discrimination and articulation could have an acoustic rather than a linguistic basis. It should be pointed out that the Wepman test cannot be assumed to be linguistically a very meaningful test for SLI children, as many of the items (*e.g.* 'clove', 'symbol', 'wretch') are unlikely to be in their passive vocabularies. Even for unimpaired young British children there are likely to be some unrecognised words ('fie', 'muss', 'vow'). Snyder and Pope (1970) analysed the responses made by six-year-olds in the Wepman test, and found that the error percentage related to sounds to be discriminated rather than knowledge of the vocabulary. However, Barton (1978) found that three-year-olds did make more discrimination errors with unknown than known words in an assessment of his own devising. The Dawn House children with delayed linguistic development and poor phonological ability may behave in this respect rather more like the three-year-olds. The Dawn House Test of Prosodic Perception is completely non-verbal. We found positive correlations between Wepman raw scores and the length and rhythm sections of the Prosody test as follows, length (N 62, rho 0.47, p<0.0001) and rhythm (N 60, rho 0.29, p = 0.02), but a non-significant correlation between Wepman scores and perception of pitch (N 63, rho 0.06, p>0.05). This association between verbal and non-verbal discrimination contradicts the idea that discrimination problems in SLI are rooted solely in inadequate phonological coding.

5. *Relationship between discrimination problems and possible aetiological factors.* Subjects with a Wepman rating of −2, or a non-standard rating of *problem* at school entry, were deemed to have inadequate speech discrimination. Chi-square tests were used to examine the relationship between adequate or inadequate speech discrimination and (i) positive or negative history of language problems in the extended family, (ii) a perinatal risk score of 0, 1, or more than 1, (iii) an environmental disadvantage score of 0 or 1, 2, or more than 2, (iv) otitis media present or absent in infancy, (v) hearing threshold above and below 15dB at school entry and (vi) language acquisition band 1, 2, or 3. None of the results reached significance.

Children with early middle-ear disease, or with hearing losses at school entry averaging 15dB or above, do not have an increased number of discrimination problems. This reinforces the conclusion at the end of Chapter 3, that middle-ear disease and hearing problems are not a significant cause of SLI in this group of children. A positive association of hearing problems and inadequate discrimination would have suggested that early ear problems caused impaired speech discrimination, which in turn caused or exacerbated language problems. Rather it seems that discrimination difficulty is an integral part of a basic language impairment in this particular population and does not result from additional handicaps of trauma, sensory deficit, health or environment.

6. *Discrimination and language skills.* Mann-Whitney U tests were used to examine differences in subjects with and without speech discrimination problems in their performance on all the language measures described in Chapter 2, other than sentence structure (LARSP) which was investigated using a chi-square test. The expectation was that poor discrimination skills would be associated with poorer language attainments (Table 5.VIII).

Most of the language measures were significantly associated with discrimination problems. The most affected measure was morphology, tested by the Grammatic Closure subtest of the ITPA, which requires the discrimination of small word changes, particularly word endings (*e.g.* from singular to plural form of nouns, or present to past tense of verbs). Somewhat surprisingly, neither of the measures of articulation, which is the language area most frequently assumed to rely on auditory discrimination, was significantly affected by poor discrimination skills. This suggests that in this SLI population, neither phonological coding problems nor speech production difficulties underlie the perceptual problem. This

TABLE 5.VIII
Speech discrimination and specific language measures

Language measures	N	Speech discrimination	
		No problem mean score	Problem mean score
Comprehension			
Vocabulary	137	88	83.2*
Grammar	97	−0.6	−1*
General~	90	18.6	27*
Language production			
Vocabulary~	126	19.5	26.9**
Structure (see below)			
Morphology	88	26.1	17.9***
Content~	76	37.7	42.6
Speech			
Maturity	141	31.6	27.3
Deviance~	140	14.6	17
Written language			
Reading age	144	78.4	78.4
Structure	137	N	N
Stage VI+		17	25
Stage V		14	24
Stage IV		12	18
Stage III−		7	20

~Lower score = better performance
* p (one-tailed) <0.05 Mann Whitney U
** p (one-tailed) <0.01
*** p (one-tailed) <0.001

raises the question of whether it is specifically discrimination of speech or non-linguistic discrimination which is associated with the language difficulties. In order to address this question, the three subsection scores of the non-verbal test of prosodic perception—pitch, length and rhythm—were combined to give a total score, and Kendall correlation coefficients used to measure how closely these scores correlated with the language measures. A significant correlation was found for only one measure, morphology (tau = 0.32, p<0.01), which was the measure also most affected by Wepman discrimination. Morphological distinction requires quite fine degrees of discrimination between pairs of words such as 'man'/'men'. Impaired language skills generally are associated with discrimination of speech rather than discrimination of non-linguistic sound.

7. *Occurrence in subgroups.* Although discrimination problems are associated with a number of linguistic areas, and with severity of comprehension deficit, no particular subgroup in this study had a significantly raised incidence of inadequate speech discrimination.

Summary of findings regarding auditory discrimination in Dawn House children
Discrimination problems are common and severe. Although they improve while the child receives special help, they remain sub-standard. They are not universal, however, and some SLI children have unimpaired and even good discriminatory powers.

None of the antecedent factors is significantly associated with speech discrimination.

Discrimination of verbal and non-verbal stimuli are associated, but it is the verbal discrimination impairment which is associated with a wide range of language attainments.

Rules governing grammatical changes within words may be particularly hard to discern for children with verbal or non-verbal discrimination problems.

There is no evidence to link errors of speech discrimination with errors of speech production. Language rather than speech skills are associated with discrimination impairment in this group of SLI children. Severity of discrimination difficulty is associated with severity of comprehension handicap.

B. Auditory short-term memory

Although there is no doubt that auditory memory is associated with language disability, the nature of this association remains controversial. A clear understanding of this relationship would not only increase our knowledge of SLI, but could have important implications for therapy and teaching.

Memory is the term used to cover a number of very different cognitive functions and processes, and the psychological models used to depict memory undergo almost constant development (for a review of models of auditory memory see Baddeley 1986). There is some agreement on the broad outline of memory processing, presented here in a much simplified summary.

Auditory verbal input enters a primary receptive area in the brain of the listener whence it fades rapidly unless it receives further attention. Information is coded phonologically at this preliminary stage, and the capacity of this speech-based (phonological) component of memory is limited. In order to retain information in its phonologically coded form, the listener can employ overt or covert rehearsal (such as the way we remember a telephone number until it is dialled). For long-term remembering (learning) the phonological code is followed by semantic coding; the information is *understood*, and meaning is extracted from the message and set into the context of other related known facts. Thus the route into the long-term memory store is via the short-term store which may also act as an output buffer for speech production, hence the importance attached to auditory short-term memory (ASTM).

The efficiency of ASTM is normally measured by asking for an immediate repetition of lists of words, syllables or, most commonly, digits. Digit span has been found to increase with age and developmental norms have been established. Brown and Fraser (1963) quoted span lengths as two digits at 30 months, three at 36 months, and four at 54 months. In adults the capacity is normally five to nine items (Miller 1956).

There has been considerable interest in the function that is tapped by digit span, and the cause of its developmental increase. It is not considered to correspond to any real (neurological) increase in capacity, but to the development of mnemonic strategies such as rehearsal and grouping (Chi 1976), to improving speed of identification (Huttenlocher and Burke 1972, Dempster 1981) or to enhanced operational efficiency which, by reducing the amount of operating space required, frees capacity for storage (Case *et al*. 1982). Hulme *et al*. (1984) argued that verbal memory is time-based rather than capacity-based, and that the increase in span is a direct reflection of increasing speed of articulation. Their experimental subjects, aged from four years to adult, could recall as much as they were able to articulate in about 1½ seconds. However, evidence that phonological coding is used by deaf children (Conrad 1970) and also by congenitally speechless subjects (Bishop and Robson 1989) prevents too literal an interpretation of the findings of Hulme *et al*. (1984) with regard to speed of articulation, and implies a more abstract and centrally represented phonological code.

ASTM *and language impairment*

There is ample evidence connecting verbal short-term memory span with the normal acquisition of language (Brown 1973, Olson 1973). It is considered a necessary subskill for the development of verbal reasoning, for learning new articulations (Locke 1969), and for acquiring vocabulary (Gathercole and Baddeley 1990*b*). However there are comparatively few studies of memory in developmental language disorders, other than those concerned with specific reading disability.

Wiig and Semel (1976) reported reduced scores on tests of short-term memory in language-impaired populations, and Graham (1980) found a significant effect of span on comprehension of language, suggesting that ASTM acts as a storage buffer while decoding of language takes place. Menyuk and Looney (1972) devised a sentence repetition test for SLI children and normal children matched for language age. Whereas normal children made errors in relation to the increasing complexity of the sentences, error rates in the SLI children increased with both structural complexity and length of sentence, seeming to implicate deficient memory span. The disordered subjects extracted the basic meaning but could not analyse the syntax beyond a simple level, nor could they repeat longer sentences which were within their productive capacity. Wiig and Semel (1980) also found that language-impaired children found semantics more accessible than syntax; they concluded that memory deficits precluded a full syntactic analysis. Kirchner and Klatzky (1985) attempted to pinpoint more exactly the nature of memory deficit in language impairment, by examining rehearsal processes. They found that 10-year-old language-impaired children were deficient in their ability to maintain and regenerate phonologically coded items, but did not differ significantly from controls in semantic encoding. These experiments all seem to implicate phonological coding; the SLI subjects are able to process some verbal information, but inefficiently. Gathercole and Baddeley (1990a) analysed the mechanism of memory deficit in language impairment. They compared a small experimental group of six SLI seven- to nine-year-olds, with two control groups matched for both verbal and non-verbal abilities in a carefully worked out sequence of experiments. After eliminating perceptual inadequacy and rate of articulation as a cause of memory deficit in their subjects, they produced interesting evidence that the SLI group did use phonological coding and rehearsal with short item lists, but abandoned these when asked to repeat longer lists. Their conclusion was that SLI children have a specific impairment in the phonological storage component of memory. They made the further bold suggestion that impaired phonological memory skills may be the direct cause of the language deficiencies in these children.

There has been more experimental work in the field of short-term memory with reading disorders than with oral language problems, and this has been mainly concerned with the ability to use phonological coding. There is good evidence for some association between reading ability and phonological coding in short-term memory (Jorm *et al.* 1986). Mann (1984) reviewed studies in this area, and concluded that poor readers have a specific impairment in memory for linguistic material (whether spoken or written) and that although poor readers do rely to some extent on phonetic representation, they do so inefficiently (see also Gathercole and Baddeley 1990a). In a further paper (Mann and Liberman 1984) the authors argued that poor phonological coding in ASTM in four-year-olds predicts poor future reading skills. This concurs with the findings of Bradley and Bryant (1983) that phonic awareness (measured in their study by the ability to segment words, and awareness of rhyme) was a reliable indicator of future reading ability.

The latter two findings support the view that reading problems and short-term memory problems have a common substrate in a phonological coding deficit. If this is true, reading difficulty should correlate both with poor phonological skills and with limited ASTM. It might also be predicted that those children with poorest digit span scores (indicating deficient phonological code) would have particular difficulty in achieving the change from using whole-word techniques of reading to the use of phonological segmentation and synthesis which normally occurs when the child has reached a reading age of approximately 7½ years.

This may be too simple a view of the complex relationship between short-term memory, phonological skills, and spoken and written language impairment. Naidoo (1972) was one of the first workers to suggest that 'specific' reading disorders might be allied to broader language problems. Bishop and Adams (1990) examined longitudinal data from four-, five- and eight-year-olds, and found that difficulties with phonology are less predictive of future reading problems than are impairments in other language areas. They suggested that reading difficulties only persist in the continuing presence of a broader language problem. The broader concept implies a correlation between ASTM and a wide range of language abilities.

Similar questions to those concerning discrimination and SLI can be addressed by the Dawn House data on ASTM:

1. How universal are ASTM problems in this language-impaired population?

2. Does the evidence suggest that ASTM development is delayed, relative to chronological age, or a more permanent deficit?

3. Are ASTM problems associated with speech discrimination problems?

4. Are any possible antecedent factors associated with ASTM deficiency?

5. Does ASTM deficiency relate to severity of language disability?

6. Is poor ASTM more strongly related to some aspects of language disability than others, and particularly to skills which rely on phonological coding?

7. Are particular subgroups of SLI more disabled than others in the field of ASTM?

Dawn House data

TESTS

Some test of auditory memory span is included in the yearly test battery. For most children the selected test is the Auditory Sequential Memory subtest of the Illinois Test of Psycholinguistic Abilities (ITPA ASM). This is a digit-span test, in which the child is asked to repeat lists of digits, increasing in length from two to eight, spoken by the tester at the rate of two per second. It is standardised for children under the age of 10.4. Raw ITPA ASM scores are converted to scaled scores with a mean of 36, and a standard deviation of 6.

The ITPA scaled scores are standardised scores which compare the short-term memory span with the span of the normal population at the same age. The raw scores are probably more useful when considering the significance of auditory memory in developmental attainments, such as oral language and reading. Raw scores are the clearest indicator of absolute processing 'space', whether this is considered to be capacity, operational efficiency, time or coding. In the ITPA digit-span assessment, the child is awarded 2 points for a correct repetition on the first trial, or 1 point for a successful second attempt. It is possible to establish cut-off points in the raw score total which relate approximately to the number of digits that can be repeated and to a developmental level of memory. These seem to indicate clinically meaningful categories of difficulties. Experientially, staff at Dawn House are mildly concerned when a child scores below 19 on ITPA ASM, and very concerned if s/he fails to achieve a score of 12 or more. A raw score below 12 corresponds to a span of three items and an age of around three years; a raw score of 18 is approximately a span of four digits and age five years; a score of over 26 indicates a span of about five digits. These figures are similar to those quoted by Brown and Fraser (1963) for the Stanford-Binet test; the minor differences are probably accounted for by the faster ITPA presentation rate.

The ITPA test is not used with the most severely speech-impaired children, whose responses might not be intelligible, or with those who are nor familiar with number labels as this would change the nature of the test into the more difficult one

145

TABLE 5.IX

ITPA ASM in SD bands at first assess-ment

ASM standard deviations	N	%
+1 to +2	3	2
0 to +1	10	7
0 to −1	24	18
−1 to −2	47	35
−2 to −3	47	35
Below −3	4	3
Total	135	100

TABLE 5.X

ITPA ASM raw scores and age equivalence at first assessment (chronological age 5.6–12.11, mean 8.1)

ASM	Age equivalent	N	%
27+	7 yrs and over	24	17
19–26	5.0–7.0	28	20
12–18	3.6–5.0	49	35
Below 12	2.0–3.6	41	29
Total		142	100

of non-word repetition. Such children are assessed using a regularised serial pointing routine, in which arrays of toy animals with single-syllable names (duck, cow, pig, sheep, horse) are placed in a line in front of the child. After sufficient practice with non-test items to ensure that the notion of serial pointing is understood, the test items are covered from view while the tester names sequences increasing in length from two to five animals. The cover is removed after each sequence and the child points in series to the items named. The length of the lists mimics the length of the digit lists in the ITPA.

RESULTS

1. Extent of auditory memory problems. The scaled scores for 135 Dawn House children who were within the age range of the test at entry have been divided into standard deviation bands (Table 5.IX). Results indicate a considerable and widespread problem, with almost 75 per cent of children being at least 1SD below the norm (compared with 16 per cent in the normal population). Although the mean scaled score of the group was 28, more than 1SD below normal, there was a wide range of scores from 14 to 47. A small group of SLI children have good short-term verbal memory.

Scores were assigned to the nine children who were initially assessed by the serial pointing task by equating the number of items they could point to sequentially with a number of digits repeated. This was then scored as in the ITPA test, and evaluated as 'problem' or 'no problem'. They were evaluated as having a problem if an equivalent score would place them 1SD below the norm on the digit-span test. Eight of the nine came into the problem category: a predictably high rate, because this is a selected subgroup of children with special difficulties of response. Children evaluated by serial pointing have been excluded from further analyses.

The scaled scores compare memory span with normal span for age. They indicate whether a child is functioning at, ahead of, or behind age level. For developmental skills such as language and reading, it may be more informative to know the absolute developmental level that has been reached, and this can be derived from the raw scores. Table 5.X shows the raw ITPA ASM scorebands and the

TABLE 5.XI

ITPA ASM raw scores and age equivalence at interim and final assessments
(age at interim 7.0–12.0, mean 9.8)
(final age 6.9–13.10, mean 11.5)

ASM	Age equivalent	Interim		Final	
		N	%	N	%
27+	7 yrs and over	6	9	21	20
19–26	5.0–7.0	19	29	38	36
12–18	3.6–5.0	30	45	40	38
Below 12	2.0–3.6	11	17	7	7
Total		66	100	106	100

TABLE 5.XII

ITPA ASM age lags at all test times

Age minus ASM age (yrs)	Assessments		
	First (N 139) %	Interim (N 64) %	Final (N 100) %
No gap or better	9	2	3
0–2	17	6	4
2–3	15	9	8
3–4	19	11	6
4–5	19	22	8
Over 5	19	50	71
Total	100	100	100

equivalent developmental ages of 142 children who were tested at school entry, when they were aged between 5.6 and 12.11. The divisions have been chosen on clinical grounds as indicators of levels of impairment. Sixty-four per cent of pupils have sufficiently poor memory to be a cause of concern to teachers and therapists experienced in working with SLI children, 29 per cent are below the developmental level of a normal 3½-year-old.

ASTM problems in this population are both extensive and severe.

2. *Does auditory memory improve?* Since only 23 pupils at the final assessment were within the age range at which a scaled score can be computed, changes in raw score bands and changes in the gap between chronological age and memory age are shown in Tables 5.XI and 5.XII.

Taking scores below 19 (equivalent to a memory age of 5.0) as experientially indicative of a considerable problem in school-age children, the percentage of children in this range at entry, interim and final assessments is 64 per cent, 62 per cent and 45 per cent. Mean chronological ages at these assessments are 8.1, 9.8 and 11.5. The final mean score of 21 represents the score of a normal child between 5.8 and 5.11, but is obtained by the Dawn House leaver with an average age of 11.5. This is similar to the mean score of 20.3 at age 11.2 found by Schery (1985) in 161 sli middle-school subjects in the Los Angeles study. There is relatively little improvement with age, and Table 5.XII shows a widening age gap. The long-stay pupils (those with persistent language problems who are given an interim test) are particularly disabled in the area of astm.

3. *Speech discrimination and astm.* When age was partialled out, digit-span scores correlated weakly but significantly with Wepman discrimination test raw scores (coefficient 0.26, df 91, p=0.006) and total scores from the test of perception of prosody (coefficient 0.26, df 80, p=0.009). If there is a causal association between the two auditory skills, as claimed by Rosenthal (1972), improvement in one should be accompanied by improvement in the other. Sixty-two children had first and final assessments in both Wepman and itpa asm. There was no significant correlation (coefficient = 0.004) between improvement in discrimination and improvement in auditory memory measured by the change from first to final assessment. Speech discrimination and astm are both related to severity of language disability, and to each other, but the correlation is weak and the association is not enduring.

4. *Memory problems and antecedent factors.* Possible antecedent or related factors were explored in relation to astm raw scores at school entry using Mann-Whitney u test and Kruskal-Wallis one-way anova. There was no association with family history of language problems, perinatal risk, environmental disadvantage, early middle-ear problems or hearing acuity at school entry. Delayed language acquisition, using the three acquisition age bands, was highly significantly associated with poor astm (Kruskal-Wallis one-way anova, n 136, p=0.003).

This is an interesting finding in the light of those theories that implicate phonological coding in deficient astm. Some form of phonological representation must be possible before the infant can begin to retain and reproduce words, although as Waterson (1971) and others have suggested this may differ from the segmental representation held by mature speakers. A fundamental breakdown in the development of phonological representation could account for a delay in the production of first words, and also underlie a later failure to develop an efficient phonological memory.

5. *astm impairment and level of language impairment.* We looked at the same three areas of language impairment that we had in relation to discrimination difficulties—comprehension, language production and speech—using the levels of severe, moderate and minor impairment and scorebands of itpa asm raw scores, in chi-square tests of significance.

In all areas, the children with poorest memory span were more likely to be the most severely disabled, but this was not significant for speech impairment. The children with very short memory spans were significantly more likely to have severe comprehension deficits (chi-square 17.6, df 6, p<0.01) and particularly likely to have severe expressive problems (chi-square 52.76, df 6, p<0.001).

The failure to find a significant association between short-term memory (thought to depend on phonological coding) and phonological development is at

TABLE 5.XIII

Correlations between ASTM and language
measures (controlling for age at ASM)

Language measures	N	r
Comprehension		
Vocabulary	134	0.08
Grammar	93	0.13
General~	85	−0.2
Language production		
Vocabulary~	123	−0.2**
Structure†		
Morphology	88	0.24**
Content~	72	−0.27**
Speech		
Maturity	136	0.122
Deviance~	135	−0.06
Written language		
Reading age	135	0.28**

~Lower score = better performance
* $p<0.05$
** $p<0.01$
† Kruskal-Wallis one-way ANOVA, chi-square 45.5, N 135, $p<0.0001$

first surprising, but supports the view that children with impaired speech production, may have well developed internal phonological representations, as did the speechless subjects discussed by Bishop and Robson (1989).

6. *Auditory memory and specific language skills.* Individual language functions within the three broad areas of impairment were examined in relation to ASTM using the 10 language measures. Correlations were measured between ITPA ASM raw scores and the continuous variables. Chronological age was partialled out of the three measures using age gaps, of phonological development (EAT raw score) and of reading age. A Kruskal-Wallis one-way ANOVA was used to compare the four sentence structure categories (LARSP stages) with ITPA ASM raw scores.

Results showed significant correlations between ASTM, all expressive language measures, and also reading (Table 5.XIII). The most significant association, as predicted by the work of Menyuk and Looney (1972) and Wiig and Semel (1976), was found between short memory span and poor development of syntax (LARSP). It has been suggested (Menyuk 1964) that children with a span of only two or three morphemes will not be able to learn syntactic rules beyond a very simple level. It is presumably significant that this is about the level in normal development (aged three onwards) that complex sentences begin to develop. Seven Dawn House children never achieved digit spans of more than two or three items. All of these children had very severe language problems. One, AD (the exemplar of the Severe

149

TABLE 5.XIV

ITPA ASM, memory age and reading age at first assessment

ASM	Memory age	Reading ages		
		>7.0	6.7–7.0	≤6.6
19+	5yrs and over	20	13	19
12–18	3.6–5.0	12	13	20
11–	2.0–3.6	5	5	26
Total		37	31	65

Chi-square 12.5, df 4, p = 0.014

TABLE 5.XV

ITPA ASM raw scores by subgroup

Language subgroup	N	Mean (SD)
Speech	18	23 (7)
Speech Plus	23	20 (8)
Classic	41	13 (5)
Semantic	29	18 (7)
Residual	10	21 (8)
Moderate	12	20 (7)
No Language	3	scores = 11, 16 and 11
Young Unclassified	3	scores = 8, 9 and 3
Severe	3	scores = 1, 11 and 3
Total	142	

Chi-square of first four groups with ASM raw score below 12, 12–18, 19+
Chi-square 25.9, N 111, df 6, p<0.001

language subgroup), never developed complex sentences and his expressive language on leaving school, aged 12.8, comprised strings of related phrases or very short clauses. The two other members of the Severe subgroup, SD and PEA, had dramatically poor word-finding skills, and would seem to blank and lose their intended utterance between formulation and production. PEA also had a decoding difficulty which may or may not have related to his poor ASTM, making very many auditory perceptual errors in spite of good hearing acuity for pure tones. However, two of the Dawn House sample in this poorest memory category, WE and CJ, did understand and produce complex sentences although they retained marked language problems, with very poor reasoning skills.

Reading age also correlated significantly with low ASTM. Cotterell (1970) drew attention to the difficulties of teaching reading to dyslexic children who had an auditory memory below the normal five-year level. A memory span of four items is the mean for normal five-year-olds, and that is about the age, in many cultures, of the development of the conscious phonic awareness that accompanies literacy. It is also the memory span at which many Dawn House pupils seem to stick. Sixty-four

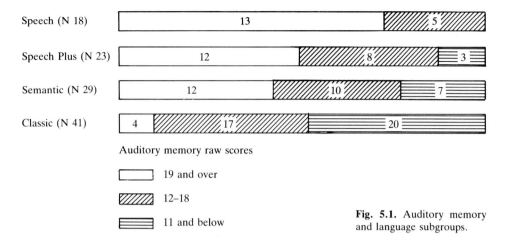

Speech (N 18) 13 5

Speech Plus (N 23) 12 8 3

Semantic (N 29) 12 10 7

Classic (N 41) 4 17 20

Auditory memory raw scores

19 and over

12–18

11 and below

Fig. 5.1. Auditory memory and language subgroups.

per cent, when they were first tested at a mean age of 8.1, had spans of four digits or less. When they were finally assessed at a mean age of 11.5, 45 per cent of them still had spans of four digits or less. In order to progress beyond a reading age of 7.0, children need to move from a whole-word reading style to one which encompasses phonic analysis. If phonic analysis depends upon a more abstract phonological coding ability, and inefficient phonological coding underlies poor ASTM, then children with poor ITPA ASM scores might be expected to plateau at a reading age of around 7.0. A chi-square test, employed to explore reading age relative to digit span, found that this was so. A significantly large number of children in the poorest auditory memory category (ITPA ASM raw score below 12) had a reading age of 6.6 or less (Table 5.XIV). This finding confirms the association between reading and auditory memory but does not indicate any causal direction.

7. *Are particular subgroups associated with poor ASTM?* The findings discussed above, of an association between ASTM and expressive language problems (particularly syntax problems) would predict an increased membership of the Classic language subgroup for children with severe ASTM deficit. Table 5. XV, which compares ITPA ASM scores between subgroups, confirms that this is so; the mean score for this subgroup being equivalent to a developmental age of 3.10, a level which seems to indicate a watershed for progress in both sentence structure and reading. Other subgroups with equally poor memory spans are the small groups with the worst performance in all language areas, those categorised as No Language, Severe and Young Unclassified (Fig. 6.1). A comparison of the raw scores of the four largest subgroups proved to be highly significant, with the Classic group having poorer than expected, and the Speech and Speech Plus language groups having better than expected ITPA ASM scores (chi-square 25.9, df 6, $p<0.001$).

Summary of findings regarding auditory memory in Dawn House children
Most Dawn House children have a considerable ASTM deficit, which is persistent.

No antecedent factors are associated with poor ASTM, but delayed onset of language is significantly associated with it, suggesting that both may derive from a common root, possibly imprecise central phonological representation.

Severity of ASTM impairment relates to severity of comprehension impairment and even more to severity of language-production impairment.

All expressive language (not speech) skills are affected, and particularly development of sentence structure.

Learning to read is also affected by poor ASTM. Children with a memory age of less than 3.10 may have great difficulty acquiring the phonic skills necessary to take them beyond a reading age of around 7.0.

Summary and discussion of auditory processing in the Dawn House sample
Both the auditory skills investigated, speech discrimination and ASTM, remain very poor in the Dawn House population. Both are associated with impaired language skills: discrimination particularly with language comprehension, and memory particularly with language production and reading.

Twenty-four of the 28 children with the lowest comprehension ability had inadequate speech discrimination, but just under half of the children with inadequate ratings had good comprehension skills, suggesting that discrimination and comprehension of language can be dissociated. Arguably, therefore, poor discrimination scores could sometimes be the result of poor comprehension, if a child only half-listens to what is being said because of a low expectation of understanding.

ASTM and language ability were not dissociated, with very small chance of good language production or adequate reading ability being paired with very poor memory span. The most severely language-impaired groups had the worst ASTM.

There was a statistically significant association between the two auditory processes, but there was no correlation between improvement made in memory and improved discrimination, suggesting that they are not causally linked but have common correlates, or are associated in some children only.

One feature that has been frequently cited in the discussion of both discrimination and auditory memory problems is the inadequacy of internal phonological representation. Phonological coding is presumed to be important for maintaining auditory input in a primary working memory until various operations can be completed. For discrimination of two unfamiliar words this might entail the phonemic categorisation and comparison of two novel strings, each consisting of three phonemes, which would require keeping six items in memory. A reverse process operates for reading unfamiliar words using a phonic approach, with a string of graphemes being first converted to phonemes and then held in memory long enough for synthesis into words. A similar process would apply to the acquisition of new vocabulary. In order to acquire and use the syntactic rules which are responsible for sentence structure, a number of words in the appropriate sequence have to be maintained in the phonologically mediated primary memory long enough for the syntactic rule to be hypothesised by the child. All of these abilities are particularly deficient in SLI children with the shortest memory spans, who were also significantly more retarded in their acquisition of language.

If ASTM deficit implies inefficient use of phonological code, it is suprising that neither delayed nor deviant phonology is significantly associated with digit span or with speech discrimination. This may relate to the range and variety of speech problems at Dawn House, only some of which are phonological in nature, others being the result of articulatory production problems. It has been shown elsewhere that adequate phonological coding can be developed at an abstract and central level without adequate speaking skills (Bishop and Robson 1989).

There is little solid support in the literature for a primary perceptual deficit as a sufficient cause of language impairment. Although Tallal's work indicates an acoustic-perceptual difference in many impaired children, it is not universally applicable and fails to explain how such children learn language at all. This is borne out by the dissociation between speech discrimination and understanding in our data. There is much more compelling evidence of a connection between language impairment and a deficient phonological memory. We found considerable evidence to link these auditory memory problems with the early development, extent and nature of language problems, and to suggest perhaps a mechanism of how particular failures occur.

It seems likely that processing (and comprehending) auditory input requires the smooth interaction of a range of linguistic and sublinguistic functions. Various writers have pointed to the loss of over-all efficiency that results from malfunction of one component (Neisser 1967, Menyuk and Looney 1972, Rabbitt 1986, Gathercole and Baddeley 1990a) resulting in maldevelopment of other language functions and inadequate language learning. If inefficient phonological memory may directly cause language impairment (Gathercole and Baddeley 1990a), the spiralling effect of consequent deficiencies in vocabulary, structure and content, complicated by individual differences such as intelligence and motivation, ensure that the relationship is not a simple one. We regard it as an important one and will discuss its significance for making progress in language skills in Chapter 7.

2. Cognitive ability

Normally, language and cognition develop *pari passu* but the nature of the relationship, much debated, is still not clear. The matter is important especially when the development of one is abnormal, both in assessing the precise nature of a child's difficulties and in deciding how best to foster growth in the defective area. Does cognition, the mental processing of incoming information, grow out of language or is language a symbolic outgrowth of the way we think? That oversimplified question reflects two opposing and extreme views. If the first is true, then the child whose language is defective will as a consequence be defective in all or some cognitive abilities. By concentrating on the remediation of language, improved general cognitive function should follow. If the second is true and the language deficit is the result of poor cognitive abilities, then remediation should concentrate on activities designed to promote cognitive processes, leading to improvements in language. In practice, all worthwhile language remediation programmes are firmly placed in the context of familiar situations which motivate and in which the development of concepts, sequences of ideas, inferences and use of language are integrated in developing language.

In the normally developing child, language surges forward on all fronts simultaneously. Although the rate of acquisition varies, one of the most significant findings to emerge from the longitudinal language development studies in Bristol (Wells and Gutfreund 1987) is the constancy of the *sequence* of development, irrespective of factors like sex, and environmental conditions such as position in family and social background, commonly associated with rate of acquisition (Puckering and Rutter 1987). However, different components of language can and do evolve at differing rates, out of step with each other as demonstrated by children with a specific language impairment. We have used some of the different patterns of imbalance to define our subgroups.

The very existence of SLI shows that some dissociation must exist between language and cognition. Children, like the subjects of this study, demonstrate mental processing in some areas of cognition which reaches at least an average level, despite considerable linguistic deficits. Modern tests of intelligence probe a range of cognitive functions, most frequently grouped into two major categories, verbal and visuospatial. Our modular approach to the description of language and the use of intelligence tests which produce a verbal IQ (VIQ) and a non-verbal or performance IQ (PIQ) enables us to examine relationships between verbal and non-verbal cognitive functions, different aspects of language and different profiles of language impairment.

The relationship between the early acquisition of language and later IQ also bears on the relationship between language and cognitive function. While most of the children in this sample were severely delayed in acquiring language, there was a fairly wide range in the age of acquisition. If the emergence of language grows out of general cognitive development, those speaking early should be more advanced in non-verbal tasks, as well as verbal tasks, than those whose language acquisition is extremely late.

Assessment of intellectual abilities at Dawn House
The assessment of a child's level of cognitive abilities forms an essential part of the investigation of speech and language delay. It helps to provide the basis for differentiating between global delay and specific impairment. Intelligence test results were recorded twice: first around the time of school entry (when the data came from reports of educational psychologists attached to referring local authorities or from examination by the school's educational psychologist), and second shortly before leaving school (when the examination was carried out by the school's educational psychologist).

TABLE 5.XVI

Verbal and performance IQ at entry

IQ range	VIQ		PIQ	
	N	%	N	%
116 or above			8	6.1
101–115	7	9.2	35	26.7
86–100	15	19.7	84	64.1
71–85	28	36.9	4	3.1
56–70	18	23.7		
55 or below	8	10.5		
Total	76		131	
Mean IQ	77.8		97.7	
(SD)	(15.1)		(9.5)	

Correlation VIQ, PIQ, r 0.38 (N 72)

When the first pupils were admitted in 1974, the Wechsler Intelligence Scale for Children (WISC), was mostly commonly used for children aged six years and above (Wechsler 1949) and the Wechsler Pre-School and Primary Scale of Intelligence (WPPSI) for younger children (Wechsler 1967). The WISC was revised and ultimately completely superceded by the WISC-R (Wechsler 1976). These three tests account for 91 per cent of IQ data at the point of entry. Other tests included the Leiter International Performance Scale, the Columbia Mental Maturity Scale, the Hiskey-Nebraska Test of Learning Aptitude and the British Ability Scales. All non-verbal IQS are subsumed under PIQ and all verbal IQS under VIQ. On final testing, only the WISC or WISC-R were used.

The Wechsler Verbal and Performance Scales can be combined to give a Full Scale IQ. In view of the large differences frequently found between the VIQ and PIQ in our sample, the computation of the Full Scale IQ would be both meaningless and misleading. No Full Scale IQS are therefore reported.

IQ at entry

A PIQ was recorded for 131 children, mean 97.7 (Table 5.XVI). Four gave evidence of average ability on three subtests although the PIQ fell just below 85. In 25 cases, an insufficient number of subtests had been given to compute a PIQ. On the basis of at least average scores on three subtests of a Wechsler scale, non-verbal ability was deemed to be average in 23, bright in one and low average in one. A VIQ was obtained for only 76 children, mean 77.8. Verbal tests involve a comprehension of oral questions (some of which employ quite complex grammar), an ability to hold these in mind, a knowledge of the relevant vocabulary and concepts, and a sufficient use of language in its semantic, syntactic and pragmatic aspects to provide the required verbal responses. Many language-disordered children, particularly the young, fail to cope. Deficient listening skills sometimes make it impossible to continue and unintelligible speech makes it impossible to score responses.

155

TABLE 5.XVII

TABLE 5.XVII

IQ and age of language acquisition

Language acquisition age band			IQ			
		VIQ			PIQ	
	N	mean	(SD)	N	mean	(SD)
Words <3 yrs or phrases <4 yrs	14	82	(17)	30	98	(9)
Words <4 yrs or phrases <5 yrs	24	82	(14)	47	98	(11)
Words ≥4 yrs, phrases ≥5 yrs	30	77	(12)	48	99	(10)
Total	68			125		

No significant differences

The correlation coefficient for VIQ and PIQ was 0.38, which although highly statistically significant is low clinically and considerably below standardisation correlations, which range from 0.56 to 0.68 (Wechsler 1976).

A VIQ very much lower than the PIQ is often regarded as indicative of a specific language problem. Is this a common feature of this sample?

Enquiry is limited to those 67 children whose VIQ and PIQ is derived from one of the Wechsler scales. Wechsler (1976) recommended the further investigation of children who displayed a difference between the two scales of 15 points or more, but as many as one in four children may have gaps as large as this (Kaufman 1976, Reynolds and Gutkin 1981). In practice, a difference of 20 points or greater is a more reliable indicator of a real verbal/performance discrepancy. The difference between verbal and performance scales has been calculated by subtracting VIQ from PIQ. The mean difference is 20.6 points in favour of PIQ. The VIQ is equal to or greater than the PIQ in three cases, 4.5 per cent. The PIQ is 1 to 19 points higher in 44.8 per cent, 20 points or more in 50.7 per cent. Discrepancies of 30 points or above occur more commonly (in 20 children) than discrepancies of 20 to 29 points (14 children).

Our finding of a very much lower verbal than performance IQ in so many children is in keeping with other studies of SLI children (Fundudis *et al.* 1979, Stark *et al.* 1983, Schery 1985) and also those of children with written language problems (Holroyd 1968, Moffitt and Silva 1987).

A VIQ lower than the PIQ by 20 points or more supports a diagnosis of language impairment: but the absence of such a gap is not sufficient evidence of the absence of a language impairment. The gap is narrower in half of the subsample with both verbal and performance IQs. It is less than 10 points in 16 children, three of whom have a slightly higher VIQ than PIQ.

LANGUAGE ACQUISITION AND IQ

Were different degrees of delay in acquiring language related to later levels of verbal and/or non-verbal ability? Table 5.XVII shows the mean performance and verbal IQs for children who were mildly delayed (using words before three or

156

phrases before four years), moderately delayed (words before four or phrases before five years) and severely delayed (words after four or phrases after five years). Mean PIQs are almost identical (98, 98 and 99 respectively). The mean VIQ (82) is the same for the mildly and moderately delayed, and lower (77) for the severely delayed but not significantly so. The possibility that the mean VIQ of the severely delayed might be significantly lower than that of the other two groups combined was examined with a non-significant result (Mann-Whitney U test).

We also looked at the PIQ/VIQ differences. For the three language acquisition age bands mean differences are 20, 17 and 24 for mildly, moderately and severely delayed speakers respectively. The gap is greatest for those whose language was severely delayed, but a Kruskal-Wallis one-way ANOVA revealed no significant differences between the groups.

There is then no evidence from this sample of SLI children that mild, moderate or severe delay in talking is associated with different levels of later verbal or performance IQ, or with the size of the difference between PIQ and VIQ. Similar results are reported for almost 800 normal children by Silva and Bradshaw (1980) when they included the age at which sentences were used, as one of nine factors considered as possible predictors of intelligence at the age of five.

IQ AND ANTECEDENT FACTORS

Antecedent factors include a family history of language problems, perinatal problems and early neurologically threatening events, environmental risk and otitis media. Interest in IQ patterns, particularly large discrepancies between verbal and performance IQ, has centred upon perinatal problems. Large discrepancies, especially where spatial skills are much lower than verbal skills, have in the past sometimes been taken as presumptive evidence of a minimal brain dysfunction. Bishop and Butterworth (1980) found little support for this. They investigated associations between perinatal risk, early neurological disease and IQ differences in a sample of unselected children. They reported a trend for children with large discrepancies to have high birth-risk scores, marginally significant at 8½ years. Large discrepancies were not associated with early neurological disease, but numbers were too small to draw firm conclusions. Using prospective data on perinatal problems and neurological status, Moffitt and Silva (1987) found no evidence that large discrepancies (22 points and above) were significantly associated with these possible aetiological factors.

Associations between our antecedent factors and VIQ, PIQ and the discrepancy between VIQ and PIQ were explored by comparing the children for whom a factor was present with those for whom it was absent (Mann-Whitney U tests for VIQ and PIQ and chi-square, df 2, for IQ differences of less than 15, 15 to 29 and 30 or greater). The mean VIQ, PIQ and IQ gap for each antecedent factor is described in Table 5.XVIII.

The presence or otherwise of the antecedent factors, considered singly, was not associated with differences in VIQ, PIQ, or the size of the gap between them.

TABLE 5.XVIII

IQ and antecedent factors

Antecedent factor		VIQ			IQ PIQ			PIQ–VIQ	
	N	mean	(SD)	N	mean	(SD)	N	mean	(SD)
Family history									
none known	30	80.5	(14)	59	98.5	(11)	30	21.0	(13)
positive	39	79.1	(14)	71	98.2	(9)	38	20.2	(15)
Neurisk*									
group A	51	80.7	(14)	88	99.3	(10)	50	20.5	(15)
group B	17	77.4	(14)	39	96.5	(9)	17	20.2	(14)
Environment									
rating 0, 1	39	81.4	(14)	76	99.2	(10)	39	19.6	(14)
rating 2+	30	77.6	(14)	54	97.1	(10)	29	21.9	(15)
Social class†									
non-manual	17	82.5	(9)	30	98.7	(10)	17	16.5	(13)
manual	48	79.1	(15)	95	98.0	(10)	47	21.3	(14)
Middle-ear scale									
rating 0, 1	53	78.8	(14)	98	97.7	(10)	52	21.1	(15)
rating 2+	16	82.9	(14)	32	100.3	(10)	16	18.7	(12)

*Neurisk—group A perinatal score <3 and no neurological illness
group B perinatal score ≥3 and/or neurological illness
† Excluding unemployed and unknown
No significant differences

Analyses of variance were carried out to explore the interactions among the set of four antecedent factors. Data on all antecedent factors and a PIQ were available for 105 children and a VIQ and PIQ/VIQ difference for 61. No F ratio for main effects reached the 5 per cent level of significance. Two interaction effects were significant, both involving the interaction between the neurological risk factor and a family history of language problems, one on VIQ (F ratio 5.49, df 1,60, $p<0.025$), the other on VIQ/PIQ discrepancy (F ratio 4.89, df 1,60, $p<0.05$). An examination of the VIQ and IQ differences of the four groups formed by combinations of family history and the neurological risk factor revealed that the lowest mean VIQ, 71, and the largest mean IQ difference, 26, were found among a small number of children, eight, with evidence of neurological risk but no history of familial language difficulty.

There is no evidence from this sample of SLI children that single antecedent factors (family history of language problems, early neurological risk, environmental risk, social class, or middle ear problems) have any significant effect upon later verbal or performance IQ. There is some suggestion, however, that the presence of neurological risk *in the absence of* a positive familial history carries a risk of low verbal IQ and a very large discrepancy between verbal and performance IQs.

IQ AND SPEECH AND LANGUAGE MEASURES ON ENTRY (Tables 5.XIX, 5.XX)
Are some aspects of speech and language more strongly related than others to the

TABLE 5.XIX

Correlation coefficients between IQ and language measures

Language measures	N	VIQ r	p	N	PIQ r	p
Comprehension						
Vocabulary	70	0.61	***	123	0.14	
Grammar	48	0.47	**	83	0.17	
General~	40	−0.81	***	77	−0.29	*
Language production						
Vocabulary~	64	−0.68	***	112	−0.25	**
Structure†	70			122		*
Morphology	53	0.58	***	84	0.26	*
Content~	39	−0.55	***	69	−0.06	
Speech						
Maturity	75	0.10		130	0.34	***
Deviance~	73	−0.10		127	−0.3	***
Written language						
Reading age	72	0.18		122	0.15	

†Structure—Kruskal-Wallis ANOVA
       VIQ chi-square 5.987, NS
       PIQ chi-square 7.916, p<0.05
~Negative correlation due to low scores indicating better performance
* p<0.05, ** p<0.01, *** p<0.001

TABLE 5.XX

Verbal and performance IQ and severity of comprehension, language production and articulation impairment (composite measures)

Language measures	N	IQ VIQ mean	N	PIQ mean
Comprehension				
minor	32	87.4	61	99.5
moderate	28	72.9	44	95.8
severe	16	69.6	26	99.6
F ratio	13.11, df 2, 73		2.02, df 2, 128	
p	<0.0001		NS	
Language production				
minor	35	83.6	44	100.9
moderate	17	76.4	33	99.9
severe	24	72.0	54	95.3
F ratio	4.69, df 2, 73		4.38, df 2, 128	
p	<0.05		<0.05	
Speech				
minor	21	77.2	27	100.7
moderate	21	78.8	27	102.8
severe	34	78.8	77	96.0
F ratio	0.08, df 2, 73		5.57, df 2, 128	
p	NS		<0.01	

IQ, particularly the verbal IQ? This question is explored by examining the correlations between IQ and individual speech and language measures. Because severity of impairment might be relevant, we also look at IQ in relation to the composite measures of comprehension, production of language and speech which are graded in terms of severity (minor, moderate and severe—see Chapter 2).

Correlation coefficients were computed between VIQ, PIQ and each measure of comprehension, language production, speech and reading, with the exception of sentence structure (Kruskal-Wallis one-way ANOVA). For those measures derived from the difference between age and language age, and for speech development, chronological age has been partialled out. Negative correlations relate to tests in which lower scores indicate better performance. The effect of the severity of impairment was explored by one-way ANOVA followed by multiple comparison of means (Scheffé tests).

Comprehension. All measures of comprehension, grammar, vocabulary and general comprehension are significantly correlated with VIQ. When VIQ and the three grades of comprehension impairment were examined, a highly significant between-groups difference was found (p<0.0001). Multiple comparisons between means revealed that the VIQ of those with minor comprehension problems was significantly higher than that of the moderately and of the severely disabled, and that there was no difference between the moderately and severely impaired. In this subsample, the VIQ of children with either a moderate or severe degree of comprehension impairment was lower than that of children with minor comprehension problems.

The PIQ was weakly associated with only one measure of comprehension, that of general comprehension. It did not vary significantly with different degrees of comprehension impairment.

Language production. All but one of the language production measures correlated significantly with VIQ. The unexpected exception was sentence structure. The degree of language production impairment was not significantly related to levels of VIQ, although the mean values were in the expected direction. Nor did any comparison among means reach a significant level. This appears surprising in view of the high correlation between most of the individual measures of expressive language and VIQ. However the composite measure of language production is based largely on the results of the LARSP which describes the development of sentence structure. Whatever the underlying reasons for the lack of association between VIQ and LARSP, they were likely to have affected associations between VIQ and the composite measure of language production.

A significant association was found between PIQ and three measures of language production, sentence structure and morphology at the 5 per cent level and expressive vocabulary at the 1 per cent level. The PIQ was affected by the severity of language production impairment (p<0.01). Comparisons among means revealed differences between minor and severe, but no difference between minor and moderate. The comparison between mild combined with moderate *vs* severe is highly significant (p<0.005). A severe language production impairment is associated with a lowered PIQ but not a minor or moderate one.

Speech. The very low coefficients with both measures of speech, maturity and deviance, suggest that these are independent of VIQ. No significant differences emerged from the analysis of variance or the subsequent comparisons between means. Degrees of speech impairment had no effect upon levels of VIQ. The lowest mean VIQ belonged to the least speech-impaired. These children are necessarily impaired in comprehension and/or language production, otherwise they would not be included in this SLI sample.

Both measures of speech, maturity and deviance correlated highly with PIQ (both p<0.001). The PIQ varies significantly with degrees of speech impairment the composite measure of which is based largely on the measure of speech development, EAT. No significant difference emerged between the mildly and moderately affected. When these are combined and compared with the severely speech-impaired, a highly significant difference is found (p<0.002). It is a severe speech impairment which is associated with a lower PIQ.

Reading. No association was found between either VIQ or PIQ and reading, a finding possibly related to the fact that most children at entry were at the very earliest stages of reading. The relationships between IQ, language measures and reading are explored in Chapter 6.

IQ AND LANGUAGE SUBGROUPS AT ENTRY

A VIQ was available for 76 children (49 per cent). It can be seen from Table 5.XXI that they are unevenly distributed among the language subgroups. This uneven VIQ distribution necessarily restricts the interpretation of analyses.

A PIQ, on the other hand, was obtained for 131 children (84 per cent) and similar proportions with a PIQ are found in all subgroups except No Language of whom only two children had been given a sufficient number of subtests to compute a PIQ.

Despite variations in the proportions of children with a VIQ, it seemed worthwhile to ask whether the groups differ with regard to both verbal and performance IQ. Kruskal-Wallis one-way ANOVA were carried out for all groups, the resulting chi-squares being significant for both VIQ and PIQ. This was followed by one-way ANOVA on the first six numerically greater groups, the Speech to the Moderate, and multiple comparisons of means (Scheffé tests).

The Speech subgroup had the highest mean VIQ (94) and the Semantic group the lowest (74), although the mean PIQ for these two groups was the same (101). When individual pairs of groups were compared, the mean VIQ of the Speech subgroup was found to be significantly higher than that of the Classic and of the Semantic. With the VIQ so strongly associated with language measures, particularly those of comprehension, it is not surprising that the Semantic subgroup, with its primary comprehension deficit, had the lowest mean VIQ of all the major subgroups. The number of VIQs recorded for Speech Plus children was very small. Although the

161

TABLE 5.XXI
Mean verbal and performance IQ of language subgroups at entry

Language subgroup	VIQ		IQ PIQ		PIQ–VIQ	
	N	mean	N	mean	N	mean
Speech	11	94	15	101	9	10
Speech Plus	5	77	19	96	4	18
Classic	18	77	39	95	18	18
Semantic	21	74	27	101	20	28
Residual	7	83	10	100	7	16
Moderate	9	82	11	103	9	22
No Language	3	45	2	*90,92		
Young Unclassified	2	*54,79	5	102		
Severe	0	—	3	90		
Total	76	78	131	98	67	21

*Individual scores

VIQ: Kruskal-Wallis one-way ANOVA, all groups, chi-square 24.34, p<0.001.
One-way ANOVA, Speech to Moderate, F 3.85, df 5, 65, p<0.01
    Scheffé tests: Speech vs Classic
                  Speech vs Semantic
                  p<0.05
PIQ: Kruskal-Wallis one-way ANOVA, all groups, chi-square 15.25, p = 0.054.
One-way ANOVA, Speech to Moderate, F 2.17, df 5, 115, NS
PIQ–VIQ: Kruskal-Wallis one-way ANOVA, all groups, chi-square 15.45, p = 0.017. No two groups differ significantly

mean VIQ (77) was the same as that of the Classic, comparison with the Speech subgroup failed to reach a significant level. Within the subset of children whose VIQ was assessed at entry, the primarily speech-impaired with their relatively normal comprehension of language obtained higher VIQ than the language-impaired, the majority of whom had moderate or severe comprehension problems.

Performance IQ differences between the groups just failed to reach a level of statistical significance, and no two pairs of groups differed significantly. Apart from the No Language and Severe, the group with the lowest mean PIQ was the Classic, whose language impairment is characterised by expressive language problems. It was seen above that the PIQ tended to be low in the presence of a severe language production impairment.

The mean difference between VIQ and PIQ was calculated for each subgroup. Numbers were small but a Kruskal-Wallis one-way ANOVA resulted in a significant between-groups chi-square, which just failed to reach the 1 per cent level of significance. The Speech group had the narrowest VIQ/PIQ difference of 10 points and the Semantic the greatest difference of 28 points.

By the time the children left the school's junior department, a reliable verbal as well as performance IQ could be obtained for almost all. The following report

TABLE 5.XXII

Verbal and performance IQ before
discharge

IQ	VIQ		PIQ	
	N	%	N	%
130 and over			2	1.9
116–129	2	2.0	11	10.0
101–115	7	6.8	29	27.1
86–100	21	20.6	47	43.9
71–85	46	45.1	16	14.9
56–70	25	24.5	2	1.9
55 and below	1	1.0		
Total	102		107	
Mean	80.75		98.2	
(SD)	(13.96)		(14.76)	

Correlation coefficient VIQ/PIQ r 0.31
(N 101)

enables us to look at changes and also to examine whether trends at entry, within the whole group and between subgroups, are still evident at a later date.

IQ before leaving

Of the 118 children who left the junior department of Dawn House, 11, whose stay was less than two years, had been given the WISC or WISC-R within 18 months of departure and their IQ results are included in the entry analyses. The tests were not repeated because of practice effects. Reported now are data from 108 children, for 101 of whom both a VIQ and PIQ were available.

There was remarkably little difference between the mean IQs at entry and at leaving. The mean VIQ, 80.75, was 3 points higher than at entry, while the mean PIQ, 98.2, remained virtually unchanged as was the correlation coefficient between verbal and PIQ, 0.31, still low by comparison with the standardisation sample. The mean difference between VIQ and PIQ was now slightly lower at 18.4. Large VIQ/PIQ differences were still evident, although the proportion of children with a gap of 30 points or more in favour of PIQ was smaller than at entry, 23 per cent compared with 30 per cent. There were 14 children whose VIQ was equal to or greater than their PIQ (Table 5.XXII).

Of the 102 children whose final VIQ was recorded, entry and final data were available for 47. Did the final VIQ of these differ from the final VIQ of the 55 for whom there was no entry VIQ? The mean final VIQ of the former was 81.9 compared with 79.8 for the latter, a small and not significant difference. If similar trends for change can be assumed for all, it is unlikely that those whose entry VIQ was not recorded differed materially in verbal cognitive ability from those with a recorded entry VIQ.

Of the 25 children whose non-verbal ability could only be estimated at entry, a final PIQ was available for 20 who were leavers. Their mean PIQ (98.4) was not dissimilar to the mean PIQ of those with entry data. There seems to be no reason to suppose that the non-verbal ability of children for whom it was estimated differed from those with a full PIQ.

Because of the small number of children for whom a VIQ had been obtained at entry, final VIQ could be compared with entry VIQ in only 47 cases. The mean verbal gain was 4.5 points with a standard deviation of 10. Gains were made significantly more frequently than no gain or losses (Wilcoxon Matched Pairs Test, z = 2.80, p = 0.0025, one-tailed).

Records of both entry and final PIQ were available for 86 children. The mean difference between entry and final PIQ was 0.7 with a standard deviation of 12.6. This suggests what the Wilcoxon Matched Pairs Test confirmed, that the number of children whose final PIQ was higher than their initial PIQ was not greater than those whose final PIQ was lower (z = 0.51, p = 0.3, one-tailed).

Stark *et al.* (1984) reported an almost identical, significant mean WISC-R verbal gain of 5 points, for their group of 29 SLI children after an interval of three to four years. The much larger mean gain of 10 points, made by their control group, is at least partly explained by the fact that the 14 control children examined at follow-up were not representative of the original normal group and not comparable in PIQ to the SLI children. However other findings in that study led Stark and her colleagues to suggest that although verbal skills of SLI children improve they do so at a slower rate than normal.

In her report of IQ changes in 120 SLI children, Ripley (1986) found that children with the lowest initial VIQ tended to make the greatest gains. This seems to be the case here too. There were 10 leavers with an initial VIQ of 60 or less. Three of these were children in the No Language group for whom a reliable final VIQ could not be obtained. The remaining seven children made gains of 4, 11, 15, 19, 20, 27 and 27 points, mean 17.5.

Some changes in IQ, both verbal and non-verbal, are to be expected over a period of time if only because of the uncertain reliability of the tests themselves and also (particularly in the case of the VIQ, which for most children was well below the standardisation mean) because of a tendency for scores to regress towards the mean. If in addition to these factors, different patterns of language impairment are associated with different rates of cognitive growth, one might expect these to be reflected in differences between the language groups on the final assessment.

FINAL IQ AND LANGUAGE SUBGROUPS

At entry significant differences were found between some groups. Prior to leaving, a VIQ was recorded for many more children than at entry, but the early pattern of differences was sustained. Between-group differences were highly significant (Kruskal-Wallis one-way ANOVA, chi-square 34.29, p<0.001). One-way ANOVA for the first six groups, Speech to Moderate, followed by Scheffé multiple comparison of means tests, identified a significant VIQ difference between the Speech group and both the Classic and Semantic, and between the Residual and the Classic

TABLE 5.XXIII

Mean verbal and performance IQ of language subgroups prior to leaving

Language subgroup			IQ			
		VIQ		PIQ		PIQ–VIQ
	N	mean	N	mean	N	mean
Speech	12	94	12	100	11	8
Speech Plus	16	82	16	98	16	16
Classic	35	78	35	94	35	17
Semantic	17	77	18	103	17	26
Residual	8	94	8	106	8	12
Moderate	7	79	8	98	7	19
No Language	2	*61, 72	5	91	2	*25, 63
Young Unclassified	2	*59, 65	2	*91, 104	2	*26, 45
Severe	3	*54, 58, 62	3	*80, 91, 114	3	*18, 32, 60

*Individual scores

VIQ: Kruskal-Wallis one-way ANOVA, all groups, chi-square 34.29, p<0.001
One-way ANOVA, groups Speech to Moderate, F 5.61, df 5, 89, p<0.001
    Scheffé tests: Speech vs Classic
                Speech vs Semantic
                Residual vs Classic
                p<0.05
PIQ: Kruskal-Wallis one-way ANOVA, all groups, chi-square 10.57, NS.
One-way ANOVA, groups Speech to Moderate, F 1.43, df 5, 91, NS
PIQ–VIQ: Kruskal-Wallis one-way ANOVA, all groups, chi-square 17.40,
p = 0.02.
Group differences: Speech vs Semantic, p<0.01
                Speech vs Speech Plus and Classic, p<0.05
                (Mann-Whitney U tests)

subgroups. The Speech subgroup retained its position with the highest mean VIQ, a position now shared with the Residuals. The mean VIQ of the Speech subgroup continued to be significantly higher than those of the Classic and Semantic groups. Early differences between the speech- and language-impaired continued to persist.

Although the Speech, Semantic and Residual groups have higher mean PIQs than other groups, analyses revealed no significant between-groups or paired-group differences, a repetition of findings at entry (Table 5.XXIII).

Differences between VIQ and PIQ are not the same for each subgroup. A significant between-groups difference was found (Kruskal-Wallis one-way ANOVA, chi-square 17.40, p = 0.02). Comparisons between the first four groups showed that the verbal/performance difference was narrower among the Speech than the Semantic group (Mann-Whitney z 2.91, p<0.01). Among the primarily language-disordered, the IQ gap was wider among those with comprehension impairments, the Semantic, than those whose impairments lay in the areas of expressive language and speech, the Speech Plus and Classic (Mann-Whitney z 2.21, p<0.05). This underlines differences between three subgroups of children whose language is primarily impaired. It also emphasises the effects of moderate as well as severe comprehension deficits which affect verbal cognitive functions, but not spatial, non-verbal function.

There were 10 children with a verbal/performance difference of more than 40 points, with VIQs ranging from 54 to 88 and PIQs from 100 to 147. Two of these had exceptionally large gaps. One, a boy in the Severe subgroup and described as typical of that group (p. 51), with a VIQ of 54 and PIQ of 114, continued his education in another school for language-disordered children; the other, who entered with an acquired receptive aphasia and whose VIQ and PIQ were 72 and 135 respectively, joined the remedial department of a comprehensive school. The 10 children belonged to one or the other of all subgroups, with the notable exceptions of the Speech and the Residual, both of which were characterised by near normal language at entry. Large differences between the VIQ and PIQ are found only among the linguistically impaired, being largest when the impairment affects comprehension.

Summary

THE WHOLE SAMPLE

At the time of entry, a VIQ had been obtained for 76 children (mean 77.8) and a PIQ for 131 (mean 97.7). The correlation between VIQ and PIQ was a low 0.38 (N 72). A mean difference of 20.6 points between VIQ and PIQ, favouring the latter, was found for the 67 children whose IQ data stemmed from one of the Wechsler tests. Large differences of 30 points or more were found in 30 per cent: but large gaps were not typical of all. One in four had a difference of less than 10 points. While large differences favouring the PIQ are supportive of the presence of a speech and language impairment, they are not a necessary feature.

At the time of discharge, the mean VIQ was 81 (N 102), and the mean PIQ 98 (N 107). The correlation between VIQ and PIQ was still low, 0.31, (N 101). The mean difference between VIQ and PIQ was 18.4 but large differences of more than 30 points were less common than at entry, 23 per cent.

An average verbal gain of 4.5 points was made for the 47 children whose VIQ was assessed both at entry and before discharge. Gains were significantly more frequent than no change or loss. Children with the lowest VIQ at entry tended to make the greatest gains but these were not specific to any particular group. The mean difference between entry and final PIQ was 0.7 for 86 children. The low correlation between VIQ and PIQ both at entry and discharge suggests some dissociation between verbal and non-verbal cognitive functions which persists after years of remediation and after many children have so progressed verbally that they have joined mainstream schools. Gains made verbally are not matched in general terms by non-verbal gains.

IQ AND AGE OF TALKING

No association was found between the age at which children began to talk and verbal and non-verbal cognitive abilities. Children not using words before four years or phrases before five years, the very late speakers, were more linguistically disabled at entry than those speaking earlier. A strong relationship between cognitive and language development would predict lower PIQs at entry in this group. In fact the mean PIQ was 1 point ahead of that of earlier speakers.

IQ AND MEASURES OF SPEECH AND LANGUAGE

We did find strong associations between the VIQ and all measures of comprehension. Both moderate and severe problems of comprehension were associated with a lower VIQ than mild.

All measures of language production, except syntax, were significantly related to VIQ. No significant difference of VIQ was found between mild, moderate and severe degrees of language-production impairment. This may have been partly due to the small number of children with low levels of syntax production and a VIQ. The possibility should also be entertained that there exists a degree of dissociation between verbal cognitive functions probed by intelligence tests and a child's ability to structure his own language. If this is so, it would accord with the Chomskian view of a cognitive capacity specific to the structure of language. It is of interest in this respect that although correlating significantly with VIQ, the correlation coefficient for VIQ with the comprehension of grammatical structures is lower than with vocabulary or general comprehension.

There was no association between speech maturity or deviance and VIQ. Nor was any difference of VIQ found between different degrees of articulatory impairment.

Performance IQ was unaffected by different degrees of comprehension impairment. Severe, but not mild or moderate, problems in language production (syntax) were associated with a lower PIQ. Why productive syntax and predominantly spatial skills should be linked in this way is difficult to understand. On the surface, there appears to be no common mental operation or cognitive ability. It is possible that each covaries with a third unknown factor.

Findings similar to language production emerge from the analyses of speech impairment and PIQ. Again only severe impairment is associated with lower PIQ. The possibility of some third covarying factor, perhaps visuomotor or aetiological, might explain this association.

IQ AND SUBGROUPS

The variability of IQ in relation to degrees of impairment has implications for our language subgroups which were created from each child's profile of comprehension, language production and speech.

The Speech subgroup, children with a primary speech impairment whose language problems are minor, had the highest mean VIQ both at entry and discharge. At entry, their VIQ was significantly higher than that of the Classic and the Semantic, a pattern which was maintained with greater group numbers at discharge. With the lowest VIQ, but with numbers too small for statistical comparison, were the children with severe problems in all areas—comprehension, expression and speech—the No Language, Young Unclassified and Severe.

PIQ did not differentiate between the groups either at entry or at discharge. Of the first four subgroups which are also numerically greater than the remainder (the Speech, Speech Plus, Classic and Semantic) the Semantic group had the highest mean PIQ, though not significantly so. This group also had the lowest mean VIQ both at entry and discharge.

Within the major subgroups, differences between VIQ and PIQ in individual children were least in the Speech and greatest in the Semantic, both at entry and at discharge. At discharge, the mean PIQ/VIQ discrepancy for this last group was 26. They differed significantly in this respect from the Speech Plus and Classic.

Although the VIQ distinguished between the linguistically nearly normal, the Speech and the major linguistically impaired groups, it did not differentiate between the Speech Plus, the Classic and the Semantic. Their mean VIQs were not dissimilar, but their language impairments were: and it would be a great mistake to treat the three groups in the same way. The Semantic are the children who operate at higher levels in their production of language and speech than in their comprehension of language. Many speak fluently and intelligibly. Yet they are very disabled and perhaps more so because they may appear to be more normal linguistically than they are. Non-verbally they are likely to function comfortably within the normal range. But their habit of misunderstanding, misinterpreting or simply failing to understand means that their comprehension problems permeate all parts of the curriculum. They may acquire decoding skills and appear to 'read' quite well but fail to understand what they read. Within the school these children are recognised as a cohesive group with problems and remedial needs peculiar to them.

Analyses of IQ data in the subgroups underline differences between the primarily speech-impaired, the Speech subgroup, and the primarily language-impaired as reported in order studies (Griffiths 1969, Hall and Tomblin 1978, Weiner 1985, Ripley 1986). The Speech, with near normal language, have a higher VIQ and a smaller VIQ/PIQ discrepancy. Verbal and non-verbal cognitive functions are developing more or less at the same pace and similar levels, while imbalance is a common persisting problem among the primarily language-impaired.

3. Laterality

Hand preference is frequently examined in children with language-learning disorders, because of the relationship thought to exist between handedness, neurological development and organisation, and cerebral functional asymmetry.

The last 30 years have seen an explosion of interest and information in this field with the development of behavioural techniques such as dichotic listening and tachistoscopic viewing. These have enabled researchers to investigate asymmetrical function in the normal brain, adult and child, adding to early and concurrent data from brain-damaged individuals, mostly adult. The purpose of this introduction is to serve as a background to the questions posed in this chapter. For comprehensive reviews the reader is referred to Bryden (1982), Bradshaw and Nettleton (1983), Beaton (1985), Springer and Deutsch (1985), Bishop (1990) and to a summary by Goodman (1987).

Cerebral lateralisation

In most right-handed individuals, speech and language are mediated by the left cerebral hemisphere, sometimes referred to as the dominant one, while visuo-spatial and non-verbal functions are subserved by the right. The division of function is not necessarily absolute. In a typical right-handed adult, the left hemisphere predominates in language which involves high-order cognition (Zangwill 1960, Masland 1981, Goodman 1987) and sequential processing (Bradshaw and Nettleton 1983). The left brain speaks and is involved in the phonological, semantic and grammatic aspects of language (Ojemann and Mateer 1979). In mediating auditory input, the left plays a predominant role with verbal material (Kimura 1961, 1967), the appreciation of rhythm (Robinson and Solomon 1974) and the perception of complex tonal sequences (Halperin *et al*. 1973). Not all language functions are subserved by the left hemisphere. The right seems able to support an auditory passive lexicon and to have some semantic capacity in the comprehension of instructions. The right also seems to have a limited syntactic competence, insofar as judgements about grammar have been demonstrated in the absence of the comprehension of syntactically constrained sentences (Baynes and Gazzaniga 1988). The right is also involved in some of the prosodic aspects of language, loudness and pitch (Nachshon 1978).

It is clear that the disordered functions of the speech- and language-impaired are those served predominantly by the left hemisphere in most individuals, although this does not necessarily apply to the left-handed and perhaps not entirely to children.

Handedness and cerebral lateralisation

Early observations of aphasia, hemiplegia and handedness had led to a contralateral rule, namely that the right-handed are left-brained and the left-handed right-brained for speech and language. With this went the notion that the development of language is best served by the early establishment of clear unilateral dominance, *i.e.* the mediation of speech by one hemisphere, usually the left. It would then follow that failure to develop cerebral dominance and definite hand preference could lead to delays or difficulties in acquiring language, ideas reflected in Nice's (1918) study of the development of speech in ambidextrous children. Later clinical experience, augmented by the study of wartime head-wounds, indicated a much more complex relationship between hand and hemisphere. Zangwill (1960) reviewed studies of aphasia, recovery from aphasia, the site of lesions and the handedness of patients and their families. He was led to conclude that contralaterality of language lateralisation and handedness could be reasonably assumed only for the right-handed of dextral stock, that the left hemisphere is more likely than the right to be dominant among the left-handed, that recovery from aphasia is more likely in the left-handed or those with left-handed relatives, and that unilaterality of language function is more pronounced in the right-handed: the last two conclusions suggesting a degree of bilateral representation in at least some left-handed individuals.

Since then, evidence from clinical sources and behavioural techniques has led to estimates of left cerebral language lateralisation varying between 91 and 98 per cent among the dextral, the latter figure relating to the strongly right-handed possibly of dextral stock. There is general agreement that most left-handers (about 70 per cent) are left-brained for language, although estimates vary from 52 to 71 per cent. Of the remainder, about half show bilateral representation. Bilateral representation appears to occur rarely if ever among dextrals (Touwen 1972, Rasmussen and Milner 1977, Alekoumbides 1978, Bradshaw and Nettleton 1983, McManus 1985, Springer and Deutsch 1985).

So deviations from the normal pattern of left language lateralisation are more likely to be found among the left-handed. But the relationship between handedness and functional cerebral lateralisation remains weak, particularly in the case of the non-dextral. The relationship would be strengthened if it were known in which of the right- and left-handed, right, left or bilateral representation occurs. Familial sinistrality and strength of hand preference have a bearing upon this question. There is considerable and conflicting evidence about both. Bradshaw and Nettleton (1983) thought that the better controlled studies indicate that non-familial sinistrals are more likely to demonstrate abnormalities of lateralisation. Kinsbourne (1979) suggested that the strongly right-handed who are also right-footed and right-eyed are most likely to be left-lateralised.

Pathological left-handedness
A raised incidence of left-handedness is commonly found among some pathological groups: the mentally retarded (Burt 1937, Hicks and Barton 1975), the epileptic (Satz 1972, Silva and Satz 1979) and the autistic (Colby and Parkinson 1977). To explain such findings and at the same time recognise the lack of evidence for cognitive differences between dextrals and sinistrals, Satz (1972, 1973) proposed a model of pathological left-handedness (PLH). This arose from a suggestion advanced by Hecaen and Ajuriaguerra (1964) that some sinistrality may result from early damage to the left hemisphere, causing a naturally right-handed child to change from right to left. Satz, assuming left-handedness in 8 per cent of the population and an equal distribution of lesion in the right and left hemispheres, constructed a model which accounted for a reported twofold increase in pathological groups. According to this model, there must also exist pathological right-handedness (PRH, shifted left-handers), but the number of PLH would far outnumber PRH, since right-handedness is so much more common. Satz calculated the ratio to be approximately 11.5:1.

Such a model could explain why among the cognitively impaired and sometimes also the language impaired, a raised incidence of non-dextrality is found and at the same time why most sinistrals do not differ cognitively from dextrals.

Bishop (1980a, 1984) extended the PLH hypothesis. She argued that if a continuum of neurological abnormality is accepted, mild impairment might be sufficient to shift the balance of skill from the naturally preferred to the non-preferred hand. Such mild impairment need not produce gross neurological signs. Working on the assumption that the non-preferred hand of the PLH is likely to be particularly clumsy, Bishop (1980a) identified the 20 per cent who were most clumsy with the non-preferred hand, as a target group among an unselected sample of 170 children aged eight or nine. The remainder served as controls. As she predicted, there was a significantly higher incidence of left handedness among the target children. The idea that the PLH are of dextral stock also received support. As for aetiology, there was no evidence that birth stress might account for the impairment, but Bishop did find a higher incidence of neurological disease (e.g. convulsions, meningitis and head injury) in the target group.

Bishop (1984) was able to replicate some of these findings using retrospective data, including speech, from a national sample of about 12,000 children who had been examined at seven and 11 years as part of the National Child Development Study. Once more, Bishop identified a target group and found that target left-handers (but not dextrals) included a significantly higher proportion of children with very poor speech.

Handedness in children with language disorders
If patterns of handedness and cerebral asymmetrical function are related and affect the development of speech and language, one might expect to find a significantly greater number of non-dextrals among children with language disabilities, oral and written. Most information on this topic comes from studies of children with reading difficulties or dyslexia. A raised incidence of mixed and/or left-handedness among children with reading difficulties has been reported (Burt 1937, Orton 1937, Ingram and Reid 1956, Harris 1957, Ingram 1959, Annett 1970, Naidoo 1972, Thomson 1979), but not by everyone (Coleman and Deutsch 1964, Belmont and Birch 1965, Clark 1970, Rutter *et al.* 1970, Sparrow and Spatz 1970). Bishop (1983) cited 17 studies, most of which produced negative results.

Annett and Turner (1974) noted that negative results tended to emerge from studies of handedness and reading ability in samples drawn from normal populations, whereas clinic samples often gave a raised incidence of non-dextrality. They neatly demonstrated that negative and positive results could arise from the same body of data. Over 100 right- and 100 left-handed children aged between five and 11 were examined for hand preference and skill and for verbal and non-verbal ability and reading. Pure right, mixed right, mixed left and pure left were compared for ability and reading with no significant differences. These authors then identified all children with a specific reading disability and examined handedness. Of the 16 children so identified, four were right-handed and 12 were left-handed.

171

Studies of children with speech and language impairments are also equivocal. Ingram (1959) commented on the lack of definite preference in children with developmental speech disorders, but Fundudis *et al.* (1979) found no raised incidence of unusual patterns of hand, eye or foot preference in their sample of 84 speech-retarded children aged seven and eight. On the other hand, Morley (1965) found significantly more left-handedness among children with speech problems, both with and without cerebral palsy, and a greater but non-significant degree of ambilaterality among children with 'developmental aphasia' when these groups were compared with controls. Drillien and Drummond (1983) found that almost twice as many speech-disordered three-year-old children as controls (39 per cent against 21 per cent) did not demonstrate definite hand preference.

The problem of conflicting evidence was addressed by Neils and Aram (1986*b*) who pointed to the heterogeneity of disorders among SLI children and argued that not all of them were likely to have a similar neurological basis. Comparing a sample of 75 SLI children aged four to five with a control group, no significant differences were found in either hand preference or skill, although left-handedness was more common among the language-disordered. Then, on the basis of semantic and phonological factors, which emerged from a factor analysis, they divided their subjects into six linguistically homogeneous groups. Left-handedness was found significantly more frequently among the most severely impaired group than among the mildly impaired. This suggested that handedness may be related to the type of language disorder. Although their data did not permit them to infer that atypical patterns of language lateralisation were present among the non-dextrals (Neils and Aram 1986*b*), this was considered to be a possibility.

Dawn House study
One might expect to find unusual patterns of hand preference in children with specific speech and language disorders. Does our SLI sample display expected frequencies of right- and left-handedness? Are they strongly lateralised for hand, eye and foot? Are similar frequencies of right- and left-handedness found in the subgroups? A greater frequency of left-handedness, strong or weak, can at best be regarded as only suggestive of anomalies of cerebral lateralisation, but information about familial sinistrality, perinatal history and early adverse neurological events permits questions about the possibility of some pathological left-handedness.

HAND, EYE AND FOOT PREFERENCE
In this sample of children with severe speech and language disorders, does the frequency of patterns of hand, eye and foot preference differ from that to be expected from a normal population?

Although individuals are commonly described as being either right- or left-handed, usually depending upon which is the writing hand, handedness varies in strength from strong unilaterality, right or left, to ambilaterality in which neither right nor left predominates. Ambilaterality does not imply that right and left are

TABLE 5.XXIV

Hand preference, 115 boys and 24 girls aged 5.3 to 11.8 (mean 7.10)

Hand preference	Boys		Girls		Total	
	N	%	N	%	N	%
Strong right	64	56	15	63	79	57
Weak right	29	25	7	29	36	26
Ambilateral	8	7	0	—	8	6
Weak left	5	4	0	—	5	3
Strong left	9	8	2	8	11	8
Total	115		24		139	

TABLE 5.XXV

Foot and eye preference

Preference	Foot		Eye	
	N	%	N	%
Right	99	77	76	57
Left	21	17	48	36
Mixed	8	6	9	7
Total	128		133	

used randomly or with equal skill, but that some activities are accomplished with the right, others with the left, there being consistency of usage for specific tasks.

Preferences were examined during a child's first term in school but occasionally this had been done at the admission interview. For handedness, two trials of six tasks were given: drawing or writing, cutting with scissors, throwing, threading a needle, screwing on a lid and dealing cards. Hand preference was assigned to one of five categories: strong right when the right hand was used 11 or 12 times, and weak right, eight to 10 times; strong and weak left were similarly identified and all other scores classified as ambilateral. Eye preference was determined by two sighting tasks, through a cardboard tube and through a hole 1½ inches in diameter cut out of a piece of cardboard and held at arm's length. The children were recorded as being right- or left-eyed if these were consistently used; otherwise they were recorded as mixed. Kicking a ball at a target twice with the same foot was recorded as either right- or left-footed, otherwise mixed.

Handedness was noted for 139 children, eyedness for 133 and footedness for 128, their ages ranging from 5.3 to 11.8, mean 7.10 years with a standard deviation of 19.9 months (Tables 5.XXIV and 5.XXV).

It is difficult to evaluate the distribution of preference categories without a control group. Differences in numbers and types of tasks, and different methods of scoring and criteria for classification, mean that caution must be exercised in making comparison with other studies.

We have been fortunate to receive some very recent data on hand preference relating to 125 English children aged between seven and 11 years. Connolly and Bishop (1991) abstracted five of the items used in this study: using a pencil, using scissors, throwing, threading a needle and dealing cards. Striking a match was substituted for the sixth task (screwing on a lid). With two trials on each task, scores range from 0 (all left) to 12 (all right). Attempting to apply our criteria for classification, a score of 8 to 12 was deemed to indicate right-handedness, 0 to 4 left-handedness and 5 to 7 ambilaterality.

In that sample, 89.6 per cent were right-handed compared with 83 per cent (strong and weak combined) in this study; 6.4 per cent ambilateral compared with our 6 per cent; 4 per cent left-handed compared with our 11 per cent (strong and weak). The SLI children included slightly fewer right-handed but almost three times as many left-handed children. The extent to which these differences arise from differences in procedures is unknown. Despite attempts to equalise the two batteries of tests, they are not identical and the systems for scoring performance on individual items are not the same.

Although our SLI sample appears to include a much larger proportion of left-handed children than Connolly and Bishop's normal sample, left-handedness was reported to occur in a very much higher percentage (29 per cent) of another sample of SLI children (Robinson 1987). No details were given of the basis on which handedness was determined, and again one is faced with probable procedural differences which make it impossible to make direct comparisons.

Right-footedness was recorded in 77 per cent, left-footedness in 17 per cent and mixed footedness in 6 per cent. Estimates of foot preference among unselected populations of children range from 86 to 89 per cent for right-footedness, 7 to 11 per cent for left-footedness and 3 to 4 per cent for mixed when this has been included (Clark 1970, Rutter *et al.* 1970, Whittington and Richards 1987). Compared with findings from studies of unselected children of the same age range and where the same test and criteria have been employed, there is less right- and more left-footedness among our SLI children.

The frequency of our eye preference patterns (57 per cent right, 36 per cent left and 7 per cent mixed) coincides closely with population estimates which range from 60 to 68 per cent right, 30 to 35 per cent left and 5 to 8 per cent mixed (Cuff 1931; Crider 1935; Clark 1957, 1970; Whittington and Richards 1987).

CONCORDANCE OF HAND, EYE AND FOOT

Information about all three preference features was available for 127 children. Concordance of hand, eye and foot preference for the right occurred in 44 children (34.6 per cent) and for the left in three (2.4 per cent), making a total concordance rate of 37 per cent.

There are few studies with which to compare these findings, and comparison is difficult because of differences in tests, categories of preference and criteria. Morley (1986) reported that of 661 unselected children and adults, 54 per cent were

TABLE 5.XXVI

Concordance of hand, foot and eye with age, 127
children aged 5.3 to 11.8

Age	Concordant		Not concordant	
	N	%	N	%
5.3–8.11	30	33.0	61	67.0
9yrs and over	17	47.2	19	52.8
Total	47	37.0	80	63.0

completely right-sided and 3 per cent left-sided, a total of 57 per cent. She also found percentages ranging from 27 per cent to 42 per cent of right-sidedness among children with speech and language problems, the lowest frequency being found among those with an 'articulatory dyspraxia'. In a study of dyslexic boys, aged between eight and 13 years, in which both tests and criteria were similar to those in the present study, concordance was found in 45 per cent of the control groups, unselected for reading, and in just under one third of a severely dyslexic group (Naidoo 1972). Our concordance frequencies appear to be low, resembling those of the speech- and language-impaired and the severely dyslexic in the studies quoted.

When rates of concordance are examined in relation to age, the frequency rises from 37.5 per cent below seven years to 47.2 per cent after nine years. Clymer and Silva (1985) found that 47 per cent of 825 seven-year-old children taking part in the Dunedin Multidisciplinary Child Development Study, displayed congruence of strong right or left hand, eye and foot preference. In this study, that percentage was not reached until the age of nine years. Below nine years there was strong unilateral concordance in only 33 per cent of our sample. This suggests that in addition to being less frequent, strong unilaterality may be slower to develop (Table 5.XXVI).

HANDEDNESS AND GENDER

When differences are found between boys and girls, they are usually in the direction of an excess of males among the left-handed or those with left-handed tendencies (Burt 1937, Clark 1957, Annett 1970). A problem for evaluating differences between the sexes in this study is the very much greater number of boys than girls (115:24). The proportions of strong and weak right-handedness are not too dissimilar and those of strong left-handedness were the same but no girl was either weakly left or ambilateral (see Table 5.XXIV). This may be due to the small number of girls. It may also be a reflection of a stronger unilaterality among girls.

Concordance of hand, eye and foot, either right or left, was found in 14 out of 23 girls compared with 33 out of 104 boys, a significant gender difference (chi-square 5.67, df 1, p<0.02). Girls in this SLI sample are more likely than boys to be strongly unilateral. Porac and Coren (1981), in their study of population laterality characteristics, found evidence of greater strength of unilaterality among females than males. They also found among females a significantly higher incidence of

TABLE 5.XXVII

Hand preference and age

Hand preference	5.0 to 6.11		Age 7.0 to 8.11		9yrs and over	
	N	%	N	%	N	%
Strong right	25	53.2	27	49.1	27	73.0
Weak right	16	34.0	15	27.2	5	13.5
Ambilateral	3	6.4	3	5.5	2	5.4
Weak left	1	2.1	3	5.5	1	2.7
Strong left	2	4.3	7	12.7	2	5.4
Total	47		55		37	

concordance across four indices of laterality, hand, foot, eye and ear. Our gender differences are broadly similar and may simply be in keeping with normal population patterns.

HANDEDNESS AND AGE

Change of hand preference is attributable partly to maturation and partly to social pressures to conform. Many children exhibit a clear unilateral preference by the end of their first year but some instability is not uncommon below the age of five, when preference is usually fixed (Gesell and Ames 1947, Subirana 1969, Sinclair 1971). Thereafter, shifting is infrequent and usually involves decreasing ambilaterality and increasing strong dextrality (Harris 1958, Whittington and Richards 1987). Socio-cultural influences may be the most important determinants during the school years, but some right and also left shifts may also be indices of slowly maturing preference patterns.

The frequency of hand preference patterns in three age bands, 5.0 to 6.11, 7.0 to 8.11, 9.0 and above, remain quite constant for ambilaterality and for weak and strong sinistrality. Strong dextrality shows an increase at the expense of weak right-handedness by the age of nine years. Combining all other categories of handedness, the incidence of strong dextrality at nine years and above is significantly higher than that below nine years (chi-square 4.49, df 1, $p<0.05$). When compared for the effect of age, boys did not differ from girls (Table 5.XXVII).

The diminishing proportion of weakly dextral children at nine years and above, along with the increase in strong dextrality, contributes to the increased congruence of hand, eye and foot noted above. This suggests that the important factor is the slowly developing dominance of right-handedness. Similar trends were reported by Harris (1958) who found a rise in strong right-hand dominance between seven and nine years among reading-disabled children and not among unselected schoolchildren.

HANDEDNESS IN SUBGROUPS

Although the distribution of categories of hand preference does not appear to

TABLE 5.XXVIII

Handedness in subgroups

Language subgroup	Total	Strong right	Weak right	Ambilateral	Weak left	Strong left
Speech	15	8	3	0	1	3
Speech Plus	23	8	9	2	1	3
Classic	43	26	10	3	0	4
Semantic	26	18	5	0	2	1
Residual	8	4	3	1	0	0
Moderate	12	7	5	0	0	0
No Language	3	2	0	1	0	0
Young Unclassified	6	4	1	0	1	0
Severe	3	2	0	1	0	0

depart from that found in unselected populations, subgroups may differ from each other (Neils and Aram 1986*b*).

Each subgroup was examined for the proportion of dextral, strong and weak right, and non-dextral, ambilateral, weak and strong left combined, but no subgroup departed significantly from the expected proportions (P = 0.83 for dextrality). Strong left-handedness appeared to occur rather more frequently among the Speech and Speech Plus but the incidence in neither group was significantly higher than that found in the whole sample (binomial tests).

There is no evidence that the subgroups differ with regard to hand preference (Table 5.XXVIII).

HANDEDNESS AND FAMILY HISTORY

A positive history of familial sinistrality is thought to predispose an individual towards left-hand usage. If so, one would expect to find sinistrality in the families of the left-handed more frequently than in the families of the right-handed. We ask whether familial sinistrality is found with similar frequency among children in the different categories of hand preference.

Information was collected about hand preference by the school's social worker on her pre-admission visit to the home. A positive family history was recorded if one or more of the child's parents and siblings was said to be wholly or partly left-handed. Of the total sample of 156, 35 children (22.4 per cent) had at least one parent, sister or brother completely or partly left-handed. Among the 139 children for whom data on hand preference were available, a positive history was reported for 29 children (20.8 per cent). Comparison may be made with two very different studies reporting the presence of strong or partial sinistrality in the nuclear family. Both Naidoo (1972) and Pipe (1987) found that just under one third of a normal control group belonged to families with a positive sinistrality history. Pipe reported a higher proportion, 41 per cent in her sample of developmentally retarded children and Naidoo reported a similar percentage, 45 per cent among dyslexic boys. The incidence of positive family histories of sinistrality in this sample of SLI children is

TABLE 5.XXIX

Handedness and a familial history of sinistrality in the immediate family

Hand preference	(Total N) T	Family history of sinistrality	
		Negative N	Positive N
Strong right	(79)	64	15
Weak right	(36)	28	8
Ambilateral	(8)	7	1
Weak left	(5)	4	1
Strong left	(11)	7	4

No significant differences in proportions expected and observed (binomial tests)

lower than that reported in normal samples, and very much lower than that reported in learning-disabled groups.

The number of children with a positive history in each category is shown in Table 5.XXIX. A series of binomial tests was run, taking the proportion with a negative history among the 139 children as the basis for the expected proportion ($P = 0.8$). There was a slight but non-significant tendency for a positive history to occur more frequently among the strongly left-handed, but in no category of hand preference did the frequency of familial sinistrality deviate significantly from the expected proportion. This is very different from a report by Bishop (1980a) of familial sinistrality in 170 unselected children whose hand preference was determined by one task only, the hand used for writing. She found that about two thirds of the right-handed had a negative history and about the same proportion of control left-handers had a positive history. Bishop (1980b) warned against confounding family size with familial sinistrality, and demonstrated that when siblings are included the incidence of familial sinistrality rises with an increase in the number of siblings. In her own study (1980a) she avoided this pitfall by deriving a familial sinistrality score from sinistrality in parents and grandparents only, a measure not taken in this study.

The incidence of a positive history of sinistrality appears to be rather low. There is a slight but not significant tendency for the strongly sinistral to come more frequently than the others from families with additional left-handed members. Nor was there any tendency for the strongly or weakly dextral to belong less frequently to families without sinistral members.

PATHOLOGICAL LEFT-HANDEDNESS

Models of pathological handedness are based on the idea that handedness may be shifted and cerebral hemispheric function altered by traumatic events occurring in the perinatal period or in infancy. One might expect such shifts to occur in populations such as children with language disorders, with shifts to the left occuring

TABLE 5.XXX

Hand preference and frequency of neurological
risk factor

| Hand preference | Risk factor | |
	Negative N	Positive N
Strong right	57	22
Weak right	27	9
Ambilateral	1	7*
Weak left	4	1
Strong left	6	5
Total	95	44

Binomial tests (P = 0.7 for each category)
*p<0.01

more frequently than to the right. A very clumsy non-preferred hand may be a better indicator of PLH than hand preference (Bishop 1980, 1984). We have data on preference only but we pursue the question of the possible presence of pathological handedness by examining hand-preference patterns and their association with perinatal and early neurologically threatening events which had been combined to produce a neurological risk factor (Table 5.XXX).

Dextrals, strong and weak right, were compared with non-dextrals, ambilateral, weak and strong left, for the frequency with which the risk factor had been recorded. The risk factor was significantly associated with non-dextrality, almost twice as many as expected having an adverse history (chi-square 5.59, df 1, p<0.02). An inspection of the risk factor in each category of handedness suggested that the raised incidence was limited to the ambilaterals. The binomial test was carried out for each group, using the over-all proportion of negative histories as the expected proportion (P = 0.7). Observed and expected proportions were almost identical in each of the dextral groups and the weak left. Negative risk factors among the strongly sinistral were fewer than expected, but not significantly so. The distribution of positive and negative risk factors among the ambilaterals was highly significant (p<0.01), with seven of the eight having a positive risk history.

The hypothesis of pathological handedness states that PLH is to be found in the absence of familial history of sinistrality, in those of dextral stock. In this sample, the most likely candidates were children with a history of neurological risk and a negative family history (N 32). Using this proportion as the expected proportion (P = 0.23), in each category of handedness, binomial tests were carried out. Expected and observed proportions were not dissimilar in each category except the ambilateral. Among these, there were three times as many children as expected with a negative family history and a history of neurological risk (p<0.01).

The ambilateral group, in which right and left hands were preferred for almost an equal number of tasks, could be described either as right-handed with strong

179

TABLE 5.XXXI

Hand preference by family history (FH) of sinistrality and neurological risk factor

Hand preference	(Total N)	FH neg. Risk neg. N	FH neg. Risk pos. N	FH pos. Risk neg. N	FH pos. Risk pos. N
Strong right	(79)	49	15	8	7
Weak right	(36)	21	7	6	2
Ambilateral	(8)	1	*6	0	1
Weak left	(5)	3	1	1	0
Strong left	(11)	4	3	2	2
Total	78	32	17	12	

*Binomial test (FH negative, risk positive, *vs* the rest)
P = 0.23, p = 0.0054

left-handed tendencies or left-handed with strong right-handed tendencies. If there is a pathological element in the determination of their hand preference patterns, this could be expressed in a pathological shift to left-hand usage in the naturally right (PLH) or to right-hand usage in the naturally left-handed (PRH). The absence of a positive history of sinistrality in six of the seven ambilaterals with a neurological risk factor supports the PLH hypothesis. The remaining child with a risk factor has a positive familial history and theoretically could be PRH (Table 5.XXXI).

The subgroups of these seven children were identified. Two belonged to the Speech Plus, two to the Classic, one to the Moderate, one to the No Language and one to the Severe group. While the children were all language- as opposed to primarily speech-impaired, they did not belong to a particular subgroup of language impairment.

There appears to be some support for the presence of a degree of pathological handedness in a small number of children who displayed ambilateral patterns of hand preference, not definite left-handedness.

Summary

The distribution of hand-, foot- and eye-preference patterns in this sample of SLI children does not appear to differ from that which might be found in an unselected population. No significant differences were found in the frequencies of dextrality and non-dextrality among the speech and language subgroups.

Concordance of hand, eye and foot is found in only 37 per cent which seems low in comparison with normal samples. Concordance may be slow to develop.

There are no weakly left or ambilateral girls, handedness tending to be more definitely unilateral. Girls were significantly more frequently strongly lateralised with concordant hand, foot and eye preference.

The higher frequency of strong right-handedness and of concordance of hand, eye and foot after nine years suggests that unilaterality may be slow to develop in some children and that it is right- not left-sidedness which is slow.

There is no excess of non-dextrality or of familial sinistrality which might suggest anomalies of cerebral lateralisation. Indeed the incidence of familial sinistrality appears to be low. The significant association between our neurological risk factor and ambilaterality, in the absence of familial sinistrality, suggests the presence of a degree of pathological left-hand usage in a small number of ambilateral children who may have been natural right-handers shifted partially to the left.

4. Behaviour

A wide range of studies, some based on samples of representative general populations (Sheridan 1973, Fundudis *et al.* 1979, Richman *et al.* 1982, Silva *et al.* 1984, Butler and Golding 1986), others based on clinic samples (Morley 1965, Garvey and Gordon 1973, Cantwell *et al.* 1979, Baker and Cantwell 1982) have demonstrated the presence of an increased incidence of behavioural disorders in children with speech and language delays and disorders. Despite variations in subject characteristics (age, IQ, type and severity of delay or disorder), in sample sources and in data collection procedures, behavioural problems and disorders have been found to occur more frequently than expected in speech- and language-delayed children; and conversely, language delays occur more frequently than expected in children with behavioural disorders.

Why should psychiatric and language disorders be associated? Reviews of the evidence indicate that although psychiatric disorders such as autism and childhood schizophenia may underlie language disorder, they rarely cause it. The more common antecedents are mental retardation, deafness, and brain damage (Cantwell and Baker 1977, Rutter and Lord 1987). The findings of Fundudis *et al.* (1979) illustrated the greater severity and frequency of behavioural disorder among language-retarded children among whom intellectual and/or neurological disability is common. Their pathologically deviant group of speech-retarded children gave evidence of most problems. Although still occurring more frequently than among a control group, the frequency decreased among children with residual speech problems, being least among those deemed to have a specific speech delay. In studies of children with SLI such as the present one, in which low intelligence, deafness and gross brain damage have been excluded, it is more likely that the language disorder leads directly or indirectly to behaviour problems (Baker and Cantwell 1982).

High on the list of problems have been attentional deficits, poor peer relationships, solitariness, difficulties with management due to tempers, disobedience and aggressive behaviour, anxiety, undue fears and inhibitions (Griffiths 1969, Garvey and Gordon 1973, Sheridan 1973, Cantwell *et al.* 1979, Fundudis *et al.* 1979, Baker and Cantwell 1982, Richman *et al.* 1982, Silva *et al.* 1984, Stevenson *et al.* 1985, Paterson and Golding 1986, Ripley 1987).

It is not difficult to understand why language disorders may give rise to problems such as these. A child's inability to comprehend completely and correctly

181

what s/he is told, whether individually or as a member of a group, not only leads to confusion and bewilderment but may also result in the child becoming the butt of laughter when a response is obviously inappropriate, effecting a lowered self-esteem.

Peer relationships are directly affected by verbal communication difficulties and also, though not so obviously, by limitations in non-verbal body language. SLI children, particularly those with expressive language problems (Ripley 1987), are poor at interpreting the non-verbal aspects of communication, and are not themselves adept at using such means of expression as facial expressions, gesture and other body language. Exclusion from group activities is often the result of the language-disabled child's difficulty in understanding and carrying out verbally transmitted game rules, together with clumsiness, and poor hand-eye and foot-eye co-ordination. Lovell *et al.* (1968) observed that the four-year-old language-disordered child's participation in group activities was affected by his limited pretend play and need for concrete props. Slapstick humour is best appreciated by the literal-minded child, who cannot understand the pun and other verbal jokes relished by children in mid-childhood, and who is thus excluded from sharing another important social experience.

Submissiveness and lack of leadership have also been noted. Siegel *et al.* (1985) observed, in free-play and guided-task situations, the interactive behaviour of normal and SLI three- to five-year-old boys grouped into three types of dyad: normal/normal, normal/SLI, and SLI/SLI, each matched for age, social class and IQ. In normal/SLI pairs, normal children were more likely to control interactions and use controlling strategies when the SLI child was engaged in solitary play. When paired with each other, SLI children were less likely to engage in solitary play and were more responsive than when paired with normal children. The normal child, attempting to elicit responsiveness from the SLI child, tried to establish dominance and control, a state of affairs which bore the seeds of conflict.

The speech- and language-impaired child, less able to deal with conflict and disagreement verbally, may react sometimes by using physical force or by socially withdrawing if the odds are against him. Many children show remarkable persistence in making themselves understood, but this usually requires a patient and sympathetic audience. Time is often limited in the ordinary classroom and occasionally also at home. Children give up and retreat or vent their frustration in anger. A positive attitude to communication is important in the assessment and treatment of disorders, as well as for facilitating social relationships. It is difficult to assess and give remedial help to a child who is reluctant to communicate verbally, whether orally or manually. A comment from a report about a child before admission sums up the emotional response to speech impairment. 'J. was very pleasant and co-operative during testing but he displayed signs of increasing frustration and distress when he could not make himself understood. He shouted, looked desperate saying he had a headache and did not want to carry on. His teacher adds that in the classroom, he sometimes resorts to miming a word, which amuses his peers and humiliates him, so he tries to avoid these situations by not coming forward.'

Parents of disabled children have a natural tendency to over-protect, with all the consequent effects on emotional and practical independence. Parental anxiety and concern are almost impossible to conceal from children, who become even more aware of their own limitations.

Behaviour and type of language disorder
Although results of different investigations are somewhat equivocal, not least because of lack of uniformity in the classification of language disorders, it appears that not all specific speech and language disorders carry the same risk of behavioural problems. The greatest agreement concerns the group of children with disordered speech but essentially normal language. In addition to comprehensive and detailed examinations which included a psychiatric evaluation, of 196 speech-and/or language-disordered children (mean age 5½ years) Baker and Cantwell (1982) asked teachers to complete a rating scale describing the children's behaviour. Behaviour problems were reported by teachers to be less than half as common among children with speech impairments, 22 per cent, compared with 52 per cent of children with both speech and language difficulties, and 56 per cent with pure language impairment. Parental reports supported this general picture. Poor peer relationships existed in approximately one third of speech- and language-impaired children: about twice the proportion of those with articulation problems only. Hall and Tomblin (1978) also found differences between the speech- and the language-impaired, favouring the former. However, in a follow-up of 49 SLI children, Griffiths (1969) judged social development to be satisfactory among most, especially the speech defective, but found more symptoms of emotional maladjustment in this group. She suggested that the attendance of the speech-disordered at mainstream schools might expose them to greater pressures than many of the language-disordered, who continued in special education.

Griffiths (1969) found few social or emotional problems among her small group of children with a severe compehension disorder. Silva *et al.* (1987), in their longitudinal study of children with a language delay at three years, identified three areas: comprehension, expressive and general language delay. When the children were examined at seven, nine and 11 years, those children with early comprehension delay and general delay had significantly higher scores on the Rutter Behaviour Scales completed by parents and teachers (Rutter 1967, Rutter *et al.* 1970), when compared with the remainder of the sample. However, these were children with a relative delay rather than a severe comprehension disorder. In a study of 11 five- and six-year-old children with receptive language disorders, attending a special school for children with language disorders, Petrie (1975) found evidence in all of some inhibition, reserve, withdrawal or depression on the Stott Bristol Social Adjustment Guide (BSAG). Retesting one year later revealed considerable improvement, suggesting that adjustment improved in an appropriate educational environment. Correlations between age, IQ and BSAG scores suggested that older, brighter language-disordered children may have greater adjustment problems than the younger and less bright.

Unlike the Dunedin study (Silva *et al.* 1987), in which delay was defined in terms of scores falling at the lowest percentile levels on tests of language, Stevenson *et al.* (1985) used the median as a cut-off point for dividing a representative population of three-year-old children into high and low achievers on tests of passive vocabulary, expressive vocabulary and structure. Only low structure scores at three years predicted behaviour deviance, predominantly of a neurotic nature, measured on the Rutter teacher's scale at eight years. The relationship between low structure scores and behaviour deviance held even when behaviour at three years was controlled.

Ripley (1987) described a counselling service in a special school for SLI children. Children were referred to her by school staff, largely because of aggressive behaviour and poor social relationships. Of the four subgroups to which the children were assigned, the highest percentage of referrals came from children described as having deviant articulation and those with an expressive dysphasia, those children with the greatest gap between comprehension and the articulatory or linguistic means of expression.

Ripley's findings appear to be quite different from those reported by Baker and Cantwell (1982), who found fewer problems among the specifically speech-impaired than among the language-impaired. However, whereas the teacher ratings reported by Baker and Cantwell were made for their total sample, Ripley's cases were a selected subsample composed of children who had been referred to her and who were not necessarily representative of all the speech- or language-impaired children in the school. Again, there is a wide age difference between the two samples. In Ripley's sample, there were no children below the age of nine years, the majority being between 12 and 14 years. The children in the Baker and Cantwell sample ranged in age from 1.9 to 14.3 years (mean 5.6). It is possible that behaviour problems occur more frequently among children with persisting, severe articulation disorders as they reach adolescence.

Dawn House study
The longitudinal nature of the study enabled us to record adverse behaviours, associated with specific speech and language impairments three times between pre-entry and the child's final year at school.

We examined behaviours in the speech and language subgroups for differences between those with speech disorders and near-normal language, and those with language disorders. Finally we identified those children considered to be most at risk of behavioural disorder.

DATA
The behaviours recorded relate to poor attention (poor concentration, short

attention span or distractibility); lack of confidence (dependence upon adults and constant seeking of approval or reassurance); poor peer relationships; solitariness (an avoidance of or reluctance to join in group activities, not necessarily the same as poor peer relationships); antisocial behaviour (aggression, disruptive or destructive behaviour or bullying); outbursts of temper; being teased or bullied; and frustrations with language problems and speech. After entry to Dawn House, two further problems were noted: being easily upset by difficulties and a negative attitude to communication. Although classes in Dawn House are very small, with much individual and supportive teaching, some children become upset or tearful at failure in the classroom, playground or residential unit. Children are encouraged to communicate orally, or by using a manual signing system if necessary. Most children have a positive attitude to communicating with peers and adults and persevere in making themselves understood. Some children in our study, however, rarely joined in conversations or spontaneously offered news of any kind, and gave up if attempts to communicate were not immediately successful.

These behaviours were not graded but simply recorded as present or absent, from observations made by parents and staff. Although not desirable, their presence at any one time should not be interpreted as constituting a behaviour *disorder* or even a major problem. At the end of this section we shall identify more serious long-term problems.

Information was collected at three points: (i) prior to entry to Dawn House, (ii) during a child's second year at Dawn House, to allow any initial adjustment problems to settle down, and (iii) during the final year at school. Pre-entry information was obtained from parents during a prestructured interview by the school's social worker and from staff (mainly teachers) of the schools, language units, preschool units, nursery schools and other establishments attended by the children. At Dawn House, reports by teachers, speech therapists and child-care staff provided the required information.

Parental and school reports of behaviour prior to Dawn House entry
All behaviours except tempers were noticed more frequently at school or nursery school than at home. Problems most commonly occurring in school were frustrations (expressed by emotional outbursts as children failed to make themselves understood), poor attention and concentration, a lack of confidence, poor peer relationships and aggression. Apart from attention, the same items are highest on the home list, although the order of frequency differs slightly.

Agreement between home and school, shown in the last column of Table 5.XXXII, was generally low. Children behave differently at home and at school, and parents and teachers are also likely to regard some misbehaviours as more important than others. Poor concentration and a short attention span are much more noticeable in the classroom than at home and this may apply to solitariness also. However, parents and school staff agreed that about one in four children showed a lack of confidence, and that about one in five showed poor attention,

TABLE 5.XXXII

Reports of behaviours from home and school, prior to entry to Dawn House; 156 children aged 4.2 to 11.8, mean 6.1

Behaviour	Home		School		Home and School	
	N	%	N	%	N	%
Poor attention	40	25.6	81	52	30	19.2
Poor peer relationships	48	30.8	67	43	30	19.2
Solitariness	18	11.6	45	28.9	8	5.1
Teased/bullied	15	9.6	24	15.4	6	3.9
Lack of confidence	65	41.7	71	45.5	41	26.3
Frustration with speech/language	50	32	85	54.5	32	20.5
Aggression	48	30.8	60	38.5	32	20.5
Tempers	61	39.2	50	32	17	10.9

TABLE 5.XXXIII

Behaviours noted at school prior to Dawn House entry, by age; 156 children aged 4.2 to 11.8, mean 6.1

Behaviour	Age		
	<5yrs (58) %	5.0 to 6.11 (68) %	≥7.0 (30) %
Poor attention	48.3	60.3	40
Poor peer relationships	43.1	41.2	46.7
Solitariness	31.1	29.4	23.3
Teased/bullied	5.2	22	20*
Lack of confidence	38	45.6	60
Frustration with speech/language	55.2	60.3	40
Aggression	44.8	38.2	26.7
Tempers	22.4	19.1	10

*Chi-square 7.46, df 2, $p < 0.05$

TABLE 5.XXXIV

Behaviours reported during the second year of attendance at Dawn House, mean age 9.1

Behaviour	Second year (N 116) %
Poor attention	44.0
Poor peer relationships	13.8
Solitariness	4.3
Teased/bullied	1.7
Lack of confidence	55.9
Easily upset	55.0
Negative attitude to communication	15.5
Frustration with speech/language	11.8
Aggression	13.8
Tempers	9.5

poor peer relationships, aggressiveness or frustration with speech and language.

AGE

One might expect some behaviours, such as tempers, to diminish with increasing age. Since the age range is quite wide, we have looked at behaviour observed at school in relation to three age groups: under five years, from five to 6.11, and seven years and above.

Tempers did indeed diminish with age from just over one in five in children under five years to one in 10 among those of seven years or over. There was also a decrease in aggressive behaviour, frustration with speech and language and solitariness. Poor peer relationships showed no change of frequency with age, affecting over 40 per cent in all age groups. After school entry at five years, there was a rise in poor attention, lack of confidence, and being teased or bullied. Problems of attention were most frequently reported among five- and six-year-olds, while lack of confidence increased from under 40 per cent in the under fives to 60 per cent in the over sevens. However no item of behaviour showed a significant change with age except being teased or bullied, which rose from 5 per cent in the under fives to 22 per cent and 20 per cent in the two older age groups (Table 5.XXXIII).

Behaviours noted by school staff during the second year of attendance
at Dawn House

Data relate to 116 children during their second year at Dawn House (Table 5.XXXIV). These were children whose disorders required more than two years of intensive speech, language and educational treatment. Not included were 24 children who had left the school by the end of their second year and who are considered below among the 118 leavers.

Compared with data obtained prior to school entry, there was a marked decrease in the proportions of children reported to make poor peer relationships, who tended to be solitary, who were teased or bullied, showed frustration with their speech and language limitations, were aggressive or threw temper tantrums. Other problems—poor attention and distractibility, problems in dealing with failure, and lack of confidence—remained at high levels (45 per cent, 56 per cent and 57 per cent respectively). The pre-entry behaviour of the 116 second-year pupils was examined. Of 60 showing early frustrations with their speech and language, 49 no longer did so; poor peer relationships improved in 43 out of 52 and solitariness in 32 out of 33.

AGE

If some behaviours tend to diminish with age, the fact that the children are on average three years older than when the first reports were made may explain some of the decrease. Chi-square was used to explore differences of frequency in three age groups, 6.0 to 7.11, 8.0 to 9.11, and 10 years or above (Table 5.XXXV). The

TABLE 5.XXXV

Behaviours reported by school staff during the second year of attendance at Dawn House by age; 116 children aged 6.4 to 13.4, mean 9.1

Behaviour	Age					
	6.0–7.11 (30)		8.0–9.11 (54)		≥10.0 (32)	
	N	%	N	%	N	%
Poor attention	19	63.3	24	44.4	9	28.1*
Poor peer relationships	3	10	10	18.5	3	9.4
Solitariness	1	3.3	4	7.4	0	0
Teased/bullied	0	0	0	0	2	6.2
Lack of confidence	18	60	29	53.7	19	59.3
Easily upset	16	53.3	29	53.7	20	62.3
Negative attitude to communication	3	10	10	18.5	5	15.6
Frustration with speech/language	3	10	8	14.8	3	9.4
Aggression	4	13.3	7	12.9	5	15.6
Tempers	2	6.7	5	9.2	4	12.4

*Chi-square 7.76, df 2, p = 0.02

small number of problems in some items precluded the calculation of chi-square itself. Only poor attention fell significantly with age, affecting almost two thirds of the children aged between 6.0 and 7.11 but less than one third aged 10 years or above (p<0.05). All other problems occurred with similar frequency in each age group. Of some concern is the high proportion of children in all three age groups who were noted to be lacking in confidence, or who were easily upset by failure in the classrooom or on the playground.

Increasing age only partly explains the dramatic fall in most of the problem behaviours. More probable reasons may lie in differing school environments. The first batch of data comes from staff in a variety of school, preschool and other educational units, most of which belong to the mainstream of educational provision, while the second comes from staff at a single special school where the needs of the children were being met. This could have at least two effects which could result in decreasing frequencies of behaviours. First, staff in special schools may be more tolerant of some behaviours, simply because they are common or because they are regarded as part of the SLI child's difficulties. If this is so, then behaviours may be reported less frequently. The second effect is a genuine fall in behaviours (Petrie 1975). SLI children in mainstream schools are likely to experience considerable stress, socially and educationally, even when staff are sympathetic to their problems. The relief from such pressures was evident in remarks made by so many children after admission to a school where all other pupils had similar difficulties which were recognised and being treated.

BOARDING *VS* DAY ATTENDANCE

Boarding school provision in special education is controversial, one objection being the possible adverse emotional and perhaps also social effect of separation from

TABLE 5.XXXVI

Behaviours during the second year of attendance, 10 children with speech disorders and the remainder, 106 with language disorders, mean age 9.1

Behaviour	Speech group (10) N	Remainder (106) N
Poor attention	0	52*
Poor peer relationships	1	15
Solitariness	0	5
Teased/bullied	0	2
Lack of confidence	6	60
Easily upset	6	59
Negative attitude to communication	0	18
Frustration with speech/language	1	13
Aggression	2	14
Tempers	3	8

*Chi-square 7.01, df 1, p<0.01

home. Dawn House offers day places to a limited number of pupils. Of the 116 children under current consideration, 16 were day pupils. The distribution of behaviours for boarding and day children was almost identical for all items except two, poor attention (chi-square 3.25, df 1, p<0.1) and poor peer relationships (chi-square 3.21, df 1, p<0.1), these being more frequent among the day pupils. We have seen above that poor attention decreased with age and this probably explains differences of inattention. The 16 day children included nine aged less than eight years, compared with 21 out of 106 boarders. Poor peer relationships were not associated with age. The study of social interactions by Siegel *et al.* (1985) supports a suggestion that the ready availability of playmates of similar age and with similar speech and language disorders may facilitate good peer relationships, conditions inherent in the boarding environment. Added to this are the active efforts by boarding staff to foster group activities into which all children are drawn.

BEHAVIOUR AND TYPE OF DISORDER

Previous studies suggest that not all speech and language disorders carry similar risks of behaviour disorder, there being the greatest accord about differences between children whose speech is defective but whose language is normal or minimally affected, and those with disordered language. The distribution of each item of behaviour in each of the nine language groups was examined, and chi-square calculated where possible, to evaluate differences between the Speech group of 10 children and the remainder of the sample (106), all of whom had language disorders (Table 5.XXXVI).

The speech-disordered showed no negative attitudes to communication, and few problems of attention, peer relationships and solitariness, but only in the case of poor attention was the difference significant (p<0.01). However, more speech-

189

TABLE 5.XXXVII

Behaviours reported by school staff during the final year of attendance at Dawn House, by age; 118 children, mean age 11.9

Behaviour	Age						
	<10.6 (30)		10.6–11.11 (55)		≥12.0 (33)		Total (118)
	N	%	N	%	N	%	%
Poor attention	13	43.3	16	29.1	13	39.4	35.7
Poor peer relationships	6	20.0	15	27.3	8	24.2	24.6
Solitariness	1	3.3	8	14.5	5	15.1	11.8
Teased/bullied	4	13.3	4	7.3	0	0	6.8
Lack of confidence	21	70.0	40	72.7	23	69.7	71.2
Easily upset	18	60.0	39	70.9	18	54.5	63.5
Negative attitude to communication	4	13.3	12	21.8	5	15.1	17.8
Frustration with speech/language	6	20.0	11	20.0	6	18.2	19.5
Aggression	2	6.7	10	18.2	5	15.1	14.4
Tempers	2	6.7	8	14.5	3	9.1	11.0

No significant associations with age

disordered children were noted to be aggressive and temper tantrums occurred in three out of the 10 compared with eight of the remaining 106.

Among the eight language subgroups the proportional frequencies of behaviours, some of which were very small, were very similar for lack of confidence, being easily upset by difficulties, frustrations with the communication barriers of their speech and language limitations, poor peer relationships and aggressive behaviour. Solitariness—a marked preference for solitary as opposed to group activity—was noted in five children, three of whom had comprehension problems and belonged to the Semantic group. The only two children to be teased also belonged to that group, being teased not for their speech or language but their inappropriate behaviour.

Behaviour during the final year at Dawn House
We now report upon the behaviour of 118 children during their final year at Dawn House. Aged from 6.10 to 13.10 (mean age 11.9) they are now on average about 2½ years older than when last reported upon.

Poor attention was a less frequent problem during the final year than during the second year at school, affecting just over one third of the children. Negative attitudes to communication, aggressive behaviour and tempers remained at much the same level. However there was a rise in poor peer relationships, solitariness, being teased, lack of confidence and lack of resilience in the face of difficulty or failure (Table 5.XXXVII). As the children approached adolescence, changes in patterns of social grouping could be observed in the playground. Groups, more tightly knit than among younger children, formed very often around one or two more dominant children. While membership varied, the cohesiveness of grouping

190

TABLE 5.XXXVIII

Behaviours during the final year of attendance at Dawn House; 15 children with speech disorders and the remainder, 103, with language disorders; mean age 11.9

Behaviour	Speech group (15) N	Remainder (103) N
Poor attention	3	39
Poor peer relationships	2	27
Solitariness	0	14
Teased/bullied	2	6
Lack of confidence	9	75
Easily upset	5	70*
Negative attitude to communication	1	20
Frustration with speech/language	4	19
Aggression	4	13
Tempers	1	12

*Chi-square 5.36, df 1, p = 0.02

TABLE 5.XXXIX

Long-term behaviour problems in 118 children in their final year, mean age 11.9

Behaviour	Not a problem %	Present at some time %	Long-term problem %
Poor attention	33.0	39.8	27.2
Poor peer relationships	42.4	39.8	17.8
Solitariness	63.5	29.7	6.8
Teased/bullied	76.3	22.0	1.7
Lack of confidence	16.1	30.5	53.4
Easily upset	12.7	33.1	54.2
Negative attitude to communication	29.7	58.4	11.9
Frustration with speech/language	33.0	54.3	12.7
Aggression	48.3	40.7	11.0
Tempers	69.5	23.7	6.8

could operate to the social detriment of some. A rise in levels of anxiety during the last year was often evident, focusing on the knowledge that a change of school was imminent and an uncertainty about the nature of a future school.

Some behaviours appeared to vary, but none significantly, with age. Solitariness, aggression and tempers were more common among children aged 10½ years or above, while no child of 12 years or above is reported to have been teased.

When the speech-disordered are compared with the remainder who have language disorders, results echo those obtained during the second year. The speech-disordered had fewer problems of attention, peer relationships and solitariness, they had a more positive attitude to communicating and were less frequently upset by difficulties, the difference on this last item reaching the 2 per cent level of statistical significance. Once again, frustrations and aggressive behaviour were found more frequently among the speech-disordered but not significantly so (Table 5.XXXVIII).

Long-term problems
So far we have been reporting on behaviours which were noted at a particular time, and many children had ceased to show earlier behaviour problems by the time they reached their final year at school. It was stressed earlier that behaviour noted once is not evidence of a behaviour disorder. Problems which persist over a period of time are a more serious matter and these are now identified. If a behaviour was present during the final year at school and had also been present during the second year (or before school entry, in the case of children who had left the school by or before the end of their second year) this was regarded as a long-term problem.

THE FREQUENCY OF LONG-TERM PROBLEM BEHAVIOURS (Table 5.XXXIX)
Heading the list of long-term problems, with over 50 per cent of the 118 leavers experiencing them, are lack of confidence and being easily upset by difficulties. Seventy-five per cent of the leavers were experiencing one or both of these features which are suggestive of a state of anxiety. In contrast, aggression was a long-term problem in just 11 per cent, and had never been a problem in almost half. Much higher rates of anxious, neurotic type behaviour than of aggressive, antisocial behaviour were also found by Stevenson *et al.* (1985) in their follow-up of children with early language delay. Problems of poor attention affected just over one third. Long-term poor peer relationships were found in about one in five, but this had not been a problem at any time for more than 40 per cent. Visitors to the school very frequently comment on the friendliness of the children and their willingness to talk. While many children on some occasion gave vent to frustrations with their speech and language limitations, this was not a major problem for most and attitudes to communication remained generally positive.

LONG-TERM PROBLEMS AND LANGUAGE SUBGROUPS
Among the leavers were 15 children from the Speech subgroup, whose primary speech impairment was accompanied by minor language problems. On each item of behaviour, they were compared with the remainder, all of whom had primary language disorders, for the presence of long-term problems, behaviours present at any one time, or no problem (chi-square, df 2). The only item which significantly differentiated the speech- from the language-disordered was poor attention, experienced by one of the former and 31 of the latter (chi-square 6.60, df 2, p<0.05). No significant differences were found for poor peer relationships or aggressive behaviour. Expected cell numbers, too small for the calculation of chi-square in the remaining items, gave some indication of trends. The only noteworthy behaviour is solitariness which occurred as a long-term problem only among the language-disordered. An examination of the different language subgroups revealed

TABLE 5.XL

Social circumstances of 24 behaviourally at risk and the 94 remaining leavers, mean age 11.9

Social factor	Children with long-term problems	
	≥4 problems (N 24)	<4 problems (N 94)
	N	N
*Non-manual social class	5	21
Manual social class	18	71
Single parent	1	12
4+ children in family	5	28

*Three children excluded—parent unemployed

No significant differences (chi-square, df 1)

that of eight children with this problem, six were members of the Semantic subgroup (comprehension disorder) of 20 children.

CHILDREN AT RISK OF BEHAVIOUR DISORDER

If each long-term problem is given a score of 1, the maximum score for any child is 10. In fact scores ranged from 0 to 8 with a mean of 2 with a standard deviation of 1.6. A cut-off point of 4 produced 24 children (22 boys and 2 girls, one in five of the total 118) who had four of more long-term behaviour problems and might be said to have or be at risk of having a behaviour disorder. Among the leavers, the ratio of boys to girls (96:22) reflects that of the sample as a whole. However, the proportion of disturbed boys (23 per cent) is more than twice that of girls (9.1 per cent).

Children with behaviour disorders have been found to be duller than their normal peers (Rutter *et al.* 1970, Richman *et al.* 1982). The mean VIQ, 75.5, and PIQ, 95.3, of our at-risk group are lower than those of the remainder, verbal mean 81.4, performance mean 98.4† but neither verbal nor performance IQ difference approached a statistical level of significance (one-way ANOVA).

Environmental circumstances have also been found to be associated with behaviour disorders (Stevenson *et al.* 1985, Golding and Rush 1986) and perhaps adverse environmental conditions are more common among the at-risk group. When compared with national cohorts, our total sample was found to have a significantly greater number of children with single parents, come from larger families and belong to the manual classes (Chapter 3). There were however no significant differences in the distribution of each of these social factors among children with four or more long-term problems and the remainder (Table 5.XL).

Inspection of the individual children in the at-risk group suggested that many had particularly severe language problems. One indication of the severity or refractoriness of the language problems is the type of school to which the children go on leaving Dawn House. Children joined mainstream schools if speech and oral language improved to a level which, although not necessarily completely normal,

†Standard deviations of 11.4, 13.1, 14.4 and 15.3 respectively.

Fig. 5.2. Long-term behaviour problems in subgroups.

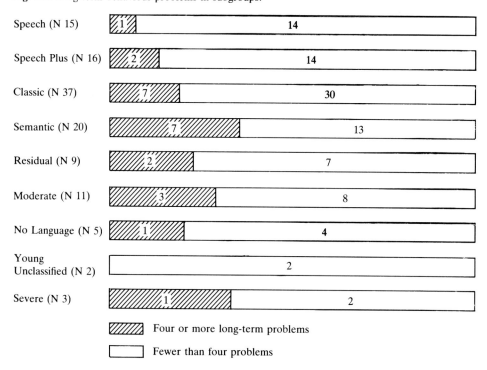

Speech (N 15)

Speech Plus (N 16)

Classic (N 37)

Semantic (N 20)

Residual (N 9)

Moderate (N 11)

No Language (N 5)

Young Unclassified (N 2)

Severe (N 3)

Four or more long-term problems

Fewer than four problems

TABLE 5.XLI

Long-term problem behaviours, among children with four or more problems and the remainder, existing in their final year at Dawn House

Behaviour	Children with long-term problems		
	≥4 (N 24) N	<4 (N 94) N	
Poor attention	16	16	****
Poor peer relationships	17	4	****
Solitariness	7	1	****
Aggression and/or temper	10	4	****
Negative attitude to communication	9	5	***
Frustration with speech/language	9	6	***
Lack of confidence and/or easily upset	23	66	*

Significance of chi-square values, df 1

* p<0.05

*** p<0.001

**** p<0.0001

allowed them to continue their education in an ordinary school. Sixty-two of the 118 leavers did so. Only eight of the 24 behaviourally at-risk children went to a mainstream school, compared with 56 of the remaining 94. Twelve with behaviour problems, 50 per cent, compared with 37 per cent of the remainder, went on to a language school. One boy, in the at-risk group, proceeded to a school for the maladjusted. Six children were placed in schools for slow learners, because of very poor academic achievement and/or social problems. Three of these are in the at-risk group. Persisting serious language problems were present in 18 of the 24 who are behaviourally at risk.

At-risk children did not appear to be equally distributed between the speech and language subgroups. They included only one of the 15 speech-disordered, a boy who had moderate comprehension and expressive language problems at leaving. They also included seven of the 20 in the Semantic subgroup, many of whose moderate or near-normal speech and expressive language can mislead people into believing that they understand much more than they do. The resulting mismatch, between the child's true level of comprehension and what is expected of him, can be very stressful. Even among those children described as having early moderate language difficulties (whose written language constituted the major disability) and those with residual problems (who had had considerable previous appropriate therapy and education) the incidence of behaviour problems was as high as in other more obviously linguistically disabled groups (Fig. 5.2).

All behaviours were found significantly more frequently among the behaviourally at-risk than among the remainder, but particularly problems of poor attention, poor peer relationships, solitariness and aggression and/or tempers ($p<0.0001$). The majority of those with a negative attitude towards communication and those who were consistently frustrated by their speech and language limitations were found among the at-risk groups. Barely reaching a level of significance, lack of confidence and/or lack of resilience were found commonly in both the at-risk group and the remainder (Table 5.XLI).

Summary
Behaviours occurring at any one of the three test-times were not graded for severity and should not be regarded as evidence of a disorder. During the children's final year at Dawn House we look back to earlier reports and regard the children with four or more long-term problem behaviours as being as risk of disorder.

Prior to admission to Dawn House, when the mean age of the 156 children was 6.1, parents and school staff reported that (apart from temper tantrums) the behaviours noted were more common at school than at home. At this stage, frustration with speech and language difficulties and poor attention were the major problems at school. Teasing or being bullied were four times more common after five years, national school-entry age, than before. Lack of confidence rose from 38 per cent of the preschool children to 60 per cent of those aged seven years or above.

By the end of their second year at Dawn House, the behaviour of 116 children (mean age 9.1), showed a marked improvement in social behaviour, frustrations and aggression, probably due to the social facilities and opportunities to mix with peers who have similar problems. The incidence of lack of confidence remained at the high level of the children seven years or older prior to Dawn House entry. At this point, poor attention diminishes with age and changes in position from being highest on the list of problems among the under eights, to third place among those aged 10 years and over.

When children with speech disorders were compared with the remainder with language disorders, no Speech child had a problem with poor attention, solitariness or a negative attitude to communicating verbally. But lack of confidence and being easily upset by difficulties or failure, now highest on the list of problems, occurred with equal frequency among the speech- and the language-disordered.

During their final year, many problem behaviours had risen among the 118 leavers (mean age 11.9). These included poor peer relationships and lack of confidence but not aggressive behaviour. It is suggested that anxiety during this year may be increased by uncertainty about future school placement, and perhaps also by the formation among the older children of more tightly knit social groups into which individuals were accepted or excluded.

The pattern of differences between the speech- and the language-disordered children, noted during their second year, was largely maintained. The speech-disordered had fewer problems of attention, poor peer relationships, solitariness and negative attitudes to communication. Significantly more Speech children were able to deal positively with difficulties or failure.

Long-term problems, occurring both during the final year at school and previously, were identified. By far the most common problems were lack of confidence and poor coping strategies, which included dependence on adult approval or attention and being easily worried or upset by failure and/or new situations: features suggestive of anxiety. One or both of these affected 75 per cent of the leavers. By contrast, antisocial behaviour was a long-term problem in just 11 per cent. Poor attention was a long-term problem in about one in four, and poor peer relationships in one in five (the latter not a problem on any occasion in more than 40 per cent).

Poor attention occurred significantly less frequently among the speech- than among the language-disordered, and solitariness (found only among the language-disordered) was most common among the children in the Semantic subgroup.

Twenty-four children (22 boys and two girls), with four or more long-term behaviour problems, were deemed to have or be at risk of having a behaviour disorder. This at-risk group constituted one in five of the 118 leavers and included proportionately twice as many boys as girls. They were not duller than the remainder of the leavers, nor were they differentiated by factors such as social class or family size. Seventy-five per cent experienced persisting serious language and/or academic difficulties. They were not evenly distributed between the language subgroups. Proportionately the highest number came from the Semantic subgroup while fewest, only one of 15, belonged to the Speech group. Children with moderate oral language but severe written language problems found in both the Moderate and Residual groups were as likely to be at risk as the more obviously language-disordered.

The children are classified according to outcome in Chapter 7. Since the reason for their admission to Dawn House was their severe speech and language impairment, the bases of judgement of outcome have been levels reached in oral and written language when they left the school. Working with the children, we are keenly aware of the implications of their ability to form social relationships, their temperament and above all their self-esteem for coping with life in general. Some who are classified as having a good or fair outcome are quite disabled by some of the problems described here. The outlook is often better for others with poor language outcome but without behaviour problems.

Whether our leavers remain within the special school system or rejoin mainstream schools, our findings underline important personal and emotional needs which staff, and the children's families, must make every attempt to meet. Lack of self-confidence, a poor self-image and a timid attitude to communicating with others, especially normal peers, can have far-reaching destructive effects. It is essential to build up self-assurance and self-respect, and to encourage a positive attitude to communication.

5. Neurological correlates[*]
Between 1978 and 1990 a total of 101 of the 156 Dawn House schoolchildren included in the main study were medically examined by the author. These 101 children form the subjects of this report and will be referred to as the 'neurostudy group'. Formal neurological examination was carried out on every child, together with detailed tests of oral, ocular, gross and fine motor skills, constructional abilities and left-right discrimination. Chromosome analysis was carried out on 20 children.

The nine speech and language groupings described in the main study were used. There were 11 children in the Speech group, 17 in the Speech Plus, 35 in the Classic, 14 in the Semantic, five in the Residual, seven in the Moderate, six in the No Language, three in the Young Unclassified and three in the Severe group.

Head circumference
The maximum occipito-frontal head circumference was measured with a tape measure and plotted on a chart (Nellhaus 1968) taking into account the child's age and sex. The standard deviation from the mean was recorded. The expected distribution was 16 per cent <1SD, 68 per cent −1SD to +1SD, and 16 per cent >+1SD. In the neurostudy children there were fewer than expected measurements

[*]The following section has been contributed by David H. Mellor MD, FRCP, Consultant Paediatric Neurologist, University Hospital, Queen's Medical Centre, Nottingham.

197

TABLE 5.XLII

Head circumference

Language subgroup	$<-1SD$ (%)	$-1SD$ to $+1SD$ (%)	$>+1SD$ (%)	Total	Not known
Speech	2 (18)	7 (64)	2 (18)	11	0
Speech Plus	1 (6)	8 (50)	7 (44)	16	1
Classic	3 (9)	25 (74)	6 (18)	34	1
Semantic	1 (8)	10 (83)	1 (8)	12	2
Residual	0	3 (60)	2 (40)	5	0
Moderate	0	5 (71)	2 (29)	7	0
No Language	1 (17)	3 (50)	2 (33)	6	0
Young Unclassified	0	3 (100)	0	3	0
Severe	1 (33)	2 (67)	0	3	0
Neurostudy	9 (9)	66 (68)	22 (23)	97	4

TABLE 5.XLIII

Left-right discrimination difficulties

Language subgroup	Normal (%)	Moderate impairment (%)	Severe impairment (%)	Total	Not known
Speech	9 (82)	2 (18)	0	11	0
Speech Plus	11 (69)	4 (25)	1 (6)	16	1
Classic	14 (45)	17 (55)	0	31	4
Semantic	8 (57)	6 (43)	0	14	0
Residual	4 (80)	1 (20)	0	5	0
Moderate	6 (86)	1 (14)	0	7	0
No Language	0	5 (83)	1 (17)	6	0
Young Unclassified	1 (50)	0	1 (50)	2	1
Severe	1 (33)	2 (67)	0	3	0
Neurostudy	54 (57)	38 (40)	3 (3)	95	6

TABLE 5.XLIV

Ocular movements

Language subgroup	Normal (%)	Moderate impairment (%)	Severe impairment (%)	Total
Speech	11 (100)	0	0	11
Speech Plus	15 (88)	2 (12)	0	17
Classic	27 (77)	5 (14)	3 (9)	35
Semantic	14 (100)	0	0	14
Residual	5 (100)	0	0	5
Moderate	7 (100)	0	0	7
No Language	6 (100)	0	0	6
Young Unclassified	3 (100)	0	0	3
Severe	2 (67)	1 (33)	0	3
Neurostudy	90 (89)	8 (8)	3 (3)	101

of $<-1\text{SD}$ and more than expected measurements of $>+1\text{SD}$ (Table 5.XLII), but the differences were not statistically significant (chi-square 3.02, df 2, p>0.1). The Speech Plus group had the highest proportion of children with head circumferences $>+1\text{SD}$, but the differences when compared with the remaining neurostudy children did not reach significance (chi-square 4.86, df 2, p>0.05).

Left-right discrimination
The children were asked to identify their own and the examiner's left or right ear, hand and leg. Children aged seven to 11 were considered to have normal left-right discrimination if they were correct with their own body and to have a moderate disorder if they were not. Children over 11 years were considered to have normal left-right discrimination if they were correct with their own and the examiner's body, a moderate disorder if they were correct only with their own body, and a severe disorder if they were incorrect with both.

Disorders of left-right discrimination were common, occurring in 43 per cent of the total neurostudy group (Table XLIII). Children in the Classic group were particularly affected, with only 45 per cent of them showing normal left-right discrimination, but the differences were not significant when compared with the remaining children (chi-square with Yates correction 1.90, df 1, p>0.1). The Speech group contained only 18 per cent with left-right discrimination difficulties, but again the differences were not significant when compared with the rest of the neurostudy group (chi-square with Yates correction 2.12, df 1, p>0.1).

Ocular movements
Ocular movements were examined and a cover-uncover test looking for latent squint was carried out. Squints were found in nine (9 per cent) of the children, which is higher than the 2 per cent prevalence usually quoted for the general childhood population (Forfar and Arneil 1978). Nystagmus was noted in five children, three of whom also had squints. No other ocular movement disorder was identified (Table 5.XLIV). The Classic group contained proportionately more children with eye movement disorders than the rest of the children, and the differences were significant (chi-square 9.26, df 2, p<0.001).

Oral movements
We checked for lip spreading and pursing, tongue forwards and lateral protrusion, upwards curling and rapid side-to-side movements and palatal movements. We also tested for nasal escape. In the neurostudy group 23 children (23 per cent) showed some impairment of oral motor function (Table 5.XLV). Most of these were in the Speech Plus and Classic groups. The differences from the rest did not reach significance in the Speech Plus group (chi-square 2.38, df 2, p>0.2), but did so for the Classic group (chi-square 6.56, df 2, p<0.05).

Fine motor skills
The children were observed carrying out the finger-nose test, rapid tapping,

TABLE 5.XLV

Oral movements

Language subgroup	Normal (%)	Moderate impairment (%)	Severe impairment (%)	Total
Speech	8 (73)	1 (9)	2 (18)	11
Speech Plus	11 (65)	3 (18)	3 (18)	17
Classic	24 (68)	9 (26)	2 (6)	35
Semantic	14 (100)	0	0	14
Residual	5 (100)	0	0	5
Moderate	6 (86)	1 (14)	0	7
No Language	4 (67)	0	2 (33)	6
Young Unclassified	3 (100)	0	0	3
Severe	3 (100)	0	0	3
Neurostudy	78 (77)	14 (14)	9 (9)	101

TABLE 5.XLVI

Fine motor skills

Language subgroup	Normal (%)	Moderate impairment (%)	Severe impairment (%)	Total
Speech	8 (73)	2 (18)	1 (9)	11
Speech Plus	11 (65)	4 (24)	2 (12)	17
Classic	28 (80)	5 (14)	2 (6)	35
Semantic	13 (93)	1 (7)	0	14
Residual	5 (100)	0	0	5
Moderate	6 (86)	1 (14)	0	7
No Language	4 (67)	0	2 (23)	6
Young Unclassified	3 (100)	0	0	3
Severe	3 (100)	0	0	3
Neurostudy	81 (80)	13 (13)	7 (7)	101

TABLE 5.XLVII

Gross motor skills

Language subgroup	Normal (%)	Moderate impairment (%)	Severe impairment (%)	Total
Speech	7 (64)	2 (18)	2 (18)	11
Speech Plus	10 (59)	6 (35)	1 (6)	17
Classic	21 (60)	8 (23)	6 (17)	35
Semantic	12 (86)	1 (7)	1 (7)	14
Residual	5 (100)	0	0	5
Moderate	6 (86)	0	1 (14)	7
No Language	1 (17)	4 (67)	1 (17)	6
Young Unclassified	2 (67)	1 (33)	0	3
Severe	1 (33)	1 (33)	1 (33)	3
Neurostudy	65 (64)	23 (23)	13 (13)	101

TABLE 5.LVIII

Gross motor skills and age at independent walking

Age	Gross motor skills		Total
	Normal (%)	Impaired (%)	
Before 18 months	49 (69)	22 (31)	71
After 18 months	13 (45)	16 (55)	29
Total	62 (62)	38 (38)	100

Chi-square with Yates correction 4.13, df 1, p<0.05

TABLE 5.XLIX

Gross motor and fine motor skills

Fine motor skills	Gross motor skills		Total
	Normal (%)	Impaired (%)	
Normal	59 (73)	22 (27)	81
Impaired	4 (20)	16 (80)	20
Total	63 (62)	38 (38)	101

Chi-square with Yates correction 16.90, df 1, p<0.001

tapping with alternating pronation and supination, piling cubes, threading beads, drawing and writing, and finger-thumb opposition test. Of the total children in the neurostudy group, 13 per cent were judged to show moderate and 7 per cent severe fine motor clumsiness for their age (Table 5.XLVI). The Speech Plus group contained relatively more children with fine motor clumsiness but the differences from the rest of the neurostudy children were not significant (chi-square 3.10, df 2, p>0.2).

Gross motor skills
The children were observed walking, balancing and hopping on one leg, crouching and recovering, heel-toe walking along a straight line and kicking a ball. Only 64 per cent of the neurostudy group were considered to have normal gross motor co-ordination for their age, with 23 per cent showing moderate and 13 per cent severe clumsiness (Table 5.XLVII). Of the speech and language groups with more than 10 children, the Semantic group contained the least proportion of clumsy children but the differences did not reach significance when compared with the rest of the neurostudy children (chi-square 3.31, df 2, p>0.1). In the total neurostudy group gross motor clumsiness was significantly more common in the children who had been late walkers (Table 5.XLVIII) and in those with fine motor clumsiness (Table 5.XLIX).

201

TABLE 5.L

Constructional skills test related to age

Age (yrs)	Normal	Moderate impairment	Severe impairment
5½	>1	1	<1
6	>2	2	<2
6½	>3	3	<3
7	>4	4	<4
7½	>5	5	<5
8	>6	6	<6
8½ and over	>7	7	<7

TABLE 5.LI

Constructional skills

Language subgroup	Normal (%)	Moderate impairment (%)	Severe impairment (%)	Total
Speech	11 (100)	0	0	11
Speech Plus	14 (82)	2 (12)	1 (6)	17
Classic	26 (74)	4 (11)	5 (14)	35
Semantic	12 (86)	1 (7)	1 (7)	14
Residual	3 (60)	2 (40)	0	5
Moderate	7 (100)	0	0	7
No Language	3 (50)	3 (50)	0	6
Young Unclassified	3 (100)	0	0	3
Severe	1 (33)	1 (33)	1 (33)	3
Neurostudy	80 (79)	13 (13)	8 (8)	101

Constructional skills

The matchstick test was used (Rutter *et al.* 1970). Five patterns (triangle, diamond, open L shape, four-pointed star and open cross shape), preconstructed from matchsticks, were shown one by one to the child, who was asked to reproduce them using matchsticks taken from a pile in front of him. Each pattern was scored 0 for failure or poor attempt, 1 for nearly correct and 2 for correct, giving a maximum score of 10 for the test (Table 5.L).

In all, 13 per cent showed moderate and 8 per cent severe constructional difficulties (Table 5.LI). Of the speech and language groups with more than 10 children, the Classic group contained the highest proportion of children with constructional difficulties and the Speech group the least, but when compared with the rest of the neurostudy children the differences were not significant. Taking all the neurostudy children, constructional abilities were not significantly associated with fine motor skills (Table 5.LII).

Cerebral palsy

Five children were found to have cerebral palsy (Table 5.LIII). In the Speech group

TABLE 5.LII

TABLE 5.LII

Constructional skills and fine motor skills

Constructional skills	Fine motor skills		Total
	Normal (%)	Impaired (%)	
Normal	65 (81)	15 (19)	80
Impaired	16 (76)	5 (24)	21
Total	81 (80)	20 (20)	101

Chi-square with Yates correction 0.04, df 1, p>0.5

TABLE 5.LIII

Some neurological syndromes

Language subgroup	N	Cerebral palsy (%)	Supra-bulbar palsy (%)	Landau-Kleffner syndrome (%)
Speech	11	1 (9)	1 (9)	0
Speech Plus	17	2 (12)	2 (12)	0
Classic	35	3 (3)	1 (3)	0
Semantic	14	0	0	0
Residual	5	0	0	0
Moderate	7	0	0	0
No Language	6	1 (17)	2 (33)	3 (50)
Young Unclassified	3	0	0	0
Severe	3	0	0	0
Neurostudy	101	5 (5)	6 (6)	3 (3)

there was a girl with a mild spastic left leg. In the Speech Plus group there was a boy with a mild spastic quadriparesis and a boy with choreoathetosis following an encephalitic illness at 15 months of age. In the Classic group a boy had a mild right spastic hemiparesis. In the No Language group a boy had a severe left spastic hemiparesis.

Supra-bulbar palsy
This was diagnosed when severe dysarthria was accompanied by drooling, nasal escape, chewing and swallowing difficulties, good lip-spreading but poor lip pursing, a small stiff tongue with poor protrusion and an exaggerated jaw jerk (Worster-Drought 1974). Six children were found to have supra-bulbar palsy (Table 5.LIII), one of which was in the Speech group, two in the Speech Plus group, one in the Classic group and two in the No Language group. Four of these children also had cerebral palsy, but the other two had isolated congenital supra-bulbar palsy.

TABLE 5.LIV

Chromosome studies

Language subgroup	N	Tested	Abnormal
Speech	11	4	0
Speech Plus	17	1	0
Classic	35	8	0
Semantic	14	2	1
Residual	5	1	0
Moderate	7	0	0
No Language	6	1	0
Young Unclassified	3	0	0
Severe	3	3	2
Neurostudy	101	20	3

Landau-Kleffner syndrome

This condition (Beaumanoir 1985) was diagnosed in three children who had shown initial normal speech and language development followed by severe regression coinciding with the onset of epileptic seizures in two of the children. EEG recordings in all three had shown epileptic discharges mainly in the temporal regions. Fits had not been difficult to control with anticonvulsant drugs but the acquired dysphasia was severe and permanent in all three children. Not surprisingly all three children were in the No Language group (Table 5.LIII).

Chromosome studies

It had been intended to carry out chomosome studies on all the children but in the event this proved difficult. Of the 20 children who had chromosome studies done, three (15 per cent) proved to be abnormal (Table 5.LIV). In the Semantic group a boy had an extra Y chromosome (47xYY). In the severe group one boy was mosaic with an extra x chromosome in one cell line and two extra x chromosomes in the other(47xxY, 48xxxY). Another boy in the severe group showed a fragile site on the long arm of chromosome 12 (46xY, fra 12q13).

Population studies on newborn babies have found a prevalence of chromosome abnormalities in the order of 0.05 per cent (Sergovich *et al.* 1969). A previous chromosome study of children attending a residential school for speech and language disorders in the south of England (Mutton and Lea 1980) found six of the 121 children (5 per cent) to have chromosome anomalies of which four affected the sex chromosomes. It appears therefore that anomalies of chromosomes—particularly of the sex chromosomes—may be causally associated with developmental speech and language disorders in a small but significant number of children.

Discussion and conclusions

Children with speech and language impairment admitted to Dawn House are carefully selected to exclude those with mental disability, primary psychiatric disorders and significant hearing loss. Nevertheless they represent a heterogeneous group with many associated problems. This study has shown that a number of problems occur more frequently than in the general childhood population. Gross motor clumsiness was present in 36 per cent, fine motor clumsiness in 20 per cent, impairment of left-right discrimination in 43 per cent, constructional difficulties in 21 per cent, poor oral motor skills in 23 per cent, ocular movement disorders in 11 per cent and cerebral palsy in 5 per cent.

The classification of speech and language disorders into nine groups raised the possibility that some of these associated features may occur more frequently in particular groups and so help to support their neurological identity. Analysis showed that ocular movement disorders and poor oral motor skills were significantly more common in the Classic group when compared with the remaining children. However no other significant group associations were demonstrated. The failure to show a greater number of significant associations could be due partly to the small numbers in some of the groups but may be more fundamental. Each of the speech and language disorder groups represents a particular kind of cerebral dysfunction. The associated disorders, such as gross motor clumsiness, represent other particular kinds of cerebral dysfunction which may only be associated with speech and language disorders in general rather than to one of the groups in particular.

Relationships were also explored between the different associated disorders in the neurostudy children. Positive relationships were found between gross motor skills and late walking and between fine motor skills and gross motor skills. These relationships were not really unexpected but lend some validity to the methods used. No relationship was found between constructional abilities and fine motor skills, suggesting that the tests used were looking at different functions.

6
READING

Some of the cognitive and linguistic correlates of reading are examined at two points in our subjects' lives, at entry to Dawn House and again at leaving. Reading has been evaluated by tests in which words or sentences are read, with the reading ages reflecting mechanical decoding skills. We also report our findings from a prose reading test which yields comprehension as well as accuracy reading ages.

The evaluation of reading skills in terms of reading ages can be misleading. It is all too easy to believe that the achievements of the SLI child with a reading age of seven years must be similar to those of a child with normal language development and the same reading age in a mainstream school: in other words to infer qualities from what is a highly selective quantitative measure. Perhaps it would be more realistic to think of the SLI reader as similar to the dyslexic child. That would be a little nearer the mark, especially if one thinks in terms of what was once known as the 'auditory dyslexic', the child whose written language problems are associated with a range of relatively minor oral language problems. But even someone with many years experience of examining and teaching dyslexic children can be quite unprepared for the problems facing SLI children in learning to read. Every teacher who joins the school's staff and has responsibility for teaching literacy skills, no matter how experienced in normal and remedial teaching, finds new problems and challenges. It is not simply a matter of slow progress, although progress is usually slow enough. There are problems in the nature of the phonological, linguistic, and conceptual deficits, in their interactions and in the unevenness of development and progress, producing difficulties which vary from child to child. Reading sometimes appears to be easier for the child with no language, the receptive aphasic, whose language learning is intimately bound up with its visual form.

The teaching of reading, like all subjects, demands highly specialised skills based on a thorough understanding of language disorders and their effects. At present no special qualification is necessary for teaching SLI children. Teachers both want and need to be informed, but at present there are few suitable courses and little or no financial support for teachers to take a course. This must be remedied if all SLI children are to receive the education best suited to them.

Reading at entry
In Chapter 2 we showed that children's standards of reading were generally low or non-existent at school entry. However, 16 were reading at or above age level, and the gap between age and reading age ranged from −20 months (*i.e.* reading 20 months above age) to 67 months (reading 67 months below age) with the gaps expectedly increasing with age. Clearly, although most were retarded in reading,

TABLE 6.I

Correlations between reading age and IQ, ASTM, measures of speech and language at entry, controlling for age at reading test

	N	r
IQ		
Verbal	72	0.18
Performance	122	0.15
ASTM	135	0.28**
Comprehension		
Grammar	91	0.07
Vocabulary	136	0.015
Production of language		
Structure~	132	−0.199*
Story retelling	106	0.12
Vocabulary	135	0.24**
Morphology	105	0.28**
Articulation		
Development	143	0.14
Deviance~	142	−0.12
(CA	144	0.56***)

~Lower score = better performance
*p <0.05
**p <0.01
***p <0.001

some were more so than others. We look at some cognitive and language factors which may be significantly associated with reading levels and enquire which if any might predict reading ability at entry when the average reading age is 6½ years.

Relationships between reading and correlates
Controlling for chronological age, we calculated correlations between reading age and VIQ, PIQ, ASTM, each of the measures of comprehension, production of language and speech. It was intended to carry out similar exercises with reading ages achieved just before the children left the school, but the age ceiling for scaled scores on many measures was too low to derive these for most children about to leave; therefore in all analyses, at both points, we used raw scores on the tests of ASTM, expressive vocabulary, morphology and speech.

At entry, reading levels were significantly associated with ASTM and three aspects of language production: sentence structure, morphology and vocabulary. Speech development and deviance, significantly associated with reading when age is not taken into account, cease to be so when the coefficients are adjusted for age. An understanding of sentence structures and passive vocabulary does not correlate with reading, with or without age adjustment. The coefficients are effectively zero. The correlation with the VIQ is 0.18, and with the PIQ 0.15, both low and not significant (Table 6.I).

TABLE 6.II

Reading age at entry by LARSP stages (sentence structure), 132 children

Reading age	LARSP group		
	1	*2*	*3*
	N	*N*	*N*
Less than 6 yrs	4	2	18
6.0–6.5	3	16	21
6.6–7.5	22	13	10
7.6 or above	13	7	3

Chi-square 39.8, df 6, p. <0.0001

The effect of auditory discrimination on reading was also examined. Auditory discrimination was evaluated either by a test of auditory discrimination, the Wepman, or (for children unable to respond to this) the Renfew Picture Pointing test. Results were combined so that the 110 children with a marked problem were distinguished from the 27 children without (see Chapter 5). To evaluate the association between auditory discrimination problems and reading, we carried out an analysis of variance with age at testing as a covariate, but no significant main effect stemmed from auditory discrimination (F 0.442, NS).

Sentence structure and reading
The production of sentence structures, not the understanding, was significantly associated with reading age. This led to a closer look at the relationship between the levels reached in the construction of sentences and reading. The 132 children with both a LARSP score and a reading age were divided by reading age into four groups:
(1) reading age of 7½ years or above (23 subjects)
(2) reading age of 6½ to 7½ (45 subjects)
(3) reading age of six to 6½ (40 subjects), and
(4) reading age of less than six years (24 subjects)
  Children assigned to LARSP Group 1 are reasonably competent in constructing sentences, making minor structural and morphological errors; at Group 2 level the stage of clause connection has been reached, although some basic structural rules are still being acquired; Group 3, combining our original Groups 3 and 4 because of small numbers, includes children who are able to string words together in a simple but correct way, but who have limited ability to express themselves, and also those who are still at a basic and inadequate level of sentence structure. The calculation of chi-square revealed a highly significant association between the stage reached in the production of syntax and the level reached in reading (Table 6.II).

Stepwise regression of reading age at entry on cognitive and linguistic variables
There are strong intercorrelations between ASTM, sentence structure and vocabu-

lary. Which would emerge as predictors of early reading when subjected to regression analysis?

A major problem in carrying out any multivariate analysis stems from variations from test to test in the number of children for whom information is available. We included as many children and independent variables as possible in analyses, ensuring that those measures which correlated significantly with the dependent variable (reading) were entered. Despite such limitations, we considered it worthwhile to carry out what can only be regarded as exploratory exercises the results of which must be interpreted cautiously.

The greatest limitation on numbers is imposed by the relatively small number with a VIQ. Only 72 children had both a VIQ and a reading age. An examination of age at testing and reading age of children with and without a VIQ, however, revealed that those with a VIQ were on average 10 months older and reading more than five months ahead of those with no VIQ, both differences being statistically significant (Mann-Whitney U tests, $z = 3.9$, $p<0.001$ for age; $z = 2.56$, $p<0.01$ for reading age). The introduction of the VIQ into any equation would automatically select a biased subsample.

We particularly wished to include measures of comprehension, language production and speech. There were 95 children with scores on ASTM, comprehension (composite measure), passive vocabulary, sentence structure, spoken vocabulary, speech development and a PIQ. Stepwise regression analyses were carried out, with and without PIQ, to determine which variables best predicted reading age, with age at testing forced into the equation first. The PIQ did not enter the equation as a significant factor, and when forced into the regression equation with all other variables had a beta value of 0.009 indicating that it had virtually no effect on reading.

With age entered first, the only two significant predictors were productive vocabulary (accounting for 6.3 per cent of variance) and sentence structure production (3.1 per cent). The remaining variables (comprehension, passive vocabulary, phonological development, and ASTM), when forced into the final equation, altogether accounted for only a further 3.1 per cent of variance and raised the total variance accounted for from 28.4 per cent to 29.1 per cent. The most parsimonious model is based on the age, expressive vocabulary and sentence construction scores of 120 children. In the final stepwise regression model, age accounted for 23.1 per cent, expressive vocabulary 7.1 per cent and sentence structure 3.2 per cent with an adjusted total variance of 31.7 per cent.

The high degree of association between categories of expressive syntax (sentence structures) and ASTM are described and discussed in Chapter 5. When both are entered as independent variables in a regression analysis, it is the measure of sentence structure which emerges as the significant predictor. However, when LARSP (the measure of syntax) was omitted from the analysis, the two independent variables to emerge as the significant predictors of reading were expressive vocabulary (5.8 per cent of variance) and ASTM (3.1 per cent of variance). Thus whether ASTM accounted for a significant proportion of reading variance depended upon the presence or absence of the measure of syntax in the analysis.

Summary and discussion

The variables significantly associated with the early stages of reading in this language-disabled sample are ASTM and aspects of language *production* involving syntax, morphology and vocabulary. Notably failing to reach a significant level of association are both measures of intelligence (verbal and performance), the comprehension measures of grammar and vocabulary, and speech (development and deviance). The exploratory regression analyses support the predictive importance of both expressive vocabulary and levels of sentence structure and suggest that ASTM is also predictive, but not in the presence of sentence-structure measures.

How do these findings agree with current work on factors identified as important in the earliest stages of reading? Beginning to read is very much a process of learning to give the correct names to their printed counterparts, be these words or letter sounds. From the beginning, learning to read must be meaningful. Reading may be tested by asking children to read words, but learning progresses by working through books, the vocabulary and language of which are familiar. Children work from what is initially unknown—the printed form—to the known—their own language. Great effort is made to ensure that vocabulary, language and situational content are familiar to normal children entering school at five years. Young readers make considerable use of contextual cues. Biemiller (1970) suggests that an initial heavy dependence on linguistic context in first-grade children gives way to a greater use of information derived from printed letter/ word forms. Syntactic information appears to play a predominant role in the use of context in the early stages of reading (Murray and Maliphant 1982). An anticipatory strategy, using information from succeeding text, appears to be more helpful in guessing unknown words than looking at past text (Beardlsey 1982), although Potter (1982) found that poor readers were less able to make use of succeeding text.

What are the implications of such findings for SLI children in the early stages of reading? Only a tiny minority of our children function at age level on tests of passive and expressive vocabulary (see Chapter 2). Without an understanding of the meaning of words to be read, the exercise degenerates to the level of 'reading' nonsense words. Passive knowledge of vocabulary is obviously important. But early success in reading is measured by a child's ability to *produce* the word. Failure to do so may arise simply from a non-recognition of the printed form. But it may also be due to real gaps in the child's spoken vocabulary or to a difficulty in recalling the word. These are the aspects of vocabulary tapped by our measure of expressive vocabulary. The Renfrew Word-Finding Test differs from many vocabulary tests in that it requires a child to label a picture verbally, not to define a given word. A response which gives attributes of the picture but not its name is counted as an error, as is a wrong name and no response. The required response is similar to that which must be made to the printed form of a word when reading. Many of our children experience enormous difficulty right at the beginning in acquiring a simple sight vocabulary as illustrated by Hyde-Wright and Cheesman (1990) who described the case history of a child with extreme word-finding and auditory memory difficulties.

In using syntactic cues, children whose use of sentence structure has developed normally, are likely to provide an appropriate class of word for an unknown one. Even if the guessed word is incorrect, the sentence is still likely to make some kind of sense. These cues are minimally available to SLI children who may not in their own spontaneous conversation make use of 'a' or 'the', and may ignore tense markers and auxiliaries like 'is', 'was', 'can' and 'do', if verbs are included at all. Their use of prepositions is very limited, and their simple sentences usually follow a pattern of subject, verb and object. Textual syntactic information may not only fail to be helpful: it may be downright confusing and semantically bewildering when sentences, so beloved of infant primers, begin with a prepositional phrase and invert subject-verb order, *e.g.* 'Out of the box jumped Tom'. A real problem for teachers of SLI children is finding readers whose syntactic structures assist in the development of both oral and reading language, the need for which led to the creation of the Language Through Reading series (I CAN 1987).

No reference has been made to an important set of cues which normal children begin to use quite early in the process of learning to read, namely phonological cues which stem from a child's recognition that words and syllables can be broken down into phonetic units which correspond to individual letters and strings of letters like *th, ch, ai*. Such cues are fundamental to the reading and spelling of languages whose written form is alphabetically based. An explicit phonological awareness, the conscious realisation that words can be decomposed into discrete sounds (phonemes) has been shown to be strongly associated with good early reading by Bradley and Bryant (1983, 1985), who also demonstrated the predictive power of the implicit phonological awareness which preschool children reveal in their play with rhymes and nonsense words.

We have no data on phonological awareness as such. Certainly in the junior department of Dawn House very few children engage in any kind of word play. Producing a single rhyming couplet, even when the rhyming word of the first line is emphasised, is beyond most. An indication of the difficulty some of our SLI children have in forming internal phonological patterns was demonstrated by Haynes (1982) in her vocabulary learning experiment reported in Chapter 7. This is an area for further investigation. It would be very useful to know when children begin to develop an implicit and explicit awareness of the phonological structure of words and relate this to the development of reading.

Reading prior to leaving
The general picture of reading at entry is not a bright one. Even in mainstream

school populations, retarded readers usually continue that way, with the gap between reading and chronological ages tending to widen rather than to narrow (Morris 1966, Hutchison *et al.* 1979, Share and Silva 1986). All studies of SLI children which have examined reading levels at follow-up have demonstrated long-term persisting educational problems, especially affecting reading and writing (Aram *et al.* 1984, Weiner 1985).

Final decisions about leaving lie not with the school but with the sponsoring local education authority in conjunction with parents. Decisions are often influenced by recommendations made by the school. Since the primary reason for admission to the school is the presence of a specific language impairment, it is the state of that impairment, not the presence or otherwise of reading problems, which is the primary consideration when discharge is discussed. If standards of speech and oral language are such that they no longer require the school's intensive therapy, persisting reading and writing difficulties are only occasionally sufficient cause for extending the special school placement. Levels of written language, and also numeracy, commonly lagged far behind age level when a child left. Local education authorities provide tuition for children with reading and writing problems, although facilities vary enormously in quality and quantity from area to area. Local remedial services are responsible for giving the skilled intensive help still required by most children returning to mainstream schools. We were well aware of the severe educational problems most children would experience after leaving.

A few of the 118 leavers did reach a level commensurate with age, and certainly some made better progress than others. This section looks at reading levels prior to leaving Dawn House, and examines those factors of speech, language, cognitive ability and auditory processing functions which appear to have a bearing upon final reading standards. Finally we look back to reading and its correlates at entry to enquire which, if any, predict reading levels on leaving.

Final reading ages
The Southgate Group Reading Tests 1 and 2 and Schonell's Graded Word Reading Test (see Chapter 2) continued to be used, but in the case of 11 children the reading accuracy age of the Neale Analysis of Reading Ability (Neale 1966) has been used. A further five were given the Word Reading Test of the British Ability Scales (Elliott *et al.* 1983).

With a mean age of 11½ years, the mean reading age of the 118 leavers was 8½ years. Reading ages were generally low. The basic mechanics of the reading process have usually been acquired when a reading age of about nine years is reached. Of the 106 leavers aged at least nine years, only 27 (23 per cent) had reached that level of reading or above. Only five children were reading at or above age level, and a further nine had a reading age less than one year below.

The reading of all children improved during their stay at school but reading seldom kept pace with time. Most of our pupils experienced difficulty, often very severe, in learning to read. Changes in reading between entry and discharge are

TABLE 6.III

Difference between reading age and age at final test in 118 children

Difference between age and reading age	N	(%)
Reading at or above age	5	(4.2)
Less than 1 yr behind	9	(7.6)
1–2 yrs behind	16	(13.6)
2–3 yrs behind	20	(17)
3–4 yrs behind	28	(23.7)
Over 4 yrs behind	40	(33.9)
Total	118	
Mean age	11½ yrs	
Mean reading age	8½ yrs	
Mean difference	3 yrs	

TABLE 6.IV

Final reading age by subgroup

Language subgroup	N	Reading age Mean	SD
Speech	15	99	11
Speech Plus	16	99	15
Classic	37	101	13
Semantic	20	110	20
Residual	9	104	12
Moderate	11	106	17
No Language	5	96	14
Young Unclassified	2	*100, 105	
Severe	3	*85, 85 94	

*Individual scores

described in terms of the difference between age and reading age at each point in time, each child's reading age being subtracted from the age when tested. The severity of reading difficulty is reflected in the diminishing proportion of children reading less than two years behind age (Table 6.III). The large number with a gap of more than four years is partly an artefact of the greater age of leavers. Such gaps only become possible in children aged over nine years. Even if the rate of learning after admission accelerates well ahead of the rate of learning prior to entry, to close the gap is extremely difficult and well nigh impossible for most.

Final reading in subgroups

An analysis of final reading ages by subgroups (Kruskal-Wallis ANOVA) suggested that there was a significant difference between the subgroups ($p < 0.05$). However, mean chronological ages also differed: and although the correlation between reading age and age was low at discharge (r 0.27) an ANOVA of the six major groups was carried out, with age as a covariate entered first. With age adjusted for, there was no significant between-groups effect (Table 6.IV).

With the wide age range of the children, and their varying length of stay at the school, the reading age is limited in its ability to indicate how well or otherwise the children functioned in reading. Chapter 7 examines outcome, reading being one of the variables on which outcome is evaluated. Children were classified into those with good, fair and poor reading outcome (terms which are relative to our sample only), using criteria relating to age, reading age and the difference between age and reading age. There were 22 children with a good reading outcome (a reading age of 10 years or above or a difference of less than a year between age and reading age). Of these, seven belonged to the Moderate or Residual groups, and a further four to the Speech group, making a total of 11 out of 35 children with minor language problems. By comparison, only 11 out of 83 children with severe language

213

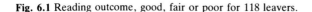

Fig. 6.1 Reading outcome, good, fair or poor for 118 leavers.

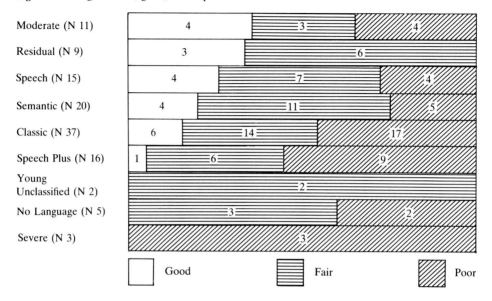

Moderate (N 11)

Residual (N 9)

Speech (N 15)

Semantic (N 20)

Classic (N 37)

Speech Plus (N 16)

Young
Unclassified (N 2)

No Language (N 5)

Severe (N 3)

Good   Fair   Poor

TABLE 6.V

Correlations between final reading age and concurrent IQ, ASTM, auditory discrimination, and measures of speech and language, controlling for age at final reading test

	N	r
IQ		
Verbal	118	0.34***
Performance	118	0.19*
ASTM	105	0.11
Auditory discrimination~	97	−0.19
Comprehension		
Grammar	93	−0.03
Vocabulary	93	0.39***
Production of language		
Story retelling	64	0.22
Vocabulary	94	0.35**
Morphology	96	0.49***
Speech		
Development	118	0.20*
Deviance~	118	−0.05
(Age	118	0.27**)

~Lower score = better performance
*p <0.05
**p <0.01
***p <0.001
(two-tailed)

impairment met the good outcome criteria. Forty-four children were deemed to have a poor outcome (with a reading age below 7½ years and a difference between age and reading age of 2½ years if aged 10 or under, or otherwise a difference of more than four years). The distribution of categories of reading outcome are detailed in Figure 6.1. The three groups whose language is the most normal—Speech, Moderate and Residual—were combined and compared with the remainder having serious language impairments. A significantly greater number of the former had a good reading outcome while fewer had a poor outcome (chi-square 7.172, df 2, p <0.05).

The greatest proportions of children whose reading was very poor by any standard are to be found among the Severe, the Speech Plus and the Classic, the last two groups including children with severe expressive and speech impairments. Although there is no good outcome among the No Language, only two of the five are poor. This may owe something to language itself being taught and learned, particularly in the early stages, through the media of a manual signing system, Paget-Gorman Signed Speech, and the written form. But it has also been observed in the classroom that once the written form has been learned by children in this group, it tends to be secure, unlike in children with expressive problems who so often forget.

Reading age at leaving and concurrent correlates
Sentence structure production, a significant predictor of reading at entry, could not be used in analyses with final reading scores. Improvement in use of syntax had the effect of drastically narrowing the range of scores, with almost 90 per cent of leavers for whom a LARSP result was available functioning in the top category of the scale.

Table 6.V shows correlations between reading ages at leaving and IQ (verbal and performance), auditory discrimination, ASTM, and measures of comprehension, language production and speech, with age at the final testing of reading partialled out. The variables now most significantly associated with reading, on average three years after entry, were primarily the VIQ and *passive* vocabulary and morphology. Expressive vocabulary continued to be significantly correlated. Additionally, coefficients with PIQ and speech development reached a 5 per cent level of significance. Age was associated with reading age as would be expected, but the value of the correlation fell from 0.56 at entry to 0.27 at discharge.

With a mean reading age of 8½ years, ASTM was not significantly associated with reading as it had been at entry. The strong association with the VIQ may be due at least partly to the fact that this measure had been obtained for all children by the time they left, compared with less than one half at entry. There were also strong correlations between VIQ and many other measures, notably PIQ, passive vocabulary, productive vocabulary, morphology and speech development. Whether or not the IQ (verbal or performance) significantly predicts reading in the presence of data on the speech and language measures, will be influenced by the degree of covariance between them.

215

Stepwise regression analyses of final reading
In all analyses, age has been entered first. We carried out an initial stepwise regression analysis of reading on VIQ, PIQ, ASTM, auditory discrimination, passive vocabulary, morphology, productive vocabulary and speech development. The only two significant predictors were passive vocabulary (accounting for 21.3 per cent of variance) and morphology (7.9 per cent, making a total of 34.8 per cent). The remaining independent variables, when forced into the equation together, accounted for a non-significant 1.5 per cent of variance.

The most parsimonious model of reading on its correlates was that of reading on age, passive vocabulary and morphology, one which included 79 children, mean age 11.9, mean reading age 8.9. After age had accounted for 7.7 per cent of variance, passive vocabulary and morphology accounted for 23.3 per cent and 7.6 per cent respectively with a total adjusted variance of 36.3 per cent.

A surprising result of the regression analyses was the failure of either verbal or performance IQ, particularly the former, to enter the equations as significant predictors of reading when accompanied by all linguistic measures. In the case of the VIQ, this seems due to its covariance with passive vocabulary. If vocabulary scores were excluded, the VIQ accounted for 12 per cent of variance and articulation now emerged to account for 4.8 per cent, but the total accounted variance, with age, is only 18.4 per cent. In the presence of passive vocabulary, VIQ fails to reach the 0.05 significance limit for entry. In no model was the PIQ a predictor of reading at discharge.

Summary
Correlating strongly with reading ages at discharge (mean 8.6) were VIQ, passive and expressive vocabulary and morphology. Also significantly correlated, but less strongly, were PIQ and articulation. The measures now most strongly associated with reading were those of comprehension as well as expression, whereas at entry the significant variables had been limited to aspects of productive language.

Articulation, not previously a significant correlate, now entered the picture. Articulation scores reflected the speech problems of children with an articulatory impairment and also, perhaps less satisfactorily, the speech of those with a phonological impairment: *i.e.* children defective in their ability to derive and apply the systemic rules which determine speech sound qualities.

All the children at this stage of reading are grappling, with varying degrees of success, with the letter-sound correspondences from which written language is constructed. Articulation cannot be equated with the phonological awareness identified as an important predictor of reading, but final articulation scores follow years of intensive therapy which included work on the sound structure of words as well as on language, and it would be surprising if increasing phonological awareness did not result.

Prior to discharge, the most consistent predictors of reading to emerge from the exploratory stepwise regression analyses are passive vocabulary and mor-

TABLE 6.VI

Correlations between final reading age and measures at entry adjusted for age at entry

	N	r
IQ		
Verbal	63	0.22
Performance	97	0.20*
ASTM	110	0.23*
Comprehension		
Grammar	70	−0.07
Vocabulary	111	0.05
Production of language		
Structure~	108	−0.16
Story retelling	83	0.04
Vocabulary	108	0.19*
Morphology	89	0.02
Speech		
Development	118	0.13
Deviance~	115	−0.05
Reading age at entry	113	0.41***

~Lower score = better performance
*$p < 0.05$
***$p < 0.001$

phology, with VIQ and articulation emerging only when passive vocabulary is omitted. There are similarities between these findings and those resulting from the test of reading accuracy and reading comprehension reported below. Both sets of results are discussed together.

Final reading age and entry measures

Were any cognitive, speech and language entry measures predictive of reading age at discharge?

As a preliminary to possible further analyses, correlations were calculated, partialling out age, between final reading ages and initial IQ, ASTM, auditory discrimination, comprehension of grammar and vocabulary, the production of sentence structures, vocabulary, story retelling and morphology, and speech, development and deviance and reading at entry. Apart from reading age at entry, only three factors were significantly correlated with final reading ages: PIQ, ASTM and expressive vocabulary, all only at the 5 per cent level of significance. Correlation coefficients with VIQ and sentence structure reached the 10 per cent level of significance (Table 6.VI).

We carried out a stepwise regression analysis of final reading age on the three significant correlates, PIQ, ASTM and expressive vocabulary. With only 88 subjects, expressive vocabulary emerged as the only significant predictor after adjusting for

TABLE 6.VII

Reading accuracy and comprehension ages and differences between them, 91 children aged 7.4 to 13.10, mean 10.9

Comprehension equal to or ahead of accuracy	N	%
24 mths or more	1	1.1
12–23 mths	5	5.5
6–11 mths	10	11.0
0–5 mths	25	27.5
Total	41	

Accuracy ahead of comprehension		
1–5 mths	21	23.0
6–11 mths	14	15.4
12–23 mths	11	12.1
24 mths or more	4	4.4
Total	50	

Reading accuracy mean 8.3 yrs, with a standard deviation of 11.7 mths
Reading comprehension mean 8.1 yrs, with a standard deviation of 13.3 mths
Correlation between reading accuracy and reading comprehension 0.70

age, and accounted for 4.2 per cent of variance. To evaluate the effect of memory without confounding PIQ covariance effects, PIQ was dropped. Numbers rose to 108. After adjusting for age, auditory memory accounted for 4.1 per cent of variance while expressive vocabulary failed to enter the regression equation. No firm conclusions can be drawn, but the results of the regression analyses suggest that ASTM and/or expressive vocabulary at entry may be predictors of levels of reading at discharge.

The highest correlation coefficient stems from final reading age and reading age at entry, echoing the results of a longitudinal study of early reading by Ellis and Large (1988). In an indirect way, those factors which best predict reading at entry may be expected to influence reading levels at discharge. These were expressive vocabulary and, almost interchangeably, sentence structure and ASTM. The exploratory regression analyses lend some support to the importance of expressive vocabulary and ASTM at entry, for levels reached in reading some years later.

Reading comprehension

So far, we have been reporting on the more mechanical aspects of reading, involving the ability to transform the printed form into words. But the primary purpose of reading is to access the information conveyed by the text. Those children who had achieved sufficient reading ability to be undaunted by being presented with a 'story' were given the Neale Analysis of Reading Ability by the school's psychologist during reviews of general progress. The results of the last test were recorded.

The Neale test consists of six prose passages, graded in interest and difficulty, for children aged between six and 13. After reading each passage aloud, the child is asked questions. These should be answered without reference to the text. The passage must not only be understood but must also be remembered. Three reading ages are derived, for accuracy, comprehension and rate of reading, the last rarely calculated for our subjects.

We report upon the reading accuracy and comprehension ages of 91 children, aged from 7.4 to 13.10 (mean 10.9), whose mean reading accuracy age was 8.3 years, with a standard deviation of 11.7 months, and whose mean reading comprehension age was 8.1 years with a standard deviation of 13.3 months.

First, we look at the difference between reading accuracy and comprehension ages, with particular attention to children with extreme differences (*i.e.* those whose reading accuracy is well in advance of comprehension) and those whose reading comprehension is well in advance of accuracy, and ask whether these are associated with different profiles of speech and language impairment.

Second, we ask whether similar or different cognitive and linguistic factors are associated with prose reading accuracy, as distinct from previous predominantly word-reading situations, and with reading comprehension.

Differences between accuracy and comprehension reading ages (Table 6.VII)
Half of the children (46 out of 91) had reading accuracy and comprehension ages which were within six months of each other, indicating that the mechanical aspects of reading and comprehension were more or less on a par with each other. The remaining 45 children were not evenly distributed between those with an accuracy advantage and a comprehension one. For the majority (29 of the 45) reading comprehension lagged behind their decoding skills. The imbalance was most marked at the extremes of difference, 24 months or more. The advantage lay with comprehension in only one case, compared with four whose accuracy was similarly ahead. Of the latter four, the reading accuracy and comprehension ages of three were considerably below age level. The remaining child's accuracy age was 15 months ahead of age, with comprehension 11 months below age. He was the only child in the sample who could be called 'hyperlexic'. The only child whose reading comprehension was far ahead of accuracy was comprehending appropriately for age, revealing a specific impairment of decoding skills.

An inspection of the language subgroup membership of the five children with extreme differences suggested that different profiles of speech and language impairment might be associated with large differences between accuracy and comprehension attainment. Three of the four with very poor comprehension relative to accuracy belonged to the Semantic subgroup, the fourth entering school as a No Language child. All had severe oral comprehension problems at entry. By contrast, the child with high reading comprehension had severe expressive and

TABLE 6.VIII

Grades on composite measures of comprehension, expression and articulation at entry, of 21 children with a difference of 12 mths or more between reading accuracy and comprehension ages

Language and speech	Accuracy > comprehension N	Comprehension > accuracy N
Comprehension		
Near normal	1	6
Moderate or severe	14	0
	p <0.001	
Expression		
Near normal	2	2
Moderate or severe	13	4
	NS	
Articulation		
Near normal	5	0
Moderate or severe	10	6
	NS	

Fisher exact probability tests, one-tailed

articulation impairments but near normal oral comprehension at entry.

The subgroup membership of the 21 children with a difference of 12 months or more between accuracy and comprehension was examined. Of the six with higher comprehension than accuracy, two belonged to the pure Speech, two to the Speech Plus, and two to the Classic subgroups. Of the 15 with accuracy higher than comprehension, one belonged to the pure Speech, one to the Speech Plus, six to the Classic, six to the Semantic and one to No Language groups. No child with a primary oral comprehension problem at entry was among those whose comprehension of reading was one year or more above accuracy.

Children had been assigned to one of nine subgroups on the basis of profiles of composite measures of oral comprehension, production of language and speech, each of which was graded near normal or with minor problems only, moderate difficulty and severe difficulty. The grades on oral comprehension, expression and articulation for the 15 children with an accuracy advantage and the six children with a similar degree of comprehension advantage are shown in Table 6.VIII. Levels of oral comprehension but not articulation or expression at entry, are, at a later time, significantly associated with the direction of the accuracy/comprehension discrepancy (Fisher's exact probability tests, one-tailed). Related to comprehension which is high relative to accuracy, is a combination of near normal oral comprehension and severe articulation problems at entry. Conversely, it is the child whose comprehension of oral language at entry is his primary problem whose reading comprehension later lags far behind the ability to cope with the decoding aspects of reading.

TABLE 6.IX

Correlations between reading accuracy and comprehension ages and
IQ, ASTM, auditory discrimination, and measures of speech and
language, controlling for age at reading test

	N	r(a)	r(c)
IQ			
Verbal	87	0.38***	0.54***
Performance	91	−0.09	0.08
ASTM	90	0.36***	0.32**
Auditory discrimination~	87	−0.05	−0.02
Comprehension			
Grammar	78	−0.01	0.21
Vocabulary	90	0.29**	0.39***
Production of language			
Structure~	87	−0.18	−0.30**
Story retelling	80	0.09	0.33**
Vocabulary	89	0.24*	0.41***
Morphology	90	0.26*	0.27**
Speech			
Development	90	0.21*	−0.13
Deviance~	89	−0.16	−0.07
(Age	91	0.44***	0.40***)

~Lower score = better performance
r(a) correlation with reading accuracy
r(c) correlation with reading comprehension
*p <0.05
**p <0.01
***p <0.001

Predictors of reading accuracy and comprehension
Would similar cognitive and language variables be associated with accuracy and comprehension?

Most of the children whose Neale reading ages were examined, were approaching discharge. Data relating to their performance at discharge have been used when calculating correlations, and in analyses based on correlations. For the remainder, interim or entry records have been used as appropriate and available.

Correlations between reading accuracy and comprehension, and cognitive, speech and language factors, adjusted for age, revealed that both were significantly associated with VIQ, ASTM and passive vocabulary (Table 6.IX). Both correlated with productive vocabulary and morphology but only at the 5 per cent level for accuracy. Only reading comprehension was strongly associated with sentence structure and story retelling, and only accuracy with speech. The understanding of grammatic structures (TROG), the only linguistic variable not significantly associated with reading comprehension, just failed to reach significance (p = 0.055). Neither accuracy nor comprehension correlated with PIQ, auditory discrimination or deviant patterns of speech.

221

TABLE 6.X

Stepwise regression analyses of reading accuracy and comprehension on speech and language measures, adjusted for age at reading test

Dependent variable	Predictors	Total % variance	Variance increase
Reading accuracy (N 83)	Age*	15.1	
	Auditory memory	24.8	9.7
	Passive vocabulary	31.4	6.6
	Speech development	37.1	5.7
Reading comprehension (N 76)	Age*	14.8	
	Passive vocabulary	29.1	14.2
	Story retelling	35.2	6.1

*Age forced into equation first

Correlations between VIQ and ASTM, passive vocabulary, story retelling and expressive vocabulary ranged from 0.42 to 0.52, and would affect results of regression analyses which included all of these as independent variables. In this sample of SLI children, the VIQ appeared to present as a non-specific measure of language and we particularly wished to examine the predictive effects of individual linguistic variables. Stepwise regression analyses have therefore been carried out for each reading measure without the VIQ, age being forcibly entered first. The inclusion of story retelling scores in the comprehension regression analyses accounts for the smaller number when reading comprehension is the dependent variable.

READING ACCURACY

ASTM emerges as the strongest predictor, accounting for 9.7 per cent of variance, while passive vocabulary and articulation continue to be significant predictors of reading accuracy (Table 6.X). With age, these three factors account for 37.1 per cent of variance and a multiple correlation of 0.63. With all variables forced into the equation, ASTM, passive vocabulary and articulation are still the only significant predictors.

READING COMPREHENSION

Passive vocabulary accounts for 14.2 per cent of variance, and story retelling 6.1 per cent. The total percentage of variance is 35.2, and the multiple correlation 0.59. With all variables forcibly entered, only passive vocabulary is significant.

With the regression equations including only language, speech and auditory memory measures, passive vocabulary was a significant predictor of both reading accuracy and comprehension. Additionally, ASTM and articulation were predictors of accuracy, and story retelling a predictor of reading comprehension.

Summary and discussion

1. *Differences between reading accuracy and comprehension*

Ninety-one children had been given the Neale Test of Reading Ability, their mean reading comprehension age (8.1) being only two months lower than the mean accuracy age (8.3). While 50 per cent gave evidence of no difference greater than six months, the remainder included almost twice as many whose reading comprehension was poorer than accuracy. Bishop and Adams (1990) also used the Neale test, in their longitudinal study of children with preschool language delay. Among those whose language problems had persisted after 5½ years they found that reading comprehension was low relative to accuracy, and was associated with generally low levels of language understanding. In that study, however, the reading accuracy of the language-delayed did not differ from that of a control group, after allowance was made for non-verbal ability. In this report, where both reading accuracy and reading comprehension were very poor, the language impairments of our subjects were much more severe than that experienced by the subjects studied by Bishop and Adams (1990).

There was a clear difference between the speech and language profiles of those children with differences of a year or more between the two aspects of reading. Very poor comprehension relative to accuracy was associated with moderate or severe oral comprehension deficits on entry. A specific accuracy deficit was related to good initial oral comprehension. Levels of expression and articulation were not significantly associated with extremes of discrepancy. The identification of children at the extremes of the accuracy/comprehension gap, irrespective of absolute levels of reading, is important for classroom management because their needs are different. It is too easy and tempting to allow the child who is mastering the letter/sound coding system and who 'reads' fluently, often with good intonation, but whose reading comprehension is poor, to proceed to more difficult readers with more complex language, concepts and plots. What is needed, at the expense of appearing to slow down progress, is to ensure that comprehension and mechanical skills keep pace with each other. On the other hand, for the child whose reading comprehension is well ahead of mechanical skills, one must try to discover the reasons for poor decoding and to work on these: in addition to the integrated approach to reading which normally occurs.

2. *Predicting accuracy and comprehension*
ACCURACY

With two exceptions, the variables which correlated significantly with reading accuracy were similar to those with reading at discharge. They included VIQ, passive vocabulary, expressive vocabulary, morphology and articulation. ASTM was strongly related to accuracy and PIQ more weakly related to reading at discharge. The samples in these analyses were not identical, not all children with Neale data being leavers, but reading ages were comparable, ranging largely from 7½ to 9½ years. The tests were different: final reading ages were derived largely from word or sentence reading tests, Southgate 1 or 2, and the reading accuracy ages came from the reading aloud of prose passages. ASTM is associated with the latter. Despite differences in samples and tests, the speech and language measures associated with reading around the 8½-year level are vocabulary, both passive and expressive, morphology, knowledge of word inflection and articulation, with ASTM specifically associated with prose reading.

Reading comprehension shares the same group of correlates as reading accuracy, with the exception of articulation and with the addition of sentence structure and story retelling.

In carrying out exploratory regression analyses, we have taken the view that VIQ, which is strongly related to so many language measures, is itself a non-specific measure of language. Its introduction into regression analyses confuses rather than clarifies the contribution of discrete aspects of language. As the first variable to enter a stepwise regression, it usurps the effect common to it and subsequently entered variables. This applies particularly to vocabulary, the acquisition of which is so difficult for the SLI child, and which must be regarded as a major specific deficit.

The predictive value of ASTM for reading accuracy but not reading comprehension may seem surprising in view of the fact that questions have to be answered without reference to the text but from memory. On several occasions, after giving the Neale test and recording the results, children with very poor relative reading comprehension were questioned again and allowed to refer to the text if they wished. Any gain in comprehension was invariably very slight. Oakhill (1984), in her study of seven- and eight-year-old children, found that poor comprehenders in a similar reading task did not improve their performance when allowed to refer to the text. We saw above that very poor relative reading comprehension was associated with poor oral language comprehension at entry and it would indeed appear to be the lack of language understanding, not memory, which is the important factor.

The role of ASTM in accuracy may be through an articulatory loop, thought to be a component of ASTM, which serves as a working storage system in decoding unfamiliar words, allowing the reader to hold sounds in mind as they are deciphered and blended into the whole word (Baddeley 1978). Poor performance on tasks of auditory memory by children with severe specific reading difficulties has been demonstrated often (Naidoo 1972, Vellutino 1979, Ellis 1981, Ellis and Large 1988), but we still do not know its precise role and whether it operates independently. In this sample of SLI children it correlates significantly with reading at all points. It also correlates highly with sentence structure and expressive vocabulary, aspects of *expressive* language. Relationships between these need to be teased out before their individual contribution to reading can be determined.

We find that reading is associated with different aspects of language at different times, appearing to reflect different stages in the acquisition of reading skills. Ellis and his colleagues (Ellis and Large 1988, Ellis 1989), in a longitudinal study of normal five- to seven-year-old children, not only identified correlates of reading at each of four stages, but tracked the dynamic interactions between them and reading in a way that enabled them to discern which factors contributed to reading at a particular stage and which benefited from earlier stages of reading. Reading and many of its significant correlates progress in a mutually beneficial manner. Thus ASTM and phonological awareness are among correlates which benefit from reading at the second stage, and in turn these factors contribute, among others, to reading at the third stage. If this is indeed the way reading skills develop, there seems to be no reason why similar principles should not apply to the reading acquisition of SLI children. If skills essential at the beginning of reading are deficient, reading from the beginning will not proceed as it should. Non-existent or distorted early reading then affects the development of factors which in turn are necessary for further reading progress. Something of a vicious circle is set up.

The severe reading problems of the SLI child are an intrinsic part of the pattern of speech and language deficits. Language learning does not proceed rapidly, nor does the acquisition of reading. The normal child begins to read upon a solid foundation of oral language. In expecting the SLI child to begin to read before s/he has the necessary linguistic skills, are we expecting the impossible? And when we recognise the language deficits, how best may the printed form be used to advance both oral language and reading? Together with a manual sign system, the printed word is a major vehicle for the teaching and learning of language for children with severe receptive language impairment, and a scheme for learning language through reading has already been devised. But there is no single easy way to facilitate the learning of reading.

The problem is, as we have seen, not a short-term one. Children who ultimately join mainstream schools still experience serious written language difficulties and continue to require skilled help. It is essential that staff in a child's new school be fully aware of the nature and source of problems. This applies to all school subjects. A specific language impairment is pervasive and long-lasting in its effects, even when good progress has been made. Problems in fully understanding and correctly interpreting incoming verbal information, problems in retaining information and in expressively formulating language, affect learning in all parts of the school curriculum.

7
OUTCOMES

In this chapter we consider the changing picture of language impairment, by comparing the pattern of abilities and disabilities found in children at the end of their education at Dawn House with that found at entry. Final test results are presented in the three linguistic areas which were used to form our subgroups: comprehension, language production and speech. Each subgroup is briefly reviewed and the final language profiles described. We summarise the outcome for each child, using a conglomerate measure which includes language, speech and reading attainments, and re-examine our data for any early predictors of outcome in the antecedents, developmental factors, associates of SLI or entry language measures. Comparative outcome is discussed by subgroup. Finally we describe the further progress of 34 ex-pupils who have passed their 18th birthdays and are now part of the adult world.

Final language abilities
During the last 20 years there has been an increasing realisation by researchers that the effects of SLI are pervasive and very long-term. The implications of this knowledge have apparently not been absorbed by society, in the United Kingdom at least, where much of the provision for children with these disabilities is still limited to infant or preschool language units in which the emphasis is on short-term intensive help and a quick return to mainstream provision. One reason for this may be the changing pattern of impairment, so that when the very obvious difficulties with speech or syntax have improved, more subtle and less eradicable problems may be overlooked. Griffiths (1969) was one of the first to follow up children who had attended a special school for speech and language impairment for between six months and 3.9 years. Griffiths examined 49 children between one and seven years after leaving; she found that 70 per cent of them had speech and language within normal limits but that most of them had considerable educational problems, particularly with reading, and few had maintained the satisfactory progress they had been making in their special school. There was also some evidence of social maladjustment, especially among the children with language as opposed to speech disabilities. Similar results have been reported in subsequent studies. Hall and Tomblin (1978) compared outcome in 18 language-impaired and 18 articulation-impaired adolescents, between 13 and 20 years after they had first attended speech clinics. Half of the language-impaired (LI) and one of the articulation-impaired (AI) group reported continuing communication problems. The LI group had also had consistently more educational problems than their peers in the AI group. Aram *et al.* (1984) reported continuing problems with language and marked educational

TABLE 7.I

Leavers before and at Dawn House leaving age, and next school

Leaving age	Type of school or unit		
	Mainstream	Language	Other
Before 12 yrs	36	9	2
12 yrs and over	26	38	7
Total	62	47	9

difficulties in 20 adolescent subjects, some of whom fell into the subnormal intelligence range. This group also had high ratings on a scale of behaviour problems compared with the normal distribution.

A difference in outcome which relates to the degree that language rather than speech is involved was found in the study by King *et al.* (1982) of 50 adolescent subjects. They divided their subjects into five clinically described groups, quite similar to our own. These were No Speech, Language Disorder/Delayed Speech, Articulation, Language & Articulation, and Articulation & Fluency. The groups reporting the greatest continuing communication problems were No Speech and Language Disorder/Delayed Speech; the least problems were in the Articulation and Articulation & Fluency groups. All groups reported some educational problems, particularly with reading, but most problems were found in the two groups with the largest language component to their difficulties, the Language Disorder/Delayed Speech and Language & Articulation groups. Only four of the sample reported social and interpersonal relationship problems and these were all originally classified in the Language Disorder/Delayed Speech group.

Dawn House data

During the period of our study, the secondary department of Dawn House has opened to admit pupils aged 12 and over whose primary needs were still for intensive speech and language therapy and special education. Earlier, children had left Dawn House either as soon as they were able to benefit from mainstream education, or when a different type of special education seemed more appropriate, or when they reached the current Dawn House leaving age sometime during or just after their 13th birthday (Table 7.I). Twenty-two children included in this study remained at Dawn House in the secondary department after their 13th birthday, and these children have been included in the category of 'leavers proceeding to a further language school'. Four children who left Dawn House precipitately for family reasons, after only short periods as pupils, have not been included in the final picture since they did not meet any leaving readiness criteria. This leaves a total list of 118 'leavers' to consider.

Speech, language and educational progress at Dawn House are monitored by annual assessment, and social and emotional behaviour is commented on in regular reports from school and care staff. Problems of comparison at two points of time are caused both by the low ceilings of speech and language tests, making some tests used at entry unsuitable for older children, and by the continuing evolution of theories of SLI which mean that the aspects of language measured gradually change. When Dawn House opened in 1974, for example, there was a focus on language structure but very little interest in the pragmatic and interactional aspects of language impairment, which came to dominate the field in the 1980s.

Speech and language outcomes

Several of the tests used at entry are not useful with older children because of content which is inappropriate for older children, and low age ceilings. These include the Reynell Developmental Scales and the Renfrew tests. Those speech and language assessments which were used at school entry and are still found to be useful with 13-year-olds are the EPVT and BPVS vocabulary scales and TROG (for comprehension of language); LARSP and the grammatic closure subtest of the ITPA (for production of language); and the EAT (for speech)*.

Comprehension

VOCABULARY

The difficulties for SLI children acquiring vocabulary have been referred to earlier in the discussion of auditory short-term memory and phonological coding (Chapter 5). In a previous study of vocabulary acquisition (Haynes 1982), nine-year-old children from Dawn House were compared with age-matched and language-age-matched normal children for their ability to acquire new vocabulary. The children listened to short stories in which two finger-puppet spacemen had a series of adventures with fantastic animals and objects, each of which was shown to the children in picture form. After hearing the stories, the children were asked to recognise the new 'words', each of which they had heard twice, in a forced choice task where the distractor items had varying degrees of similarity to the target item. Not only did the Dawn House children make many more wrong choices than the two normal groups, but their errors were random while the normal children's errors had phonological similarities to the target words. After two-word exposures in an enjoyable and involving activity, the SLI children were not beginning to form any internal phonological pattern of the word which the normal groups had either learned or of which they had already learned some features.

This considerable difficulty in word acquisition is reflected in the final passive vocabulary tests of the children in the present study. Of the 112 leavers who had a final EPVT or BPVS test, 102 had also undertaken a test at entry. A standard score could be computed for 93 of them. These combined EPVT and BPVS results in SD bands were compared with the initial results of the same children (Table 7.II); they

---

*These assessments although designed for younger children are generally relevant for older SLI children, although standard scores for the ITPA and EAT cannot be computed.

TABLE 7.II

Passive vocabulary scores at final test compared with entry

Standard deviations	Final N (%)	Entry N (%)
+1 and over	0	2 (2)
0 to +1	4 (4)	11 (12)
−1 to 0	26 (28)	39 (42)
−2 to −1	46 (49)	36 (39)
Below −2	17 (18)	5 (5)
Total	93 (100)	93 (100)
Mean standard score	80	86

TABLE 7.III

Difference between vocabulary and chronological age at final test compared with entry

VA compared with CA	Final N (%)	Entry N (%)
Over 1 yr ahead	1 (1)	3 (3)
0–1 yr ahead	3 (3)	11 (11)
0–1 yr behind	9 (9)	23 (23)
1–2 yrs behind	9 (9)	36 (35)
2–3 yrs behind	22 (22)	22 (22)
3–4 yrs behind	27 (27)	6 (6)
Over 4 yrs behind	31 (30)	1 (1)
Total	102 (100)	102 (100)
Mean age	11.8	8.2
Mean vocabulary age	8.4	6.9

showed a deterioration relative to age, with 67 per cent of the 93 subjects now more than 1SD below the norm, compared with 44 per cent of the same children at entry. The vocabulary age of 102 leavers ranged from 4.9 to 13.2 (mean 8.4) when their chronological age range was 6.9 to 13.11 (mean 11.8). Any unremitting problem will naturally show increasing age gaps as children get older (Table 7.III). A further influence on vocabulary acquisition may be reading ability. It is assumed that children's vocabularies grow more rapidly in size and range as they begin to read for pleasure, a skill attained very late, if at all, by SLI children. A positive correlation (0.4) is found between final reading age and passive vocabulary age in this study.

Are there any early predictors of better or worse vocabulary development? Entry attainments in language, reading and IQ were correlated with final vocabulary standard score, partialling out age and length of stay. The cross-lagged correlation technique described by Clegg *et al.* (1977) was used to examine the relationship as it is considered to indicate the direction of causal relationships. In this technique the

TABLE 7.IV

Crossed-lagged correlations between passive vocabulary, verbal intelligence (VIQ), comprehension of grammar (TROG), and expressive vocabulary (RWF)

	Passive vocabulary Entry	Final	
Passive vocabulary			
Final	0.7**		
VIQ (N 19)			
Entry	0.5**	0.7**	
Final	0.5**	0.4*	(Entry VIQ affects final passive vocabulary)
TROG (N 53)			
Entry	0.3*	0.4**	
Final	0.1	0.2	(Entry TROG affects final passive vocabulary)
RWF (N 52)			
Entry	0.4**	0.4**	
Final	0.2	0.4**	(Entry RWF affects final passive vocabulary)

* $p < 0.05$
** $p < 0.01$
Arrow indicates most likely direction of causality

correlations of two variables at two points of time are permutated to give six correlation coefficients. If the correlation between variable x at time 1 and y at time 2 is larger than y at 1 and x at 2, the direction of causality can be considered to run from x to y (Table 7.IV). This technique suggests that poor early VIQ (and to a lesser extent poor early comprehension of grammar) may indicate a continuing problem with passive vocabulary, but that the best indicator is a low entry vocabulary score.

GRAMMAR

The interpretation and formulation of a rule-governed grammatical system of language provides a problem for almost all Dawn House entrants. Sixty to 70 per cent of children who come into school have problems in this area. It has been hypothesised that the difficulty in acquiring grammatical rules may relate to processing capacity (Menyuk and Looney 1972, Johnston 1985). Certainly language form (grammar) seems to be an area where specific therapy and teaching techniques which limit processing demands can bring about substantial improvement. During language therapy, when attention and involvement are controlled and when demands on memory, vocabulary and semantics are reduced as far as possible, SLI children are able to understand and internalise grammatical rules and gradually incorporate them into daily use.

The assessment of the comprehension of grammar is TROG. Sentences to be

TABLE 7.V

Comprehension of grammar at final assessment compared with entry

TROG Z-scores	Final N (%)	Entry N (%)
2+	1 (2)	0
1+ to 2+	1 (2)	0
0 to 1+	12 (28)	9 (21)
−1 to 0	20 (47)	16 (37)
−2 to −1	3 (7)	12 (28)
−3 to −2	6 (14)	4 (9)
below −3	0	2 (5)
Total	43 (100)	43 (100)
Mean Z-score	−0.27	−0.89
Mean age	12.0	9.3

decoded range from simple declaratives ('the boy is jumping') to complex embedded clauses ('the circle the star is in is red'). Scores have been transformed into z scores to enable comparisons with a normal population. TROG had not been produced when many of the leavers group first entered Dawn House, but a first and final result were available for 43 subjects and these are compared in Table 7.V.

Scores better than 1SD below the norm are considered within normal limits. At final assessment only nine children (21 per cent) fell below this level, compared with 18 children (43 per cent) at entry, demonstrating a reasonable level of catching-up on grammatical comprehension skills, although problems persisted for some children.

Of the entry measures of IQ, language, auditory memory and reading, only the initial TROG score correlated significantly with the final comprehension of grammar.

GENERAL COMPREHENSION EVALUATION

Comprehension was evaluated for all leavers using similar criteria to those used in evaluating oral comprehension for subgroup definition in Chapter 2. Evaluations were based on TROG (65 children), vocabulary tests (34 children), or staff reports (19 children) as follows:

High comprehension ability

TROG	Within 1SD from the norm or better
Vocabulary	Within 1SD from the norm or better
Reports	Excellent, very good, no problems

Medium ability

TROG	−1 to −2SD
Vocabulary	−1 to −2SD
Reports	Generally good, occasional problem

Low ability
        TROG   Below −2SD
        Vocabulary   Below −2SD
        Reports   Problems, often confused

In examining comprehension scores at school entry (see Chapter 3), we found poorer performance among those children with a non-British mother or with a foreign language spoken at home. We suggested that this was most likely a delay attributable to the increased learning load in a home with two cultures or two languages. In the final assessment these children had caught up on comprehension skills to a considerable extent. Three of them were in the high comprehension group of leavers, and the other five in the medium comprehension group.

Seventy-six children (64 per cent) in the high category had average comprehension levels, and would function reasonably well in the normal classroom. Thirty-two (27 per cent) in the medium group had some problems understanding. These children would be definitely disadvantaged in many situations as their comprehension difficulties might not be readily apparent. The 10 children (9 per cent) in the low-level category would be more severely hampered, but it is likely that their problems would be obvious, and that some additional help might be offered or that expectations would be more realistic.

Production of language
STRUCTURE
Unlike the TROG test of grammatical comprehension, the LARSP procedure analyses the spontaneous production of grammatical language by children, and records the maturity of clause and phrase structures which they select to express their meaning. It is not a test, and children cannot have a negative score, although errors in systems such as verb tense and pronouns may be noted at the sentence completion stage (Stage VI).

Of the leavers with LARSP analysis at entry, 101 also had a final analysis or had previously reached the level of competence (Stage VI or VII) at an interim test time. Language structure levels of these 101 children are shown in Table 7.VI.

Over 90 per cent of the children had achieved competence in grammatical production when they left Dawn House, and only two children—one dysarthric and one Landau-Kleffner aphasic—still had limited use of language structure. However, this does not mean that the leavers had total command of English grammar. Children may be competent and fluent language-users, but still produce some grammatical errors. Such errors are logged at Stage VI of the LARSP procedure. Of the 93 children who were finally judged to be competent, over half (54) were at Stage VI of LARSP and still had some fine points of the grammatical system to master. This stage, reached in normal development between the ages of 3.6 and 4.6, had been attained by SLI school-leavers aged between 7.0 and 13.11 (mean age 11.2).

TABLE 7.VI		
Production of grammatical structure at final assessment compared with entry		
LARSP levels	*Final*	*Entry*
Group 1. Competent	93	32
Group 2. Productive	6	24
Group 3. Limited	2	25
Group 4. Basic	0	20
Total	101	101

TABLE 7.VII		
Grammatic closure final age gaps compared with entry		
CA – Grammar age	*Final*	*Entry*
Under 1 year	10 (16%)	10 (16%)
1–2 yrs	8 (13%)	8 (13%)
2–3 yrs	9 (14%)	18 (28%)
Over 3 yrs	37 (58%)	28 (44%)
Total	64	64
Mean grammar age	8.1	6.9
Mean CA	11.2	8.7

None of the entry assessments of language, IQ or reading correlated significantly with the final LARSP level. Even the initial LARSP stage was not a valid index of future attainment.

MORPHOLOGY

The grammatic closure subtest of the ITPA assesses knowledge of the structural form of words (particularly inflections used to indicate changes of tense, number, person *etc.*) in regular and irregular forms. A child who has not mastered these aspects of grammar, and therefore fails many items in this test, would also be expected to present with Stage VI errors on the LARSP profile. There is a correlation of 0.3 (p = 0.002) between final LARSP and final grammatic closure results (83 subjects). An important difference between the two assessments is that whereas the LARSP procedure analyses the child's idiosyncratic choice of structure, the ITPA forces the child to make grammatical decisions, and therefore may reveal more difficulties. Because the ceiling age of the ITPA is 10½ years, very few scaled scores measuring performance against age norms can be produced. Results are recorded as equivalent grammatic closure ages, and the increasing gaps between such age levels and chronological age are shown in Table 7.VII. Many children have remaining difficulties with fine grammatical points at the time of leaving Dawn House. (Some typical examples of errors taken from record sheets are 'mouses', 'gooder', 'stoled', 'hisself'.)

When final grammatic closure scores were compared with language measures at entry, after partialling out age, correlations of 0.5 (p = 0.0001) were found with both expressive vocabulary and with the same grammatic closure test. There was a smaller correlation of 0.3 with reading age at entry (p = 0.005). The relationship between these three linguistic skills remained a strong one. Correlations between grammatic closure and both expressive vocabulary and reading had increased at final assessment to coefficients of 0.7 (p<0.0001) and 0.6 (p<0.0001) respectively. Cross-lagged correlations did not suggest any direction of causal relationships between the three abilities.

233

As with comprehension, scores from a number of assessments were used to provide each child with an evaluation of language production at school leaving. These final evaluations were derived as follows:

LARSP	Stage VII	High
	Stage V or VI	Moderate
	Stage IV and below	Low

Grammatic closure

	Above −1sd	High
	Equivalent age 10 or more (ceiling)	High
	Equivalent age 8.0 to 10.0	Moderate
	Equivalent age below 5.6	Low

Reynell expressive scale (for three children not able to undertake other assessments)

| | Five years below CA | Low |

The final 'high' category contained two children who had expressive scores above age level on the Reynell scale, Action Picture Test and Bus Story at entry, but no further expressive language tests.

Using these measures, 63 children in the 'high' productive category (53 per cent) were using normal language structures which are grammatically correct. Fifty children in the moderate category (42 per cent) were reasonably fluent language-users but their output was still characterised by errors. The five children (4 per cent) in the lowest group were inadequate language-users.

Speech

The full Dawn House phonological assessment performed on children's continuous speech at school entry is only repeated in its full form for children with deviant patterns affecting the whole of their output. Otherwise partial reassessments are made of those areas of the child's phonological system which are not developing normally. Since such partial reassessments are not statistically comparable, only the results of the picture-naming EAT are presented, compared with patterns at entry in Table 7.VIII.

FINAL SPEECH EVALUATION

For the final phonological evaluation, EAT scores of over 50 are counted as high, 34

TABLE 7.VIII

Articulation final scores compared with entry

EAT raw score	Final (%)	Entry (%)
Over 50	73 (62)	20 (17)
34–50	27 (23)	25 (21)
16–33	14 (12)	34 (29)
Below 16	4 (3)	39 (33)
Total	118 (100)	118 (100)

to 50 as medium, and below 34 as low (see rationale for cut-off points on p. 28).

The 73 children (62 per cent) in the high group would usually sound normal to the general public, although the practised ear would notice some immature sounding words, slowness or stumbling over polysyllabic words, in some of this group. These difficulties would be most noticeable—as with the normal population —if the child was also struggling to formulate ideas, or was stressed in some similar way. The speech problems of the 27 children (23 per cent) in the medium group would be noticeable and such children would generally be considered to have defective speech by the lay public. There would be occasional problems of intelligibility. The 18 children (15 per cent) in the low speech evaluation group would present frequent intelligibility problems at best and be mainly unintelligible at worst.

Summary of final language profiles

We have produced evaluations of language comprehension, production and speech which are based on objective measures, but which also relate to functional communicative competence. Around two-thirds of the children were functioning within normal limits for language comprehension and speech when they left Dawn House. Just over half were functioning adequately in terms of language production. These are very praiseworthy achievements for children whose early communication skills were so improverished, and for whom language acquisition is the result of conscious and persistent effort. However it means that a considerable number of this group of SLI children—between a third and a half of the school leavers—still had noticeable and disabling language problems when they moved on from Dawn House Junior School.

Subgroups

At the beginning of the study we used profiles of language abilities to define subgroups of language-impaired children. We now consider the over-all progress of each subgroup together with any changes in group profile.

GROUP 1. SPEECH

At school entry, this group contained 19 children with severe speech problems but

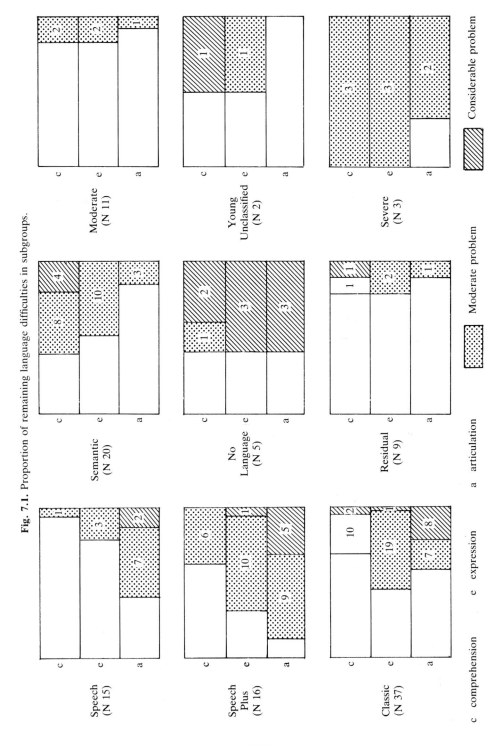

Fig. 7.1. Proportion of remaining language difficulties in subgroups.

c comprehension   e expression   a articulation

Considerable problem

Moderate problem

236

with only minor disabilities in the areas of receptive and expressive language. One child was severely dysarthric as a result of supra-bulbar palsy and one girl had a repaired cleft of the hard and soft palates and lip, but the other 17 children had no overt cause of their speech difficulties. None of the possible antecedent factors had a significantly raised incidence in this group of children. They were more likely to have a mild or moderate delay than a severely delayed language acquisition, and compared to the other subgroups they had higher verbal IQ and better ASTM. Of all the children in the study, this subgroup seemed to have the most discrete and least pervasive difficulties, although not necessarily the least severe (some remaining unable to communicate through speech).

Fifteen of these children were among our leavers. Their profile of difficulties at leaving is shown, together with those of the other subgroups, in Figure 7.1. From this it can be seen that they had largely overcome their difficulties with language, as opposed to speech, but one child had achieved only moderate competence in comprehension and production of language, and two other children (both of whom had severe dyspraxic speech difficulties) achieved only moderate expressive language ability. The profile of difficulties shadows the entry profile, with speech difficulties still the most prominent feature, occurring in more than half of the group. The Speech subgroup children remained at Dawn House between 15 months and 4.7 years (mean stay 2.10). They left Dawn House when they were aged between 8.1 and 13.8 (mean leaving age 11.3), and all except one child were able to proceed to mainstream schools. One child with persisting expressive language difficulty and behaviour problems continued at Dawn House Senior School.

Frank, who was our exemplar of the Speech subgroup in the original description of subgroups, proceeded to mainstream school after 4½ years at Dawn House. He occasionally made a minor grammatical error or stumbled over the pronunciation of a polysyllabic word, but he was generally a clear and fluent speaker. However, he still had considerable difficulties with both reading and spelling.

GROUP 2. SPEECH PLUS

There were 23 children who came to Dawn House with speech problems as severe as those in the first subgroup, but whose problems with the production of language (and also with the comprehension of language in some cases) were more severe than those in Group 1. The expressive abilities of all 23 children and the comprehension abilities of four were graded moderately impaired.

Five of the children had neuromotor impairments affecting all articulatory organs, and one boy was unable to close the palato-pharyngeal sphincter but had normal tongue and lip function. For 17 children there was no overt physical cause of their severe speech problems. Examination of the reported antecedent factors showed a higher than expected number of children in this group, 11, with adverse perinatal factors or neurologically threatening conditions, including four of the six who had neuromotor dysfunction. There was also an increased incidence (N 16) of environment risk. This group uniquely had multiple antecedent factors, often incorporating perinatal/neurological risk and/or environmental risk. It is possible that the speech problems and the language problems have separate aetiologies (p. 103), and that adverse environmental conditions could exacerbate problems in a child whose communicative development was hindered by speech-production difficulties. Auditory processing abilities were less impaired in this group than in the majority, supporting its distinction from other mainly language-impaired subgroups.

Sixteen of the Speech Plus subgroup were leavers and they retained a considerable level of impairment across the linguistic areas assessed. None of the group reached the high-competence category in all three areas of comprehension, production and speech, and in only four children (two of whom are dysarthric) was the final impairment confined to speech production.

The Speech Plus subgroup had a mean stay at Dawn House of three years 10 months (range 1.10 to 5.11), and their average age at leaving was 12.4 (9.3 to 13.6). Only four of the children left for mainstream schools before their 12th birthday. Ten needed to continue in special language schools after reaching Dawn House leaving age, and two severely dysarthric boys with good comprehension and additional physical disabilities went to schools for the physically disabled.

Our exemplar, George, spent six years at Dawn House and transferred to another language school at the age of 13.5, still needing speech and language therapy and special educational help. George's comprehension and production of language were adequate, but he had a limited vocabulary and made occasional grammatical errors. He found it difficult to express his ideas clearly. Use of a palatal training device had reduced the nasality of his speech, and his sound system was complete but inconsistently used in spontaneous speech. He was reading at a nine-year level.

GROUP 3. CLASSIC

The largest subgroup of entrants, 46, we labelled 'Classic' because their pattern of impairment is the one most frequently associated with SLI: severe expressive language impairment, lesser difficulties with comprehension, and phonological impairment ranging from moderate to severe. We avoided the term 'expressive disorder' or 'syntactic-phonologial disorder' because these labels appear to underplay the comprehension problems which in our experience are an important part of the disability.

When considering antecedent factors, more of this group than expected (29 children) had a positive family history of language disorder, and fewer than expected had perinatal, neurological or environmental risks. They were more likely to have only one or no antecedent factors present than the other groups. Their acquisition of language was particularly delayed, and they had very limited ASTM. Their performance IQs clustered below the median for the whole sample.

238

The picture is one of a very disabled subgroup of children, with a genetic factor contributing to their disability, and associated problems which make it harder for them to overcome their language-learning difficulty.

Thirty-seven of this group were leavers. Surprisingly their final profile (Fig. 7.1) looked somewhat better than the Speech Plus group. Eleven of these leavers were in the highly competent group for all three language functions (comprehension, production and speech). Although most difficulties were still found in the area of language production (N 20) the profile was flatter than expected, with comprehension and speech difficulties still featuring for many children. Three of the group had a degree of dysarthria, and one boy had a well repaired cleft palate. These all appear in the low speech-competence band.

The next school placement was mainstream school for 16 of the Classic group, language school for 18. Two boys with continuing educational rather than language problems went to a school for children with moderate learning difficulties and one hyperactive boy went to a residential school for children with social and behavioural problems. Eleven of the group were young leavers, leaving before they were 12 years old. The mean leaving age was 11.9, and ranged from 8.1 to 13.10. The mean length of stay at Dawn House was 4.4 years, with a range from 1.7 to 6.11.

Alice (see p. 48) went on to another language school just before her 13th birthday, after 6½ years at Dawn House. She had made considerable improvement but still had problems in every linguistic area. She transferred from the second language school to a comprehensive school for her final year. She is one of our group of 34 young people (AJ) whose follow-up questionnaires at the age of 18+ are reported at the end of this chapter.

GROUP 4. SEMANTIC

Difficulties with decoding and encoding meaning are characteristics of the group we have labelled 'Semantic'. Thirty such children were among our entrants having language profiles in which comprehension problems were severe or moderate, and expressive language and/or phonological abilities were less impaired. Although, with their marked comprehension difficulties which affect language use and every aspect of living and learning, these children form a relatively cohesive and recognisable group within school, no background features delineated them as group members. No antecedent or developmental factors were associated with this group, and although they were characterised by low verbal IQ, they differed significantly in this only from the Speech subgroup.

Of the 20 school leavers in this group, 12 still had comprehension problems and comprehension was evaluated at the lowest level in four youngsters. Half of the group only achieved moderate expressive language function, the other half reached a high level; only two of the 20 failed to achieve a high level of speech competence. Five group members had no problem at any language level.

The final language picture for the Semantic subgroup is one of minor or moderate residual problems, with comprehension still being the area of greatest difficulty. Ten of the group were able to proceed to mainstream schools. Five of these had a final high evaluation for comprehension and five were moderate: four moving into mainstream as young leavers. Nine children remained in language schools, including four whose comprehension level was regarded as low. One girl with low comprehension ability was transferred, against the advice of Dawn House staff, to a school for moderate learning disability. The mean leaving age was 12.2 (range 9.11 to 13.10). The mean length of stay was 3.10 (range 1.3 to 5.7).

Warren left Dawn House for mainstream school after 2½ years, aged 9.11, with good comprehension and production of language on assessment, and clear speech. He was reading above age level. Staff felt some anxiety about his tendency to withdraw his attention from the current activity, sometimes making him miss the crucial point of a lesson or conversation. For this reason he was partially and successfully integrated into a local mainstream school before being recommended for discharge. He participated in the 18+ follow-up reported below (WK).

GROUP 5. RESIDUAL

Ten children in this group and 13 in the Moderate group shared the same entry profile, in which no disability in any of the three language areas was worse than moderate. They were treated as two separate groups because the former children had all previously attended other language schools or units, and it is probable that the skills we were measuring at entry to Dawn House showed an improvement on their baseline abilities when first entering special education. One boy was removed very early from Dawn House because his parents were unable to come to terms with the separation, and he is not included in the group of nine leavers.

Only three children in this subgroup did not reach a high all-round language competence. Two of these had some subtle comprehension difficulties, one also having expressive and speech problems; one other boy had continuing problems with the production of complex sentences. All were able to transfer to mainstream school, eight doing so before their 13th birthday. The mean leaving age for the group was 10.6 (range 7.6 to 12.2) and the mean length of stay was 2.4 years (range 1.3 to 3.4).

Our exemplar, Andy (AJJ), stayed at Dawn House for three years, moving into the first year of his local comprehensive at the age of 11.8. At this age his oral language and speech skills were good, although his phonology was not fully mature. He was reading and spelling at a nine-year level and still had considerable difficulties in this area. Further developments are reported in the 18+ follow-up.

GROUP 6. MODERATE

In terms of evaluated attainments, the profile of the Moderate group looks very similar to the Residual group (Fig. 7.1). Of the 11 children in the leavers group, only three were not evaluated 'high' in each language area. The pattern of remaining difficulties was similar to that in the Residual group. However, they achieved this profile at a later age: the mean leaving age was 11.6 (range 6.10 to 13.5). They spent longer at Dawn House than the group whose specific therapy and education had begun before entry. The mean length of stay for our Moderate group was 2.11 (range 0.11 to 4.7). Five of this group remained at Dawn House until leaving age, four needed to continue in special language education and one went to a school for moderate learning difficulties.

Wesley had a very short stay at Dawn House. His moderate language impairment improved rapidly, and he left aged 6.10 after a stay of only 11 months.

GROUP 7. NO LANGUAGE

Five of the six children who entered school with no speech or language capability are leavers. Figure 7.1 shows that the outcome profiles in this tiny group are not homogeneous. The outcomes here reflect the nature of the underlying communication problems rather than the pattern at entry. Indeed a profile in which all skills are below the baseline is not in any real sense a profile at all. Three of these leavers were children with total receptive aphasia, who had developed no ability to perceive words or speech sounds at school entry aged 6.6, 7.0 and 8.4. All progressed to the level where they could understand and produce varying degrees of signed, written and spoken English, but with such a severe disability that improvement did not take them out of the low competence level (apart from one girl, our exemplar Gemma, who reached the moderate level of comprehension ability). One of the other children in this group had receptive aphasia acquired post-lingually following encephalitis at the age of four. This boy made rapid progress when he was introduced to Paget Gorman Signed Speech and regained his understanding and production of spoken language. The final child was a puzzling case who entered school with no apparent cause for his inability to use language at the age of 7.7. No reason for his silence was ever confirmed, but his fairly rapid language progress after settling into school suggests some psycho-emotional root to his problem. The last two boys had final evaluations of 'high' in each language area.

Gemma suffered from the Landau-Kleffner syndrome and entered school with no understanding of speech. She failed to develop completely adequate speech perception ability, but by the time she left Dawn House she could understand class instructions and simple sentences through the spoken medium. In new situations, or for more complex language, she remained dependent on signed and written language. She had a reading and spelling age of just over eight and was making good progress when at the age of 11.10, after three years and four months, she moved to another language school. Gemma is further reported (GS) in the 18+ follow-up.

GROUP 8. YOUNG UNCLASSIFIED

Six children aged between 5.6 and 6.7 were in the lowest category for each language area at entry, but unlike the No Language children, they had developed some communicative abilities. We felt that our measures were too gross to classify these children who had failed to reach a baseline in any area. This proved to be the case and the later language status of these six children was very varied, although only two are members of the leavers' group—one having a good language outcome and one a considerable comprehension problem. As with the No Language children discussed above, our entry measures were not adequate for classification. More sensitive measures would be needed to group children with very low-level skills into language-impairment subgroups.

GROUP 9. SEVERE

The three boys in this group differed from the previous group only in age. It was expected that children over seven years of age with such low-level language attainments would have a long-term problem. This expectation has been fulfilled. All three leavers had continuing language difficulties, poor ASTM, comprehension problems, word-finding difficulties, syntactic and phonological difficulties. They did improve slowly during the five or six years they spent at Dawn House, and achieved moderate language competence levels. Two continued education in language schools and one in a school for moderate learning disability.

Arthur (p. 51) went on to a second language school when he was 12.8 after three years and four months at Dawn House. Informal contacts with staff at the second school indicated that his communication and educational problems remained severe, although he achieved some partial integration into a local comprehensive school. We were unable to contact any of this group for the 18+ follow-up.

Prediction of outcome

Studies into SLI serve three major functions. The most valuable function may be a descriptive one. Until criteria for SLI are defined in a universally acceptable way, and subgroupings are agreed, the corpus of knowledge about the condition derives from studies such as this which describe the natural history of language impairment within one defined sample.

The second function is an investigation of aetiology. We believe that this is best accomplished by smaller specific studies which can explore particular aspects of aetiology in a thorough and systematic fashion, with planned and reliable data. In this study we have only been able to list the main theories and discuss how our data support them or otherwise.

A third function of such studies is to consider any practical applications, and to ask whether we can use the results to make decisions about future management: either of the individual child, or in the wider context of society as a whole.

In this study, because of changing practice, we have not been able to evaluate therapy or teaching. All the children have attended the same school in which a constant underlying philosophy has been served by evolving methodological approaches during the 13 years of the study. No comparisons of individual management are possible. We are, however, able to consider the long-term needs of this impaired group within society, by relating children's outcome at discharge from Dawn House to the pattern of their disorder at entry and to possible antecedent factors. If we can improve our prediction of the future pattern of problems, and the likely duration of problems in language-impaired seven-year-olds, we may be better able to match provision with need.

Outcome grading

Children come to schools such as Dawn House because of their deficiencies in language and/or speech skills which seriously impede their learning ability and progress in education, preventing them from reaching their potential in mainstream schools. Therefore we decided that good or poor outcome should be assessed in the three areas of language, speech and education. Although we consider personal and emotional strength to be extremely important in determining future success, after careful consideration this was not included as an outcome measure, as it was not a prime reason for placing the child in special education.

Our outcome measure has three components.

LANGUAGE

Earlier we described the final language profile in the areas of comprehension and production. The outcome language measure is derived from the ability, or otherwise, of leavers to return to mainstream school. Children are originally sent to Dawn House, most leaving their home and family, because their language problems are such that they cannot hope to achieve their potential in a mainstream school. The objective is to return to mainstream education. Language outcome is graded 1 (good) in children whose language abilities improve to the extent that they are able to rejoin their normal peers, understand class instructions, express themselves coherently and generally participate gainfully in normal education. Of the 118 leavers, 62 (52 per cent) were able to do this.

A poor language outcome, graded 3, was assigned to those children who, after between 18 months and seven years of intensive therapy and education, still required the special sort of help provided by language schooling. For 47 leavers (40 per cent), their language needs were still paramount.

A small group of nine youngsters (8 per cent) fell between these two positions. Their primary needs were no longer for specifically language-oriented special education, but they were not able enough to benefit from mainstream education. They required some additional support from specialist teaching or smaller groups, which was available at special schools for pupils with moderate learning disability, physical disability, emotional or adjustment problems. These children were graded 2 (fair) for language outcome.

SPEECH

The speech component of the outcome grade relates to intelligibility and the completeness of the phonological system. Since the measure for which we have a full set of data is essentially a test of articulation (EAT), children may score below

TABLE 7.IX

Components of final outcome grade

	Language	Speech	Reading
(1) Good	62	72	22
(2) Fair	9	10	44
(3) Poor	47	36	52
Total	118	118	118

the ceiling if they stumble over polysyllabic words incorporating phonemic clusters ('umbrella', 'toothbrush') or if they are using an immature form of /r/ or /th/. The speech of such children would be intelligible and accepted by many listeners as normal. Atypical speech substitutions on the contrary are very noticeable, particularly as a child gets older, even if they do not affect intelligibility. For the final outcome we take count not only of the extent of phonological development in terms of the speech sounds used correctly in context, but also of the deviant use of sounds.

1. *Good*. EAT raw score of 50 or more and no more than one atypical score: 72 children (61 per cent).

2. *Fair*. EAT raw score 33 to 49 and no more than one atypical score: 10 children (8 per cent).

3. *Poor*. EAT raw score 32 or below, or more than one atypical score: 36 children (31 per cent).

READING

The education measure is essentially a measure of reading ability. Despite the fact that most children were still in need of remedial support when they left, some had achieved serviceable levels of reading, and others still at earlier stages of reading were functioning at levels close to average for age. Many would not be out of place in most mainstream schools on the basis of their reading ages or the degree of reading retardation. There were also many who had a very serious reading problem by any criterion. In describing ultimate reading standards, we thought it would be more informative to use a graded scale which would divide the children into three groups, based on a combination of reading age (RA) and the difference between RA and chronological age (CA). The mechanics of reading are generally assumed to have been acquired when a reading age of about nine years has been reached. These skills have been consolidated at a reading age of 10. Children who have failed to reach a reading age of 7.6 have not yet succeeded in mastering the letter/sound correspondences upon which literacy depends. The use of the adjectives 'good', 'fair' and 'poor' as descriptions of our three reading groups, as indeed of all our outcome groups, are of course relative to this sample and not to a normal population.

1. *Good.* RA of 10 years or above, or a difference of less than one year between CA and RA: 22 children (19 per cent).

2. *Fair.* (a) Children aged 10 years or under—RA above 7.6 and a difference of 12 to 30 months between CA and RA. (b) Children over 10 years—RA above 7.6 and a difference of 12 to 48 months between CA and RA: 52 children (44 per cent).

3. *Poor.* (a) Children aged 10 years or under—RA below 7.6 and a difference of more than 30 months between CA and RA. (b) Children over 10 years—RA below 7.6 or a difference of more than 48 months between CA and RA: 44 children (37 per cent).

Grades for the language, speech and reading components of final outcome are shown in Table 7.IX.

COMPOSITE OUTCOME GRADES

The composite outcome grades were based on a combination of these component measures and clinical judgement. Both authors subjectively and separately graded the functional language abilities and educational prospects of all school leavers, each of whom was known to them personally. These lists were compared, firstly with each other, and then with the objective gradings of language, speech and reading described above. There was a considerable degree of harmony between subjective and objective ratings which were grouped to produce the following outcome grades.

1. *Good.* A school leaver was considered to have an over-all 'good' outcome if s/he scored 1 in each of the three components, or if both language and speech were rated 1 but reading was only 2 (fair). Thirty-eight children were rated with an over-all good outcome.

2. *Fair.* In order to qualify for a 'fair' outcome children were required to have scored 1 or 2 for language, at least one component needed to be 'good', and only one component could be 'poor'. Forty-one children were rated 'fair' according to these criteria.

3. *Poor.* A 'poor' outcome was assigned to children with two components rated 'poor', or one 'poor' and two 'fair'. Thirty-nine children fell into this category. The breakdown of grades is shown in Table 7.X.

Predictive factors

All of the factors and assessments described in this book are candidate predictors for the final (*i.e.* school-leaving) outcome of this group of children. We therefore considered all the antecedents, developmental factors, associates of SLI, and school-entry language tests for their predictive power.

The first level of analysis was to examine correlations between these variables and the final outcome grades, controlling the effect of age. For the nominal variables of gender, laterality and speech discrimination, chi-squares were used to examine the relationship (Table 7.XI). Where the dataset is incomplete, the number of subjects is shown.

TABLE 7.X

Final outcome grades based on components of language (L), speech (S) and reading (R)

Final outcome grades	LSR	N
Good	111	12
	112	26
		38
Fair	113	6
	131	2
	122	4
	123	1
	132	7
	212	3
	213	4
	231	1
	311	5
	312	8
		41
Poor	133	4
	233	1
	322	2
	313	8
	323	3
	322	2
	332	2
	333	17
		39
		118

TABLE 7.XI

Correlations of antecedents, associates and entry language measures with final outcome grades

	Outcome
Antecedents	
Family history	-0.3**
Perinatal risk	-0.2*
Environmental risk	0.2*
Middle-ear problems	NS
Development	
Walking age (N 112)	-0.3**
Language acquisition	NS
Oromotor ability	NS
Associates	
Age at entry	NS
Gender	NS
Hearing	NS
Speech discrimination (N 112)	NS
ASTM	0.4***
PIQ (N 97)	0.3**
VIQ (N 63)	0.5***
Laterality	NS
Hearing	NS
Behaviour	NS
Entry language measures	
Passive vocabulary	0.3***
Comprehension of grammar (N 70)	NS
General comprehension (N 79)	NS
Expressive vocabulary (N 115)	0.3**
Sentence structure (N 108)	0.4***
Morphology (N 89)	0.4***
Story re-telling (N 83)	NS
Phonological development	0.4***
Phonological deviance (N 117)	-0.2

*$p<0.05$
**$p<0.01$
***$p<0.001$

CORRELATION BETWEEN OUTCOME GRADES AND ANTECEDENTS

Children with a better outcome are more likely to come from a family with a history of language disorders, to have an increased perinatal risk, and to have no environmental disadvantages. This is a little unexpected; children with two potentially disabling antecedents seem to make better progress than those without. Such a finding can be interpreted as support for the multi-causal and multi-factorial model of SLI in which a variety of causes lead to different profiles of language impairment which differ also in prognosis. In our sample those children whose problems are familial, and to a lesser extent those children whose problems stem from birth trauma, both overcame their problems to a considerable extent. This is possibly because their impairment was restricted in range if not in severity. Bishop

246

and Edmundson (1987a) also found, contrary to their hypothesis, that impairment in one linguistic domain had a better outcome than a more broadly based even profile of impairment which encompassed semantic, syntactic and phonological difficulty.

In Chapter 3 we reported a raised incidence of family history of language disorder in the Classic subgroup, with an increased possibility that no other antecedent factor would be found. We also reported a suggestively higher incidence of perinatal risk or neurologically threatening condition in the Speech and No Language subgroups, although this was not statistically significant. The Speech Plus group, on the other hand, was more likely to have multiple antecedent factors including perinatal risk which co-occurred with environmental disadvantage.

If the single cause and the narrower range of impaired linguistic functions have a greater chance of eventual improvement, we should find that children in the Speech group (single aetiology, single impaired function) have a better outcome than children in the Classic and No Language groups (single aetiology, multiple impaired functions), who in turn do better than those in the Speech Plus group (multiple aetiology, multiple impaired functions).

CORRELATION BETWEEN OUTCOME GRADES AND DEVELOPMENT

Another unexpected correlation is the one between walking age and outcome. Children with a good outcome have a mean walking age of 14 months, while those children with fair or poor outcome have a mean of 18 months. This is surprising in view of our failure to find any association between age of walking and language abilities in 151 children at entry to school, or between walking age and subgroup, although there was a non-significant raised incidence of late walking in the Speech Plus subgroup (see Chapter 4). We must consider whether late walking, often taken as a measure of general late development (Fundudis *et al.* 1979), is associated not with the occurrence of language impairment, but with the rate of progress, and the chance of making good improvement.

We also found that in terms of outcome, age of walking is dissociated from family history of language problems (r. −0.2 p = 0.014). Late walkers are less likely to have a positive family history, adding credence to the suggestion of multiple routes to the disorder.

CORRELATION BETWEEN OUTCOME GRADES AND ASSOCIATES OF SLI

The associates of language impairment considered as predictors are taken from measures at school entry. The only associates that are significantly correlated with outcome are intelligence (both performance and verbal scales) and ASTM. For none of these is the dataset complete, VIQ information being the most deficient with data for just over half the subjects. It has been suggested (p. 224) that, in this group of subjects at least, VIQ is a composite measure of a range of language skills for which other assessments are available. We also found that subjects who were given VIQ testing at entry were a subset of our population having a higher mean age than

TABLE 7.XII

Correlations between entry language measures

	2	3	4	5	6	7	8	9
1. Passive vocabulary	0.4 ***	0.4 ***	0.5 ***	NS	0.4 ***	NS	NS	NS
2. Comprehension of grammar		0.4 **	0.4 **	NS	NS	0.5 ***	NS	NS
3. General comprehension			0.4 ***	0.6 ***	0.3 *	0.5 ***	NS	NS
4. Expressive vocabulary				0.4 ***	0.3 ***	0.6 ***	NS	NS
5. Structure					0.3 ***	0.4 ***	0.4 **	−0.2 *
6. Morphology						0.3 **	0.2 *	NS
7. Story retelling							NS	NS
8. Phonological development								−0.9 ***
9. Phonological deviance								

*p<0.05, **p<0.01, ***p<0.001

those who were not tested. For these reasons VIQ is not considered further as a predictor of outcome. The emergence of PIQ as a correlate of outcome is expected, confirming the findings of other studies (Aram *et al.* 1984, Schery 1985, Silva 1987) and the association reported in this study between PIQ and language skills at entry, particularly between low PIQ and severe speech impairment. Children with language-learning difficulties are educationally disadvantaged and need to use other cognitive processes to achieve success. Those children with better visual and spatial cognitive strengths may be able to compensate to some extent for their verbal deficiencies in learning, and thus achieve a better outcome.

We reported in Chapter 5 that 75 per cent of our sample have limited ASTM at school entry. It is so universal and so poor as to be considered almost a descriptive parameter of SLI. An association has also frequently been reported between ASTM and reading impairment (Naidoo 1972, Mann 1984, Jorm *et al.* 1986). The highly significant correlation between entry ASTM and outcome (r 0.4, p<0.001) suggests that ASTM is also associated with the progress of SLI.

Entry age, gender, laterality, hearing and behaviour (a conglomerate of confidence, resilience, sociability and attitude to communication) were not related to outcome grades.

ENTRY LANGUAGE MEASURES

Six of the nine entry measures are significantly related to outcome. Language at entry is clearly important in the prediction of outcome, but interpretation is

TABLE 7.XIII

Correlations of antecedents, associates and entry language measures with final outcome grades and components

	Outcome	Language	Speech	Reading
Antecedents				
Family history	−0.3**	−0.2*	−0.3***	NS
Perinatal risk	−0.2*	NS	−0.2**	NS
Environmental risk	0.2*	NS	NS	NS
Middle-ear problems	NS	NS	NS	NS
Development				
Late walking (N 112)	−0.3**	−0.2**	−0.2*	NS
Language acquisition	NS	NS	NS	NS
Oromotor risk scale	NS	NS	0.2*	NS
Associates				
Age at entry	NS	NS	NS	−0.3***
Gender	NS	NS	†*	NS
Speech discrimination	NS	NS	NS	†*
ASTM	0.4***	0.4***	NS	0.3***
PIQ (N 97)	0.3**	0.3**	0.2*	0.2*
VIQ (N 63)	0.5***	0.5***	NS	0.4***
Laterality (N 108)	NS	NS	NS	NS
Hearing	NS	NS	NS	NS
Behaviour	NS	NS	NS	NS
Entry language measures				
Passive vocabulary	0.3***	0.3**	NS	0.4***
Comprehension of grammar (N 70)	NS	NS	−0.3**	NS
General comprehension (N 79)	NS	0.2*	NS	0.2*
Expressive vocabulary (N 115)	0.3**	0.3***	0.1*	0.4***
Sentence structure (N 108)	0.4***	0.4***	NS	0.3**
Morphology (N 89)	0.4***	0.4***	0.2*	0.2*
Story retelling (N 83)	NS	NS	NS	NS
Phonological development	0.4***	0.2*	0.6***	0.2*
Phonological deviance	−0.2*	NS	−0.4***	NS

†Gender: chi-square 6.2, df 2.   Speech discrimination: chi-square 7.4, df 2
*p<0.05
**p<0.01
***p<0.001

difficult to attempt, given the difference of subject numbers and the level of correlation between these predictor variables, suggesting a considerable degree of covariance between them (Table 7.XII).

Components of outcome and predictive factors

In order to function adequately in society after leaving Dawn House, a child needs to have attained a broad degree of proficiency: so our outcome measure was built from the three components language, speech and reading. Although these are all factors which may be impaired in SLI, they can be dissociated, and the profiles of strengths and weaknesses in these areas are individually drawn. Those antecedents, associates and language measures which correlate with outcome may be associated with specific components of the composite measure, and this information could assist in planning and prediction. Table 7.XIII displays the correlations of predictors and outcome, partialling out age as in Table 7.XI, but additionally shows the correlations between predictors and components. Only environmental risk is associated with the composite outcome without being associated with any of the individual components.

The pattern of correlation between predictors and the language component is very close to that between predictors and outcome which has already been discussed, and indeed the language component is the one which correlates most strongly with the over-all outcome grade (r. = 0.75, as opposed to r. 0.66 between outcome and speech and r. 0.65 between outcome and reading). The only predictor measure correlating with language but not with outcome is the measure of general comprehension (Reynell Developmental Comprehension Scale), but data are available for only 79 children.

Speech uniquely has small but just significant correlations with early oromotor problems (a continuation of the association reported earlier between oromotor problems and speech at entry) and gender, with girls having a marginally worse speech outcome than boys. Although many more boys than girls have speech difficulties, impairment in girls may be the result of more serious underlying disabilities. The strong correlation between speech outcome and entry phonological ability is explained by the fact that both measures are derived from scores on the same test of articulation (EAT). The negative correlation between good entry comprehension of grammar (TROG, N 70) and poor speech outcome is harder to explain, but may be attributable to the different types of disability within our population. This could indicate that children with specific comprehension disability and children with specific speech disability are strongly dissociated. Children admitted to Dawn House with severe speech impairments would in this case have relatively high comprehension scores. At school-leaving age the speech scores of this group would still be poorer than average for the sample.

Unlike reading age, which was the measure chosen to evaluate reading ability in Chapter 2, the reading component in outcome is based on a combination of reading age and the gap between chronological and reading age. Those associates of language disorder and entry language measures which are correlated with final oral language skills are also correlated with final reading ability. These are ASTM, IQ, vocabulary (active and passive), sentence structure, and to a lesser extent general comprehension, morphology and phonological development. The similarity of the relationship between early measure predictors and oral language on the one hand, and written language on the other, confirms that in this population the difficulties with reading and spelling are part and parcel of the over-all language impairment. Age at entry also correlates significantly with reading outcome at the 0.1 per cent level. Children who enter school younger, and who therefore make an earlier start on the intensive programme of reading and skilled teaching available, have a better reading outcome: although this is relative to the continuing reading difficulties

TABLE 7.XIV

Final outcome by subgroups

Language subgroup	(N)	Outcome		
		Good	Fair	Poor
Speech	(15)	5	7	3
Speech Plus	(16)	2*	3	11*
Classic	(37)	9	12	16
Semantic	(20)	8	8	4
Residual	(9)	8**	1	0**
Moderate	(11)	4	7	0
No Language	(5)	1	1	3
Young Unclassified	(2)	1	1	0
Severe	(3)	0	1	2
	(118)	38	41	39

Binomial test good *vs* poor, P = Q = 0.5,
*p<0.05, **p<0.01

Fig. 7.2. Proportion of good, fair and poor outcome in subgroups.

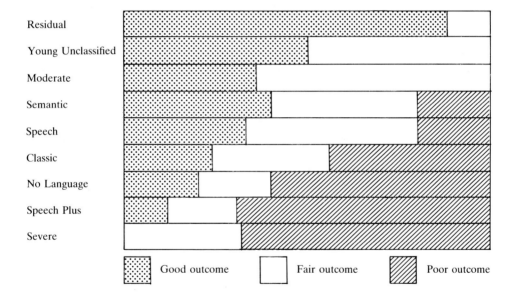

experienced by almost all pupils. A controlled study would be necessary to ascertain if an earlier start really does improve reading outcome.

Subgroups and final outcome
An examination of outcome in terms of subgroups should provide useful prognostic information for children profiled at entry to school, and may also validate or invalidate the clinical groupings that we devised to partition our SLI subjects. Did the Severe group have long-term severe problems? Were the Residual truly residual and the Moderate truly moderate?

251

TABLE 7.XV

TABLE 7.XV

Components of outcome by subgroup

Language subgroup	(N)	Language			Speech			Reading		
		Good	Fair	Poor	Good	Fair	Poor	Good	Fair	Poor
Speech	(15)	14	0	1	6	2	7	4	7	4
Speech Plus	(16)	4	2	10	3	2	11	1	6	9
Classic	(37)	16	3	18	21	4	12	6	14	17
Semantic	(20)	10	1	9	18	1	1	4	11	5
Residual	(9)	9	0	0	8	0	1	3	6	0
Moderate	(11)	7	1	3	11	0	0	4	3	4
No Language	(5)	1	1	3	2	0	3	0	3	2
Young Unclassified	(2)	1	0	1	2	0	0	0	2	0
Severe	(3)	0	1	2	1	1	1	0	0	3
	(118)	62	9	47	72	10	36	22	52	44

Table 7.XIV shows the outcome of our nine groups, and the same information is figuratively displayed showing the relative proportion of good, fair and poor outcome in the unevenly sized groups in Figure 7.2. Proportions mean very little when there are only two or three leavers in a subgroup, but all groups are displayed for the sake of completeness in this final summary of results. The subgroups are discussed in the order in which they have been presented throughout the book.

The Speech group might be expected to have good outcomes. Bishop and Edmundson (1987a) found that many children whose early language impairment was restricted to the phonological level later overcame their difficulties completely. Follow-up studies have generally found better results with articulation-impaired rather than language-impaired subjects (Hall and Tomblin 1978, King et al. 1982). Although our Speech group is the most discretely impaired of our categories, no child is admitted to Dawn House whose language is unimpaired, and they may be more disabled than the speech or articulation groups reported in other studies. Our Speech group had moderate success. Around half of the group still had poor speech indicative of a long-term problem, and over half had reading problems. However, almost all of the group made sufficient progress to return to mainstream school, and so achieved the major objective of their intensive therapy and education. Table 7.XV shows the outcome component measures for all the subgroups, and these are represented graphically in Figures 7.3 to 7.5.

The Speech Plus group comprised children with severe speech disabilities and some additional language problems. They presented as mainly impaired by reason of speech deficit, with language problems which, although significant, were less prominent. As we proceeded with the analysis it became abundantly clear that these children were disabled not just in the range of linguistic impairment but also in severity, and we have speculated that these children could have multiple disabilities and aetiologies. Their outcomes substantiate our growing awareness of the severity of their problems, and confirms our hypothesis (p. 247) that outcome

252

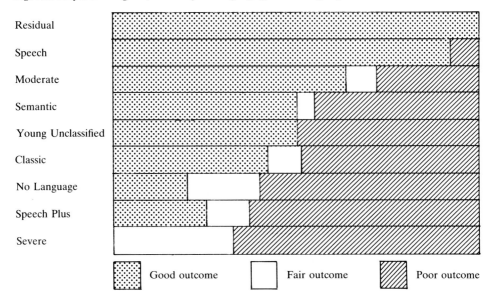

Fig. 7.3. Proportion of good, fair and poor language grade in subgroups.

Residual

Speech

Moderate

Semantic

Young Unclassified

Classic

No Language

Speech Plus

Severe

Good outcome   Fair outcome   Poor outcome

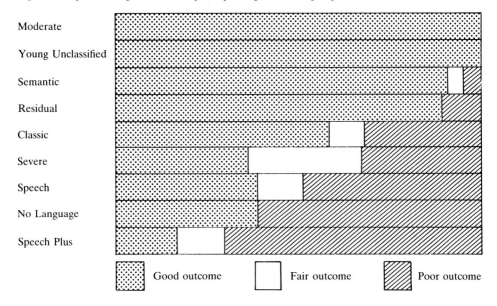

Fig. 7.4. Proportion of good, fair and poor speech grade in subgroups.

Moderate

Young Unclassified

Semantic

Residual

Classic

Severe

Speech

No Language

Speech Plus

Good outcome   Fair outcome   Poor outcome

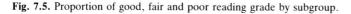

Fig. 7.5. Proportion of good, fair and poor reading grade by subgroup.

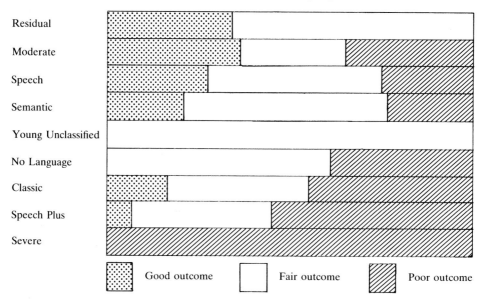

would be poor. There are significantly raised possibilities of outcome being poor rather than good (binomial test p = 0.011). The extensive and long-lasting nature of their problems is comparable only with those of the Severe group. We need to take more account of the problems of such children in our future planning.

The group whose problems we expected to be the most long-lasting and disabling was the Classic. Outcome here presents few surprises, possibly because this is the language profile most archetypal to SLI and most frequently described in the literature. Almost half had a poor language outcome and needed continuing special language provision after the age of 13. For speech attainments, this group occupied a central position in the hierarchy of subgroups, with over half having a good speech outcome. Written language continued to present major difficulties, as expected, with almost half in the poor outcome group for reading.

Some of the most puzzling children at Dawn House are those in our Semantic group. The somewhat gross definition of disability we used to define the group, in which level of comprehension is lower than expressive language skills or speech skills or both, does not tap the subtle and sometimes surprising difficulties they have, with unexpected profiles of ability and weakness, knowledge and naivety. Over-all outcome is reasonably good, 80 per cent being graded good or fair. The pattern of outcome in terms of its components is for language to be roughly half good and half poor, speech outcomes to be good (speech problems were generally only minor in this group), and for the bulk of the reading outcomes to be graded fair.

Although the Residual and Moderate groups shared a common entry profile of language abilities, we distinguished between them on the suspicion that the Residual group might consist of earlier members of the Classic group improved by several years of intensive help in other special language schools or units (see Chapter 2). If this were the case, a less disabled Moderate group should have a better outcome than the quasi-Classical, Residual group. In the event the opposite proved true, with the Residuals having the best outcomes of any of our subgroups, being superior to the Moderates in every component as well as in the over-all outcome grade. None of the Residuals had a poor outcome; eight of the nine were in the good outcome group (binominal test p = 0.004). In our review of other studies in Chapter 1, we referred to the difficulties of cross-study comparison because of the differences in subject groups. The Residual group, who came to Dawn House by way of the selection criteria of other schools and units, may represent a different and less disabled population.

The No Language group were at the bottom of our ability range on entry to Dawn House. By the time they leave, they have made progress which may be modest in absolute terms, but is considerable relative to the severity of their initial disabilities. Although the small group size means that results must be interpreted cautiously, these children appear to have better outcomes, as predicted above, than those in the Speech Plus group.

Only two of the Young Unclassified children were leavers, one with a good and one with a fair outcome. It is to be expected that children in this category who are more disabled will not yet have left school.

The three children with Severe disabilities were expected to have a long-term and disabling impairment when they were found to have the lowest abilities in comprehension, production and speech at entry to school aged over seven. This prediction was sadly correct, although two of the three did rise above the lowest grade in at least one of our final areas, and one achieved an over-all fair outcome.

Discriminant function analysis
The correlation matrix (Table 7.XIII) indicated a number of predictor variables which were associated with outcome. Covariance between predictors and unequal numbers of data made interpretation difficult, particularly for the entry language measures. Discriminant function analysis (Norusis 1985) is designed to form linear combinations of a set of predictor variables which will optimally classify subjects into groups. Although designed for use with normally distributed continuous independent variables, discriminant function analysis can successfully incorporate dichotomous independent variables (Hedderson 1987). A weighted average of variables is summed into a single index which has the maximum power to separate individual cases into the dependent groups. The relative contribution to prediction of each variable can be estimated by adding or dropping them individually from the analysis, but this is essentially a multivariate analysis which analyses the effect of a group of variables acting jointly.

Some additional data and some transformations of data were employed (as detailed below) before entering the predictor variables which correlated with outcome into a discriminant function analysis.

Additional data were incorporated for ASTM (standard scores on the ITPA auditory sequential memory scale). Since ASTM is reasonably stable in this sample of children (Pearson correlation of 0.8 between first and second tests), scores from the first test after entering school were used for 11 children who lacked preliminary test results.

Additional data were also included for passive vocabulary (EPVT and BPVS standard scores). Three children who failed by a wide margin to reach the basal standard score of 60 on the EPVT were given an estimated score of 50; four other children were assigned the group mean scores. These scores completed the data set for passive vocabulary.

Log transformations were performed on the phonological development data (EAT raw scores) to normalise the skewed distribution. Discrete variables were coded dichotomously as follows: family history, perinatal risk and environmental risk (yes/no), walking age (before or after 18 months), and LARSP sentence structure (complex clause, Stage V or below).

Of those predictor variables which correlated with outcome, VIQ was omitted because of the number of missing data, and phonological deviance (EAT atypical scores) was omitted because of abnormal distribution. The other significantly correlating predictor variables were entered into a stepwise analysis using the three levels of outcome as the dependent group variable. These were:

Family history	Yes/no
Perinatal risk	Yes/no
Environmental risk	Yes/no
Walking age	Before or after 18 months
Age at entry	
ASTM	ITPA ASM standard scores
PIQ	
Passive vocabulary	EPVT and BPVS standard scores
Expressive vocabulary	Renfrew Word-Finding scores
Sentence structure	LARSP Stage V and over, IV and below
Morphology	Grammatic closure (ITPA) standard scores
Phonological development	EAT correct scores

Because of the correlation between age and the tests of expressive vocabulary (Renfrew Word-Finding), sentence structure (LARSP) and phonological development (EAT), age was forced into analysis first to mop up covariance. Eighty-seven cases had no missing values and were processed. PIQ, walking age, passive vocabulary, sentence structure and morphology failed to enter the analysis. Morphology was then excluded from the analysis, bringing the number of cases

TABLE 7.XVI

Variables remaining in the discriminant analysis on outcome and standardised discriminant coefficients for each function

	Function 1	Function 2
Age at entry	−0.73	−0.27
Phonological development	0.67	0.08
ASTM	0.65	−0.49
Family history	0.58	−0.3
Expressive vocabulary	0.49	0.78
Environmental risk	−0.34	0.007
Perinatal risk	0.02	0.8

TABLE 7.XVII

Percentage of cases correctly classified by step

Predictors (additional to age)	%
EAT	47
EAT, RWF	54
EAT, RWF, ASM	60
EAT, RWF, ASM, FH	64
EAT, RWF, ASM, FH, peririsk	69
EAT, RWF, ASM, FH, peririsk, envrisk	70

EAT = Edinburgh Articulation Test; RWF = Renfrew Word-Finding; ASM = ITPA auditory sequential memory; FH = family history; peririsk = perinatal risk; envrisk = environmental risk

processed to 97, with no change to the variables remaining in the analysis. Since PIQ had still failed to enter the anlaysis, it was then excluded so that all 118 cases could now be processed. Two discriminant functions can be calculated for a dependent variable with three groups, the first function always being the more powerful discriminator. Table 7.XVI shows the variables which contributed to the two discriminant functions best separating the three groups. Both functions significantly contribute to group differentiation ($p < 0.00005$, $p < 0.009$). The coefficients indicate the relative contribution of the variables to the functions which discriminate between groups. The linear combination of these variables accounts for 57 per cent of the variance between outcome groups.

One measure of the effectiveness of discriminant analysis is the comparison between the group classifications predicted by the discriminant functions and actual group membership: *i.e.* how many cases would be classified correctly using only scores from the variables in the analysis. In our sample, outcome would be correctly predicted as good, fair or poor for 70 per cent of cases from the seven variables in the analysis, reducing the error of random classification by 55 per cent. Table 7.XVII shows the percentage of cases classified correctly at each step of the

257

analysis. Using only age and the three 'best' predictors—the EAT, Renfrew Word-Finding, and auditory sequential memory—we could correctly classify 60 per cent of cases.

Prediction may not be equally important for all groups. It may be particularly valuable to know, for example, which children are most likely to return to mainstream school, or which children might have very long-term problems. Discriminant analysis can be used selectively to improve prediction of one or more groups. If we use the analysis described above to look at only the extreme groups, those with good and poor outcome, only one discriminating function is computed (one less discriminating function than number of groups). Perinatal risk fails to enter into this two-group analysis, and the other six variables correctly classify 87 per cent of the 77 children into good and poor outcome.

Summary
Entry tests of language and ASTM, which correlates with several linguistic skills, are the best predictors of school-leaving outcome. This tallies with Schery's (1985) finding that pretest ability accounted for 69 per cent of the post-test variance in 718 subjects aged three to 16.

We have been constrained by the need to select tests which have been widely used with our sample in order to maximise data, and also by the need to use scorable tests, rather than more sensitive profiles, to allow statistical analysis of the results.

We cannot present a complete picture of the language-impaired child which will give the best prediction of future ability. We can only evaluate the language abilities for which we have tests. Nevertheless, within the limitations of our data we have measured a range of linguistic skills, and those that clearly have predictive value are phonological development (for speech outcome only), and expressive vocabulary. No test of comprehension has been found which indicates future outcome.

As predictors, antecedent factors are generally less important than the pre-measure language ability, but an awareness of familial language impairment is useful in predicting not only outcome but subgroup of disorder.

The final predictor of outcome, ASTM, contributes to both of the discriminant functions which separate the outcome groups. ASTM has frequently been a significant factor in the analyses described in this book, associated with severe language acquisition delay, and a range of linguistic skills, notably with language production and with learning to read. Particularly poor ASTM was found in the archetypal Classic subgroup of impairment and in the three extremely disabled children in the Severe group. We now have evidence that it is also implicated in the persistence or otherwise of disability.

Outcome can be predicted in 70 per cent of the intake to school on the basis of the preliminary language assessments, measurement of ASTM and a detailed case history.

TABLE 7.XVIII

TABLE 7.XVIII

Details of 34 ex-pupils who participated in 18+ follow-up

	Sex	Age	Age leaving Dawn House	Dawn House outcome	Information source
AN	M	18.5	8.2	1	Subject and father
EM	M	19.6	12.3	3	Mother
LAS	M	18.9	8.6	2	Subject
LES	M	21.4	13.2	3	Mother
LT	M	20.10	13.3	3	Subject (letter)
MI	M	20.10	10.1	1	Mother
PA	M	22.3	11.0	1	Subject
SC	F	22.10	12.8	3	Subject
WP	M	20.9	12.7	2	Father
AJ	F	19.2	12.11	3	Subject
WK	M	20.2	9.11	1	Subject
SOP	M	20.2	12.5	2	Mother and subject
DS	M	19.6	10.3	1	Mother
RJ	F	19.9	10.1	1	Mother and subject
WI	M	21.0	10.0	1	Subject
FJ	F	20.8	12.4	3	Mother and subject
HS	M	19.4	11.1	2	Subject
STP	M	18.7	8.1	1	Mother
EI	M	20.11	11.9	1	Father and mother
MS	M	19.3	10.1	2	Mother
PJ	F	18.6	12.2	2	Father
SB	M	18.7	11.1	3	Mother
TP	M	20.2	12.0	1	Subject
AJJ	M	20.5	11.8	1	Mother
BB	M	20.9	12.7	2	Mother
GS	F	20.1	11.10	3	Mother
SS	F	20.4	13.0	3	Subject
SN	M	20.10	10.11	1	Subject
TM	M	19.0	10.10	1	Subject
CK	M	20.5	11.3	3	Subject
PT	M	19.7	11.4	2	Mother and subject
BP	M	19.6	13.3	2	Subject and mother
DW	F	18.10	12.5	2	Mother
WE	M	18.9	12.7	2	Father

Outcome: 1 good, 2 fair, 3 poor

Follow-up of 18-year-old ex-pupils

With the growing awareness of the long-term nature of language problems, interest has increased in the social and employment prospects of young adults who have suffered early language impairment. As a corollary to this study of 156 SLI children, it was decided to contact as many of our ex-pupils as possible who had reached the age of 18, and to catch up on their educational, career and social progress by means of a telephone questionnaire.

Intelligibility was likely to be a continuing problem for some of these young people, preventing a satisfactory exchange of information over the telephone. Separate letters were therefore sent to the subjects and their parents outlining the nature and purpose of the survey, and suggesting that they discuss between themselves who should take the telephone call. Of the 43 ex-pupils of the appropriate age, contact was established with 26 young men and eight young women. All of them agreed to take part, and telephone calls were made between July and October 1987 (Table 7.XVIII). Interviews were conducted by the two authors. Thirteen of the subjects answered the questions personally, one by letter rather than telephone; in 15 cases a parent took the call, and in six cases the youngster and a parent each contributed some information.

Information was sought in three areas: (i) continuing education and academic progress, (ii) training for work and employment, and (iii) residual problems and social life.

Continuing education
SCHOOL AND PUBLIC EXAMINATIONS
All this group of young people had left Dawn House before the secondary department was opened. All except two girls and two boys had been boarders at Dawn House. Eleven had remained in special education, seven at further residential schools for language-impaired children, and four at day schools for children with moderate learning difficulties—at that time designated ESN (M) schools. One boy attended a Quaker boarding-school and the remaining 22 went to local comprehensive schools.

On the whole the transfer to new schools had been made happily, but there were some academic and social adjustment problems. Two academically able boys (DS and SN) had transferred into the final year of primary school in order to travel with a peer group into secondary school, but this had proved a bad time to join well established groups and they had been unhappy until moving to the comprehensive school. AJJ and HS, who had reading and spelling difficulties, had also been unhappy in the remedial groups at their local comprehensive schools. This was attributed to the fact that they were the only children with a specific rather than general learning difficulty, and although friendly and sociable boys at Dawn House, they had not found any friends among the remedial group. Teasing was a problem in 17 subjects. This is rare at Dawn House, where there is a common vulnerability, and where, when it occurs, teasing is not usually directed at language-related weaknesses but at physical characteristics, quickness to temper or tearfulness.

Tables 7.XIX and 7.XX list the number and nature of external examination successes achieved by these pupils. At the less academic level (Certificate of Secondary Education, CSE) there is a preponderance of practical over academic subjects, but a surprising 12 passes in English, and even one pass in a foreign language. Those youngsters who were able to take the more academic GCE (General Certificate of Education) O- and A-level examinations gravitated towards maths and the sciences; one young man was obliged to change his choice of career from the police force to scientific research when he repeatedly failed English Language O-level.

TABLE 7.XIX

Type of school attended after Dawn House and external examinations

Type of school	Subjects	Passed (range)
Local comprehensive		
(N 22)	7	No exams
	15	59 CSE (1–7)
	5	28 GCE O (1–12)
	3	9 GCE A (2–4)
Language boarding		
(N 7)	3	No exams
	4	7 CSE (1–3)
Educationally subnormal (moderate)		
(N 4)	3	No exams
	1	1 CSE
Private boarding		
(N 1)	1	4 CSE

TERTIARY EDUCATION

Almost two-thirds of the group had continued their education after reaching statutory school-leaving age, whether at college, university or on day release from employment or Youth Training Scheme courses. The commonest provision was a mix of continuing basic educational skills and vocational training. Ten subjects obtained externally moderated qualifications (Table 7.XXI). Twelve other youngsters underwent some vocational training without achieving any externally recognised qualifications, in the following skills: gardening, brick-laying, catering, lettering and graphic design, community care, painting and decorating, motor mechanics, farmwork, cabinet making and adult literacy.

Generally the only courses at Further Education colleges available to SLI students were those designed for the slow learner, compared with whom SLI students are usually more able and at the same time more vulnerable because of the communication difficulties. More than one of our ex-pupils had become disenchanted and deeply disappointed that after looking expectantly to college life, they were repeating work previously undertaken at school, but at a slower pace. These reactions have been echoed in a recent report of vocational opportunities for SLI students which describes not only the problems faced by the youngsters themselves but also by tutors, careers officers and work-experience employers who were unfamiliar with the nature and implications of communication disorders (Baginsky 1990). Very rarely were any speech therapy services available at this level, either for helping the young people directly, or for staff to turn to for information and advice.

Training and employment

Twenty-five young people were employed, including two in a part-time capacity and two temporarily in a government-sponsored training scheme. There were three

TABLE 7.XX

Examinations passed by ex-Dawn House pupils in final school placement

CSE			GCE O-level			GCE A-level	
English		12	English		3		
Maths		6	Maths			Maths	2
			Maths	3			
			Additional maths	3			
					6		
Computer Studies		1	Economics		1	Economics	1
Science			Science				
Physics	4		Physics	3		Physics	2
General science	3		Chemistry	2		Chemistry	2
Applied science	1		Physics with chemistry	1			
Engineering science	1		Biology	1			
Human biology	1				7		
		10					
Humanities			Humanities				
Geography	4		Geography	3		Geography	1
History	1		History	1			
French	1		Environmental				
Religious education	1		studies	1			
General studies	1		General studies	2		General	
European studies	1				7	Studies	1
Social studies	2						
Humanities	1						
		12					
Music		1					
Physical Education		2					
Drama		2					
Art, design, technology			Art, design, technology				
Art	7		Art	2			
Craft and design	2		Engineering				
Technical drawing	4		drawing	1			
Design and			Engineering workshop				
problem-solving	1		theory and practice	1			
Design and metal-work	1				4		
Woodwork	3						
Motor vehicle studies	1						
		19					
Life skills and home economics							
Homecraft	1						
Cookery	2						
Needlework and							
creative textiles	1						
Childcare and							
development	1						
Roadcraft	1						
		6					
Total		71			28		9

TABLE 7.XXI
Tertiary education and qualifications for pupils in 18+ follow-up

Type of education	N	Qualifications obtained
Further Education or Technical College	8	C&G communication skills Community care certificate Pre-vocational education certificates (2)
University/polytechnic	3	BA (economics) BSc (Hons) chemistry* BSc (aeronautical engineering)*
Day/block release on Youth Training Scheme	7	C&G electrical installation C&G electronics C&G communication skills C&G catering
Day/block release other employment	2	C&G electrical engineering
Agricultural college/centre	2	C&G horticulture
No further education	12	
Total	34	

*These degrees have been awarded since the questionnaire was completed
C&G = City and Guilds Examination Board

full-time students in higher education and one full-time catering student. Five subjects were unemployed: two had been out of work for just three weeks, one being made redundant because of a shortage of work in his firm, and one dropping out of a contract which would have taken him too far from home. They both expected to be back in work shortly. Of the other three unemployed, two had only had a number of short-term jobs and were not seriously chasing work currently. One young man who was incapacitated by depression had spent three years at home without any work or training. Eight of the group currently employed had spent some periods out of work, ranging from one month to 18 months.

Six young people in work expressed some dissatisfaction with the type of job they had been able to find. Table 7.XXII lists the employment status and job aspirations of all the ex-pupils. Compared with the socio-economic status of their families, there has been an increase in manual as opposed to non-manual work (even assuming that the three students at university or polytechnic would eventually be engaged in non-manual work), but this is not statistically significant (Table 7.XXIII).

Of 21 ex-pupils who had participated in government training schemes, 17 were working at the time of the survey, seven in jobs stemming directly from their training. Of the 13 who had not been on a training scheme, eight were currently employed (a slightly smaller proportion). This just reaches statistical significance (chi-square 3.9, df 1, $p<0.05$). The job opportunities provided by the training schemes were quite lowly; four ex-pupils were trained in skilled occupations, nine in partly skilled and eight in unskilled. Other methods of finding a job, not mutually exclusive, were: career office (4), family or friends (4), job centre (3),

263

TABLE 7.XXII

Current employment position and aspirations

	Job	*Youth training*	*Preferred career*
NA	Nurseryman	Nursery work*	Farming
EM	Bar work		
LAS	Gardening	Horticulture	
LES	Kitchen porter	Warehouse porter	Driver
LT	Building labourer	Shop assistant	Bricklayer
MI	Electrician		
PA	Crane driver	Electronic workshop	Lab. technician/electronics
SC	Classroom aide	Classroom assistant	
WP	Unemployed	Building labourer	Building/engineering
AJ	Part-time catering assistantt	Cooking	
WK	Unemployed	General assistant in hologram firm	Computer work
SOP	Unemployed	Gardening	Gardening
DS	Engineering storekeeper	Office work*	Civil Service
RJ	Clothing factory: brusher-off		
WI	Student—degree course		
FJ	Part-time kitchen assistant	Care assistant Kitchen assistant*	
HS	Student—catering course		
STP	Student—degree course		
EI	Unemployed		
MS	Greengrocery assistant	Painting	Greengrocer
PJ	Part-time catering assistant	Catering	Child-care work
SB	Fibreglass moulder	Fibreglass moulding*	
TP	Garden ornament painter	Painting*	
AJJ	Vehicle recovery driver		Long-distance HGV driver
BB	Building labourer (temp.)	Gardening	Car mechanic
GS	Kitchen assistant	Kitchen assistant*	
SS	Soap packer		
SN	Student—degree course		
TM	Unemployed	Warehouseman Apprentice jockey	Outdoor work
CK	Livestock farming		
PT	Market trader		
BP	Cabinet maker		
DW	Clerical work	Clerical work*	
WE	Catering assistant (temp.)		

Youth training includes government sponsored and local schemes
*Training led directly to present job

advertisement (3), own initiative (2), school (1), college (1), disablement training office (1), and local training service (1). Table 7.XXIV compares the type of employment being undertaken and diagnostic category in school. In terms of socio-economic status the highest achievers come from the Speech, Moderate and Residual categories, and the lowest achievers from the Classic, Speech Plus and No Language groups.

There were very different levels of job satisfaction expressed by individual reports.

TABLE 7.XXIII

Socio-economic status of the ex-pupils and their families

Groups	Families	Subjects
Top professional	4	0
Managerial	3	1
Skilled non-manual	3	2
Skilled manual	17	5
Partly skilled	6	9
Unskilled	1	8
Unemployed	0	5
(Students)	0	4
Total	34	34

Difference between manual and non-manual groups NS

TABLE 7.XXIV

Jobs by language subgroup

Speech			TP	Garden ornament painter
DS	Engineering storekeeper		CK	Livestock farming
STP	Student—degree course		WE	Catering assistant (temp.)
DW	Clerical work		*Semantic*	
PT	Market trader		SC	Classroom aide
Speech Plus			WK	Unemployed
LT	Building labourer		WI	Student—degree course
SS	Soap packer		BB	Building labourer (temp.)
TM	Unemployed		*Residual*	
Classic			EI	Unemployed
NA	Nurseryman		AJJ	Vehicle recovery driver
EM	Bar work		SN	Student—degree course
LAS	Gardening		*Moderate*	
LES	Kitchen porter		MI	Electrician
WP	Unemployed		PA	Crane driver
AJ	Part-time catering assistant		BP	Cabinet maker
RJ	Brusher-off in clothing factory		*No Language*	
FJ	Part-time kitchen assistant		SOP	Unemployed
HS	Student—catering course		SB	Fibreglass moulder
MS	Greengrocery assistant		GS	Kitchen assistant
PJ	Part-time catering assistant			

Ruth (RJ) was a member of the Classic subgroup and had a good outcome. She had aberrant social behaviour while at Dawn House and had previously attended a school for children with language and emotional problems. Her antisocial behaviour diminished while at Dawn House but she remained a loner. After Dawn House she went to a mainstream school and then to a college of further education, where she was very happy studying lettering and graphics. She longs for a job in the art world, but has an unskilled factory job.

265

Paul (PT) was a member of the Speech subgroup. His outcome was judged to be fair as he had continuing moderate speech and written language difficulties. However, he obtained seven CSE passes at the comprehensive school he went to when he was 11.4. After leaving school he had two industrial jobs (injection moulding and vehicle body-building) which he did not enjoy. He and his brother are now self-employed and have been running a stall on the local market for over two years. He seems to be successful and is very happy in his work.

Warren (WK) has been described before as the exemplar of the Semantic subgroup. His outcome was good. He is not currently employed and not actively seeking work. He hopes to work eventually with computers. He feels rather disillusioned with life, convinced that in the several jobs that he started he was relegated to the lowest level of chores while less able lads obtained advancement. We can only say that Warren did show considerable ability at Dawn House, but that this could be masked if he still makes some odd semantic errors.

Sara (SS) was in the Speech Plus group, and her outcome grade was poor. From Dawn House she went to another language school because she still had language, speech and reading problems. Being of a happy and gregarious nature, she seemed undeterred by her problems. After a year's work on a Youth Training Scheme, she found a permanent packing job in the same local factory as her mother. She likes working there and does not want to change her job.

Carl (CK) benefited from his life on the family farm which meant that he had been training for his career since he was about three years old! A member of the Classic subgroup, his outcome had been poor with continuing serious problems with speech and written language. He had enough ability to take him from school to agricultural centre where he gained some further practical skills. He went on to work on a number of local farms. He now breeds and manages stock on his own account, reads the farming papers and has friends in the close local community. Carl is enthusiastic about his work and his life.

Peter (PA), who was in the Moderate subgroup, left Dawn House with a good outcome. He finished comprehensive school with seven CSE passes and went to work as a technician in an electronics laboratory, gaining a City and Guilds qualification in electrical engineering on day release. He was made redundant and now works as a crane driver, but hopes to return eventually to some sort of work in electrical engineering.

Sam (SB) was a Landau-Kleffner syndrome boy in the No Speech group, and had a poor outcome. He passed one CSE at his final language school, and gained some experience of repairing boats. This led to a Youth Training Scheme placement and eventually a permanent job in fibreglass moulding. He is glad to have work and is not looking for change.

Residual problems, social life and leisure activities
REMAINING LANGUAGE PROBLEMS

Only three young people or their parents considered that there were no residual

TABLE 7.XXV

Residual language difficulties by original subgroup of SLI

Language subgroup	N	Comprehension	Expression	Speech	Reading	Writing	Spelling
Speech	4	0	2	4	0	1	3
Speech Plus	3	1 (2)	2	1	0	1	3
Classic	14	5 (6)	9	8 (9)	7 (8)	9	8
Semantic	4	2	1	2 (3)	1	1	2
Residual	3	2	2	2	1	2	2
Moderate	3	1	1	2	0	1	2
No Language	3	3	2	3	3	2	1
Total		14 (16)	19	22 (24)	12 (13)	17	21

Numbers in brackets indicate a different report from subject and parent

problems with spoken or written language. One of these, LAS, had previously been classified as having a Classic language impairment. Although he considered that he had no further difficulty, the interviewer still found his speech unclear and a little hard to understand, but LAS himself did not perceive this as a problem. MI also reported no difficulties. His problems at school entry had been classed as Moderate, being mainly problems of written language. He had left Dawn House at the age of 10 and had gone on to pass three GCE o-levels and seven CSEs. One of the Semantic group, WI, also reported no further problems with spoken or written language. At the time of the survey, he was one of the students pursuing a degree course at university. The other 31 ex-pupils all reported numerous continuing difficulties (Table 7.XXV). The level of reported difficulties in 90 per cent of young people between the ages of 18 and 22 is very high; higher than the level reported by Hall and Tomblin (1978), half of whose 18 SLI 20-year-olds had communication problems, or by King et al. (1982), who found that 42 per cent of 50 subjects aged between 14 and 20 continued to have communication problems. Both of these studies relied on parental report, the former a written questionnaire and the latter, like the present study, a telephone interview. The different levels of continuing disability may directly relate to different subject groups. Criteria for selection given by Hall and Tomblin (1978) indicate a less severely disabled population than that at Dawn House. King et al. (1982) did not specify the original entry criteria for their subjects, but they suggested that their subjects might be less severely affected than those who attended a sister school to Dawn House with similar selection criteria, described by Griffiths (1969).

Since these are subjective reports, not objective assessments, it is possible that our ex-pupils had a heightened awareness of their disability and were unduly self-critical. However, whenever the reports of subjects and parents differed, the parents always noted more problems than the young people did themselves. King et al. (1982) reported a parental perception of 42 per cent continuing communication problems. They also asked parents how many of their young people would classify themselves as still communication-disabled. This elicited the reduced figure of 24 per cent. It seems that young adults are more likely to play down than to exaggerate their problems. We have no estimate of the severity of the problems reported by our subjects; many may be slight. Problems identified by the young people include the pronunciation of 'big words' (AJ), and difficulty filling in forms and using the phone (LT). One subject (HS) wryly suggested, 'Some people think—that guy sounds a little odd'. Another (DS) was said to have difficulty following films. Even if some of the difficulties are relatively minor, the fact that they are perceived as disabilities could have deleterious effects on self-confidence and social skills, and thence on employment opportunities. In a single case study of a 16-year-old boy with a history of language problems, Weiner (1974) concluded that residual deficits in speech and language skills had adversely affected his communication, educational achievement and social adjustment.

LIVING CONDITIONS

Most of the young people, 29, were still living under the parental roof. Two full-time students were in university accommodation, the third shared a flat. One boy lived near home with relatives, and one girl whose parents had moved abroad lived with family friends. Two youngsters had tried independent living but had returned to their parents' homes, one because he was lonely, one for financial reasons. The picture is one of continuing dependence.

FRIENDSHIPS

To some extent this dependence is echoed in the description of social activities, where family support and involvement are still important. Although 20 of the group said that they went out regularly with friends, 14 others went out only rarely and nine of these had only family friends. FJ's mother described her daughter as having only middle-aged friends, while WE, aged 18, was said to associate only with younger lads. Another young man (SB), who had a severe communication impairment, went to the pub with much older men who accepted him and made few demands on him conversationally. Only seven had particular friends of the opposite sex at the time of the survey. There was a difference in the replies of parents and subjects to a question about social problems. When young people were asked if they had any difficulties making and meeting friends, only two out of 17 reported general social problems and one lad 'found females difficult'. When the same question was asked of parents, 13 out of 21 reported problems, expressing considerable concern over social isolation. Two parents contradicted what the young person had previously reported. This was overridingly the area of greatest concern to parents.

LEISURE AND HOBBIES

Hobbies and leisure interests can make life generally more fulfilling and are also one way of making social contacts. We divided the reported leisure interests into

TABLE 7.XXVI

Leisure interests of 34 ex-students

Home-based (N 13)	Outside home (N 7)	Social (N 13)
Television (6)	Walking (3)	Snooker (3)
Gardening (4)	Driving (3)	Playing football (2)
Reading (4)	Motorcycling (2)	Playing tennis (2)
Cooking (3)	Cycling (2)	Sports club (2)
Pop music (2)	Swimming	Badminton
Knitting (2)	Running	Teaching swimming
Painting (2)	Fishing	Ballroom dancing
Tinkering with cars (2)	Weight training	Playing in youth band
Collecting coins	Watching football matches	Chess
Collecting stamps	Watching stock-car races	Bell-ringing
Model trains	Visiting churches	Darts
Plastic modelling		First-aid group
Writing computer games		St John's Ambulance group
Tapestry		Bingo
Breeding chickens		Nightclubs with friends
		Political club
		Radio car club
		Pub with friends (2)

three categories, those which can be undertaken alone and at home, those which take place outside the house but which can still be solitary, and those which normally require the participation of others. The individual hobbies are listed in Table 7.XXVI. There seems to be a normally wide range of leisure pursuits; only one young man who was having some emotional difficulties had no hobbies. However 13 of the youngsters had only hobbies which were home-based, and a further seven had additionally only hobbies which did not require companions. Three parents commented that unless they took an initiative the young people were unlikely to become involved in any activity.

SOCIAL PROBLEMS

The social problems reported by 14 families may be an underestimate in view of the tendency of subjects to report no difficulties. Social problems must certainly be taken seriously. We considered factors other than communication difficulty that might be influencing this outcome, *e.g.* separation from home to attend boarding school in childhood, gender, and general immaturity. When the 14 subjects with reported difficulties were compared with the 13 who went out most frequently with friends of their own age and/or had sociable leisure interests, no differences were found in these areas (Table 7.XXVII). We then looked at behaviours measured during their stay at Dawn House, to see if any indicated a future social difficulty (Table 7.XXVIII). Of the five behaviours we considered—peer relationships, solitariness, confidence, attitude to communication and coping with difficulties—the one that best separated the two extreme groups was attitude to

TABLE 7.XXVII

Social difficulties, gender, age and residential schooling

| | Boarding | | Day | Mean age | Gender | |
	Dawn House	(Post Dawn House)			Boys	Girls
Social problems (N 14)	12	(4)	2	19.7	10	4
Social success (N 13)	11	(2)	2	18.8	9	4

No differences

TABLE 7.XXVIII

Later social difficulties and behaviour at school

| | | | Problems at Dawn House | | |
	Peer relations	Solitariness	Confidence	Attitude to communication	Coping with difficulties
Social problems (N 14)	3	2	10	7*	10
Social success (N 13)	1	1	10	0*	8

*Binomial test, P = Q = 0.5, p<0.01

TABLE 7.XXIX

Language subgroups and later social problems

	Speech	Speech Plus	Classic	Semantic	Residual	Moderate	No Language
Social problems (N 14)	0	0	9	1	1	1	2
Social success (N 13)	3	2	3	2	1	2	0

communication (p = 0.008, binomial test). This is interesting especially as similar numbers of children—six in the socially successful group and five in the problem group—had had marked intelligibility problems. When Schery (1985) looked for indicators of good progress in 718 Los Angeles children, she found that one of the better predictors of gain was the child's socio-emotional status. Those children in our study who do not let their speech and language difficulties stand in the way of communicating may have a great advantage.

Finally, we considered whether better or worse social skills were associated with subgroups of language impairment (Table 7.XXIX). The numbers are small but suggestive of long-term social problems being associated with language rather than speech impairments, and as one would expect, with severe rather than moderate communication disability.

Summary of follow-up

Language impairment, in its severest manifestations, is a life-long problem. None of our ex-pupils is free from some difficulty with spoken or written language or social consequence, even though some of the problems are now relatively minor.

Although these problems interfere directly with learning and education, SLI children who are given intensive and appropriate help can go on to make considerable achievements.

With adequate help, a small percentage may reach high academic levels. Many others can attain reasonable educational success and have the satisfaction of achieving their full potential, although in many cases learning and reading will never bring much pleasure.

Judgement of oneself as an adequate person, and full mastery of language, are not easy to disentangle. It is difficult to retain high self-esteem if one cannot fully understand the import of what is said, and cannot express feelings and share ideas with others adequately. None of the youngsters with predominantly speech problems, some of whose difficulties remained severe, figured in the list of those with major social problems. These problems are caused by impairment of the subtleties of *language*, and society needs to recognise how much of a disability this is.

This study has emphasised not only the severity and persistence of problems in SLI, but also the possible achievements that can be made in the face of great odds. In a fair society, wider recognition of the nature and extent of this disabling condition and an awareness of the questions which remain to be answered must lead to improved funding for continuing research, and to adequate long-term educational and therapeutic provision being accepted as a basic human right for all language-impaired individuals.

REFERENCES

Abberton, E. (1980) 'Diagnostic implications of phonological analysis.' *ICAA Conference: The Assessment and Remediation of Specific Language Disorders.* London: I CAN.

Ajuriaguerra, J. de, Jaeggi, A., Guignard, F., Kocher, F., Maquard, M., Roth, S., Schmid, E. (1976) 'The development and prognosis of dysphasia in children.' *In* Morehead, D. M., Morehead, A. E. (Eds) *Normal and Deficient Child Language.* Baltimore, MD: University Park Press.

Alekoumbides, A. (1978) 'Hemisphere dominance for language: quantitative aspects.' *Acta Neurologica Scandinavica,* **57**, 97–140.

Allen, D., Rapin, I. (1980) 'Language disorders in preschool children: predictors of outcome—a preliminary report.' *Brain and Development,* **2**, 73–80.

Annett, M. (1967) 'The binomial distribution of right, left and mixed handedness.' *Quarterly Journal of Experimental Psychology,* **29**, 327–333.

—— (1970) 'The growth of manual preference and speed.' *British Journal of Psychology,* **61**, 545–558.

—— Turner, A. (1974) 'Laterality and the growth of intellectual abilities.' *British Journal of Educational Psychology,* **44**, 37–46.

Aram, D., Nation, J. (1975) 'Patterns of language behavior in children with developmental language disorders.' *Journal of Speech and Hearing Research,* **18**, 229–241.

—— —— (1980) 'Preschool language disorders and subsequent language and academic difficulties.' *Journal of Communication Disorders,* **13**, 159–170.

—— Ekelman, B., Nation, J.E. (1984) 'Preschoolers with language disorders: 10 years later.' *Journal of Speech and Hearing Research,* **27**, 232–244.

Babson, G.S., Behrman, R.E., Lessel, R. (1970) 'Fetal growth: live born birth weights for gestational age of white middle class infants.' *Pediatrics,* **45**, 937–944.

Baddeley, A.D. (1978) 'Working memory and reading.' *In* Kolers, P. A., Wrolstad, M.E., Bouma, H. (Eds) *Processing of Visible Language. Vol. 1.* New York: Plenum Press.

—— (1986) *Working Memory. Oxford Psychological Series 11.* Oxford: Oxford University Press.

Baginsky, M. (1991) *Vocational Education Opportunities for Students with Specific Speech and Language Impairment.* Slough: NFER.

Baker, L., Cantwell, D.P. (1982) 'Language acquisition, cognitive development and emotional disorder in childhood.' *In* Nelson, K.E. (Ed.) *Children's Language, Vol. 3.* Hillsdale, NJ: Lawrence Erlbaum.

Barron, R.W., Baron, J. (1977) 'How children get meaning from printed words.' *Child Development,* **48**, 587–594.

Barton, D. (1976) *The Role of Perception in the Acquisition of Speech.* University of London: PhD thesis.

—— (1978) 'The discrimination of minimally different pairs of real words by children aged 2.3 to 2.11.' *In* Waterson, N., Snow, C. (Eds) *The Development of Communication.* Chichester: Wiley.

Bax, M. (1987) 'Paediatric assessment of the child with a speech and language disorder.' *In* Yule, W., Rutter, M. (Eds) *Language Development and Disorders. Clinics in Developmental Medicine, Nos 101/102.* London: Mac Keith Press with Blackwell Scientific; Philadelphia: J.B. Lippincott.

—— Hart, H., Jenkins, S. (1983) 'The behaviour, development and health of the young child: implications for care.' *British Medical Journal,* **286**, 1793–1796.

Baynes, K., Gazzaniga, M.S. (1988) 'Right hemisphere language: insights into normal language mechanisms.' *In* Plum, F. (Ed.) *Language Communication and the Brain.* New York: Raven Press.

Beardsley, G. (1982) 'Context cues in early reading.' *Journal of Research in Reading,* **5**, 101–112.

Beaton, A. (1985) *Left Side, Right Side: A Review of Laterality Research.* London: Batsford Academic and Educational.

Beaumanoir, A. (1985) 'The Landau-Kleffner Syndrome.' *In* Roger, J., Dravet, C., Bureau, M., Dreifuss, F.E., Wolf, P. (Eds) *Epileptic Syndromes in Infancy, Childhood and Adolescence.* London: John Libbey.

Belmont, L., Birch, H.G. (1965) 'Lateral dominance, lateral awareness and reading disability.' *Child Development,* **36**, 57–71.

272

—— Marolla, F. (1973) 'Birth order, family size, and intelligence.' *Science*, **182**, 1096–1101.
Bennett, F.C., Ruuska, S.H., Sherman, R. (1980) 'Middle ear functioning in learning disabled children.' *Pediatrics*, **66**, 254–260.
Benton, A.L. (1964) 'Developmental asphasia and brain damage.' *Cortex*, **1**, 40–52.
Bernstein, B. (1961) 'Social structure, language and learning.' *Educational Research*, **3**, 163–176.
—— (1965) 'A socio-linguistic approach to social learning.' *In* Gould, J. (Ed.) *Penguin Survey of the Social Sciences*. London: Penguin.
Biemiller, A. (1970) 'The development of the use of graphic and contextual information as children learn to read.' *Reading Research Quarterly*, **6**, 75–96.
Bishop, D.V.M. (1980*a*) 'Handedness, clumsiness and cognitive ability.' *Developmental Medicine and Child Neurology*, **22**, 569–579.
—— (1980*b*) 'Measuring familial sinistrality.' *Cortex*, **16**, 311–313.
—— (1983) 'How sinister is sinistrality?' *Journal of the Royal College of Physicians of London*, **17**, 161–172.
—— (1984) 'Using non-preferred hand skill to investigate pathological left-handedness in an unselected population.' *Developmental Medicine and Child Neurology*, **26**, 214–226.
—— (1987) 'The causes of specific developmental language disorder ("developmental dysphasia").' *Journal of Child Psychology and Psychiatry*, **28**, 1–8.
—— (1990) *Handedness and Developmental Disorder. Clinics in Developmental Medicine, No. 110.* London: Mac Keith Press with Blackwell Scientific; Philadelphia: J.B. Lippincott.
—— Butterworth, G.E. (1979) 'A longitudinal study using the WPPSI and WISC-R with an English sample.' *British Journal of Educational Psychology*, **49**, 1–13.
—— —— (1980) 'Verbal-performance discrepancies: relationship to birth risk and specific reading retardation.' *Cortex*, **16**, 375–389.
—— Edmundson, A. (1986) 'Is otitis media a major cause of specific developmental language disorders?' *British Journal of Disorders of Communication*, **21**, 321–338.
—— —— (1987*a*) 'Language impaired 4-year-olds: distinguishing transient from persistent impairment.' *Journal of Speech and Hearing Disorders*, **52**, 156–173.
—— —— (1987*b*) 'Specific language impairment as a maturational lag: evidence from longitudinal data on language and motor development.' *Developmental Medicine and Child Neurology*, **29**, 442–459.
—— Rosenbloom, L. (1987) 'Childhood language disorders, classification and overview.' *In* Yule, W., Rutter, M. (Eds) *Language Development and Disorders. Clinics in Developmental Medicine, Nos 101/102.* London: Mac Keith Press with Blackwell Scientific; Philadelphia: J.B. Lippincott.
—— Robson, J. (1989) 'Unimpaired short-term memory and rhyme judgement in congenitally speechless individuals: implications for the notion of "articulatory coding".' *Quarterly Journal of Experimental Psychology*, **41a**, 123–140.
—— Adams, C. (1990) 'A prospective study of the relationship between specific language impairment, phonological disorders and reading retardation.' *Journal of Child Psychology and Psychiatry*, **31**, 1027–1050.
Bradley, L., Bryant, P. (1978) 'Difficulties in auditory organisation as a possible cause of reading'. *Nature*, **271**, 746–7.
—— —— (1983) 'Categorising sounds and learning to read: a causal connexion.' *Nature*, **301**, 419–421.
—— —— (1985) *Rhyme and Reason in Reading and Spelling.* Ann Arbor: University of Michigan Press.
Bradshaw, J.L., Nettleton, N.C. (1983) *Human Cerebral Asymmetry.* New Jersey: Prentice-Hall.
Breznitz, Z., Friedman, S.L. (1988) 'Toddlers' concentration: does maternal depression make a difference?' *Journal of Child Psychology and Psychiatry*, **29**, 267–279.
Brown, R. (1973) *A First Language.* Cambridge, MA: Harvard University Press.
—— Lenneberg, E.H. (1954) 'A study in language and cognition.' *Journal of Abnormal Social Psychology*, **49**, 454–462.
—— Fraser, C. (1963) 'The acquisition of syntax.' *In* Cofer, C.N., Musgrave, B. (Eds) *Verbal Behaviour and Learning.* New York: McGraw-Hill.
Bruner, J.S. (1964) 'The course of cognitive growth.' *Journal of American Psychology*, **19**, 1–15.
Bryant, P.E., Bradley, L. (1980) 'Why children sometimes write words which they do not read.' *In* Frith, U. (Ed.) *Cognitive Processes in Spelling.* London: Academic Press.
Bryden, M.P. (1982) *Laterality.* New York: Academic Press.
Burt, C. (1937) *The Backward Child.* London: University of London Press.

Butler, N.R., Bonham, D.G. (1963) *Perinatal Mortality*. Edinburgh: E. & S. Livingstone.
—— Alberman, E.D. (1969) *Perinatal Problems*. Edinburgh: E. & S. Livingstone.
—— Peckham, C., Sheridan, M. (1973) 'Speech defects in children aged 7 years: a national study.' *British Medical Journal*, **1**, 253–257.
—— Golding, J. (1986) *From Birth to Five*. Oxford: Pergamon Press.
Cantwell, D.P., Baker, L. (1977) 'Psychiatric disorder in children with speech and language retardation: a critical review.' *Archives of General Psychology*, **34**, 583–591.
—— —— Mattison, R.E. (1979) 'The prevalence of psychiatric disorder in children with speech and language disorder.' *Journal of the American Academy of Child Psychiatry*, **18**, 450–461.
Carey, S. (1978) 'The child as word learner.' *In* Halle, M., Bresnan, J., Miller, G.A. (Eds) *Linguistic Theory and Psychological Reality*. Cambridge, MA: MIT Press.
Case, R., Kurland, D.M., Goldberg, J. (1982) 'Operational efficiency and the growth of short-term memory span.' *Journal of Experimental Child Psychology*, **33**, 386–404.
Cataldo, S., Ellis, N.C., (1988) 'Interactions in the development of spelling, reading and phonological skills.' *Journal of Research in Reading*, **11**, 86–109.
—— —— (1989) 'Learning to spell, learning to read.' *In* Pumphrey, P.D., Elliott, C.D. (Eds) *Primary School Pupils' Reading and Spelling Difficulties: Current Research and Practice*. Basingstoke: Falmer Press.
Chalmers, D., Stewart, I., Silva, P., Mulvena, A. (1989) *Otitis Media with Effusion in Children—the Dunedin Study. Clinics in Developmental Medicine, No. 108*. London: Mac Keith Press with Blackwell Scientific; Philadelphia: J.B. Lippincott.
Chi, M.T.H. (1976) 'Short-term memory limitations in children: capacity or processing deficits?' *Memory and Cognition*, **4**, 559–572.
Clark, M.M. (1957) *Left-Handedness*. London: University of London Press.
—— (1970) *Reading Difficulties in Schools*. Harmondsworth: Penguin.
Clegg, C.W., Jackson, P.R., Wall, T.D. (1977) 'The potential of cross-lagged correlation analysis in field research.' *Journal of Occupational Psychology*, **50**, 177–196.
Clymer, P.E., Silva, P.A. (1985) 'Laterality, cognitive ability and motor performance in a sample of seven year olds.' *Journal of Human Studies*, **11**, 59–68.
Colby, K.M., Parkinson, C. (1977) 'Handedness in autistic children.' *Journal of Autism and Childhood Schizophrenia*, **7**, 3–9.
Coleman, R., Deutsch, C. (1964) 'Lateral dominance and left-right discrimination: a comparison of normal and retarded readers.' *Perceptual and Motor Skills*, **19**, 43–50.
Connolly, K., Bishop, D.V.M. (1991) 'The measurement of handedness: a cross-cultural perspective.' (*Submitted for publication.*)
Conrad, R. (1970) 'Short-term memory processes in the deaf.' *British Journal of Psychology*, **61**, 179–195.
Cotterell, G. (1970) 'The dyslexic child at home and at school.' *In* Franklin, A.W., Naidoo, S. (Eds) *Assessment and Teaching of Dyslexic Children*. London: I CAN.
Cox, A.D., Puckering, C., Pound, A., Mills, M. (1987) 'The impact of maternal depression in young children.' *Journal of Child Psychology and Psychiatry*, **28**, 917–928.
Crider, B. (1935) 'Unilateral sighting preference.' *Child Development*, **6**, No. 2.
Cromer, R.F. (1974) 'The development of language and cognition: the condition hypothesis.' *In* Foss, B.M. (Ed.) *New Perspectives in Child Development*. Harmondsworth: Penguin.
Crystal, D. (1976) *Child Language, Learning and Linguistics*. London: Edward Arnold.
—— (1979) *Working with LARSP*. London: Edward Arnold.
—— (1986) 'Prosodic development.' *In* Fletcher, P., Garman, M. (Eds) *Language Acquisition, 2nd Edn*. Cambridge: Cambridge University Press.
—— (1987) *Clinical Linguistics*. London: Edward Arnold.
Cuff, N.B. (1931) 'A study of eyedness and handedness.' *Journal of Experimental Psychology*, **14**, 164.
Dalzell, J., Owrid, H.L. (1976) 'Children with conductive deafness: a follow-up study.' *British Journal of Audiology*, **10**, 87–90.
Davie, R., Butler, N., Goldstein, H. (1972) *From Birth to Seven*. London: Longman.
Davis, J.M., Elfenbeim, J., Schum, R., Bentler, R.A. (1986) 'Effects of mild and moderate hearing impairments on language, educational and psychosocial behaviour of children.' *Journal of Speech and Hearing Disorders*, **51**, 53–62.

Dempster, F.N. (1981) 'Memory span: sources of individual and developmental differences.' *Psychological Bulletin*, **89**, 63–100.

Donaldson, M. (1978) *Children's Minds.* Glasgow: Fontana/Collins.

Douglas, J.W.B. (1964) *The Home and the School.* London: McGibbon & Kee.

—— Blomfield, J.M. (1958) *Children under Five.* London: Allen and Unwin.

Downs, M. (1981) 'Contribution of mild hearing loss to auditory language learning problems.' *In* Roeser, R.J., Downs, M. (Eds) *Auditory Disorders in Schoolchildren: the Law, Identification and Remediation.* New York: Thieme-Stratton.

Drillien, C., Drummond, M. (1983) *Developmental Screening in the Child with Special Needs in a Population Study. Clinics in Developmental Medicine, No. 86.* London: SIMP with Heinemann; Philadelphia: J.B. Lippincott.

Edwards, M.L. (1974) 'Perception and production in child phonology: the testing of four hypotheses.' *Journal of Child Language*, **1**, 205–219.

Eilers, R.E., Oller, D. (1976) 'The role of speech discrimination in developmental sound substitutes.' *Journal of Child Language*, **3**, 319–330.

Elliot, A.J. (1981) *Child Language.* Cambridge: Cambridge University Press.

Eisenson, J. (1984) *Aphasia and Related Disorders in Children, 2nd Edn.* New York: Harper and Row.

Ellis, N.C. (1981) 'Visual and name coding in dyslexic children.' *Psychological Research*, **43**, 201–218.

—— (1989) 'Reading, phonological skills and short-term memory: interactive tributaries of development.' *Journal of Research in Reading*, **13**, 107–122.

—— Large, B. (1988) 'The early stages of reading: a longitudinal study.' *Applied Cognitive Psychology*, **2**, 47–76.

Ellis, R.W.B., Mitchell, R.G. (1968) *Disease in Infancy and Childhood.* Edinburgh: E. & S. Livingstone.

Entus, A.K. (1977) 'Hemispheric asymmetry in processing of dichotically presented speech and non-speech stimuli by infants.' *In* Segalowitz, S.J., Gruber, F.A. (Eds) *Language Development and Neurological Theory.* New York: Academic Press.

Ervin-Tripp, S. (1973) 'Some strategies for the first two years.' *In* Moore, T.E. (Ed.) *Cognitive Development and the Acquisition of Language.* London: Academic Press.

Essen, J., Peckham, C. (1976) 'Nocturnal enuresis in childhood.' *Developmental Medicine and Child Neurology*, **18**, 577–589.

Ferguson, C.E., Farwell, C.B. (1975) 'Words and sounds in early language acquisition.' *Language*, **51**, 419–439.

Fischel, J.E., Grover, J.W., Whitehurst, J., Caulfield, M.B., DeBaryshe, B. (1989) 'Language growth in children with expressive language delay.' *Pediatrics*, **82**, 218–227.

Fischler, R.S., Todd, N.W., Feldman, M.C. (1985) 'Otitis media and language performance in a cohort of Apache Indian children.' *American Journal of Diseases of Children*, **139**, 355–360.

Fletcher, P. (1986) 'Characterising language impairment in terms of normal language development: advantages and limitations.' Paper presented at the *Symposium on Research in Child Language Disorders*, University of Wisconsin, Madison.

—— Garman, M. (1986) *Language Acquisition, 2nd Edn.* Cambridge: Cambridge University Press.

Fogelman, K. (1983) *Growing up in Great Britain.* London: Macmillan.

Forfar, J.O., Arneil, G.C. (1978) *Textbook of Paediatrics, 2nd Edn.* Edinburgh: Churchill Livingstone.

Francis, H. (1984) 'Children's knowledge of orthography in learning to read.' *British Journal of Educational Psychology*, **54**, 8–23.

Freeman, B.A., Parkins, C. (1979) 'The prevalence of middle ear disease among learning impaired children.' *Clinical Pediatrics*, **18**, 205–212.

Friedrich, U., Dalby, M., Staehelin-Jensen, T., Bruun-Petersen, G. (1982) 'Chromosomal studies in children with developmental speech retardation.' *Developmental Medicine and Child Neurology*, **24**, 645–652.

Friel-Patti, S., Finitzo-Heiber, T., Conti, G., Brown, K.C. (1982) 'Language delay in infants associated with middle ear disease and mild, fluctuating hearing impairment.' *Pediatric Infectious Diseases*, **1**, 104–109.

Fundudis, T., Kolvin, I., Garside, G. (1979) *Speech Retarded and Deaf Children: Their Psychological Development.* London: Academic Press.

Furukawa, C. (1988) 'Conductive hearing loss and speech development.' *Journal of Allergy and Clinical Immunology*, **81**, 1015–1020.

Garvey, M., Gordon, N. (1973) 'A follow-up study of children with disorders of speech development.' *British Journal of Disorders of Communication*, **8**, 17–28.

Gathercole, S., Baddeley, A. (1990a) 'Phonological memory deficits in language disordered children: is there a causal connection?' *Journal of Memory and Language*, **29**, 1–25.

—— —— (1990b) 'The role of phonological memory in vocabulary acquisition: a study of young children learning new names.' *British Journal of Psychology*, **84**, 439–454.

Gaudena, A. (1982) 'The social nature of private speech of preschoolers during problem solving.' *International Journal of Behavioural Development*, **40**, (2).

Gesell, A., Ames, L.B. (1947) 'The development of handedness.' *Journal of Genetic Psychology*, **70**, 155–175.

Golding, J., Butler, N.R. (1986a) 'The first months.' *In* Butler, N.R., Golding, J. (Eds) *From Birth to Five*. Oxford: Pergamon Press.

—— —— (1986b) 'Sore throats, ear discharge and mouth breathing.' *In* Butler, N.R., Golding, J. (Eds) *From Birth to Five*. Oxford: Pergamon Press.

—— —— (1986c) 'Squints and vision defects.' *In* Butler, N.R., Golding, J. (Eds) *From Birth to Five*. Oxford: Pergamon Press.

—— Rush, D. (1986) 'Temper tantrums and other behaviour problems.' *In* Butler, N.R., Golding, J. (Eds) *From Birth to Five*. Oxford: Pergamon Press.

—— Tissier, G. (1986) 'Soiling and wetting.' *In* Butler, N.R., Golding, J. (Eds) *From Birth to Five*. Oxford: Pergamon Press.

Goodman, R. (1987) 'The developmental neurobiology of language.' *In* Yule, W., Rutter, M. (Eds) *Language Development and Disorders. Clinics in Developmental Medicine, Nos 101/102.* London: Mac Keith Press with Blackwell Scientific; Philadelphia: J.B. Lippincott.

Gordon, A.G. (1988) 'Some comments on Bishop's annotation "Developmental dysphasia and otitis media".' *Journal of Child Psychology and Psychiatry*, **29**, 361–363.

Gottlieb, M.I., Zinkus, P.W., Thompson, A. (1979) 'Chronic middle ear disease and auditory perceptual deficits.' *Clinical Pediatrics*, **18**, 725–732.

Graham, N. (1980) 'Memory constraints in language deficiency.' *In* Jones, F. M. (Ed.) *Language Disability in Children*. Baltimore, MD: University Park Press.

Greene, J. (1972) *Psycholinguistics: Chomsky and Psychology*. Harmondsworth: Penguin.

Griffiths, C.P.S. (1969) 'A follow-up study of children with disorders of speech.' *British Journal of Disorders of Communication*, **4**, 46–56.

Grunwell, P. (1975) 'The phonological analysis of articulation disorders.' *British Journal of Disorders of Communication*, **10**, 31–42.

—— (1981) *The Nature of Phonological Disability in Children*. London: Academic Press.

—— (1982) *Clinical Phonology*. London: Croom Helm.

—— (1985) *Phonological Assessment of Child Speech (PACS)*. Windsor: NFER-Nelson.

Gubbay, S.S. (1975) *The Clumsy Child*. Philadelphia: W. B. Saunders.

Hadders-Algra, M., Touwen, B.C.L., Huisjes, H.C. (1986) 'Neurologically deviant newborns: neurological and behavioural development at the age of six years.' *Developmental Medicine and Child Neurology*, **28**, 569–578.

Haggard, M., Hughes, E. (1990) 'Objectives, value and methods of screening children's hearing – a review of the literature.' *IHR Internal Report Series A (4)*. London: HMSO.

Haggerty, R., Stamm, J.S. (1978) 'Dichotic auditory fusion levels in children with learning difficulties.' *Neuropsychologia*, **16**, 349–360.

Halperin, Y., Nachshon, I., Carmon, A. (1973) 'Shift of ear superiority in dichotic listening to temporally patterned nonverbal stimuli.' *Journal of the Acoustic Society of America*, **53**, 46–50.

Hall, D.M.B., Hill, P. (1986) 'When does secretory otitis media affect language development?' *Archives of Disease in Childhood*, **61**, 42–47

Hall, P.K., Tomblin, J.B. (1978) 'A follow-up study of children with articulation and language disorders.' *Journal of Speech and Hearing Disorders*, **43**, 227–241.

Harris, A.J. (1957) 'Lateral dominance, directional confusion and reading disability.' *Journal of Psychology*, **44**, 283–294.

—— (1958) *Harris Tests of Lateral Dominance*. New York: Psychological Corporation.

276

Haynes, C. (1982) *Vocabulary Acquisition Problems in Language Disordered Children*. University of London: MSc thesis.

Hecaen, H., Ajuriaguerra, J. de (1964) *Left-handedness*. New York: Grune and Stratton.

Hedderson, J. (1987) *SPSS-X Made Simple*. Belmont, CA: Wadsworth.

Hicks, R.E., Barton, A.K. (1975) 'A note on left-handedness and severity of mental retardation.' *Journal of Genetic Psychology*, **127**, 323–324.

Holm, V.A., Kunze, L.H. (1969) 'Effect of chronic otitis media on language and speech development.' *Pediatrics*, **43**, 833–839.

Holroyd, J. (1968) 'When WISC verbal IQ is low.' *Journal of Clinical Psychology*, **24**, 457.

Hulme, C., Thomson, N., Muir, C., Lawrence, A. (1984) 'Speech rate and the development of short-term memory span.' *Journal of Experimental Child Psychology*, **38**, 241–253.

Hutchison, D., Prosser, H., Wedge, P. (1979) 'The prediction of educational failure.' *Educational Studies*, **5**, 73–82.

Hutt, E., Donlan, C. (1987) *Adequate Provision? A Survey of Language Units*. London: I CAN.

Huttenlocher, J., Burke, D. (1972) 'Why does memory span increase with age?' *Cognitive Psychology*, **8**, 1–31.

Hyde-Wright, S., Cheesman, P. (1990) 'Teaching reading vocabulary to a language-delayed child.' *Child Language Teaching and Therapy*, **6**, 1–12.

I CAN (1987) *Language through Reading*. London: I CAN.

—— (1988) *Units for Primary School Children with Speech and Language Disorders*. London: I CAN.

Ingram, D. (1976) *Phonological Disability in Children*. London: Edward Arnold.

—— (1981) *Procedures for the Phonological Analysis of Children's Language*. Baltimore, MD: University Park Press.

Ingram, T.T.S. (1959) 'Specific developmental disorders of speech in childhood.' *Brain*, **82**, 450–467.

—— Reid, J.F. (1956) 'Developmental aphasia observed in a department of child psychiatry.' *Archives of Disease in Childhood*, **31**, 161–172.

Jensen, T.S., Boggild-Andersen, B., Schmidt, J., Ankerhus, J., Hansen, E. (1988) 'Perinatal risk factors and first-year vocalisations: influence on preschool language and motor performance.' *Developmental Medicine and Child Neurology*, **30**, 153–161.

Johnston, J.R. (1985) 'Fit, focus and functionality: an essay on early language intervention.' *Child Language, Teaching and Therapy*, **1**, 125–134.

Johnston, O. (1980) 'Ill health and developmental delays in Adelaide four-year-old children.' *Australian Paediatric Journal*, **16**, 248–254.

Johnston, R.B., Stark, R.E., Mellits, D., Tallal, P. (1981) 'Neurological status of language-impaired and normal children.' *Annals of Neurology*, **10**, 159–163.

Jorm, A.F., Share, D.L., MacLean, R., Matthews, R. (1986) 'Cognitive factors at school entry predictive of specific reading retardation and general reading backwardness: a research note.' *Journal of Child Psychology and Psychiatry*, **27**, 45–54.

Kahmi, A.G. (1985) 'Questioning the value of large N, multivariate studies: a response to Schery (1985).' *Journal of Speech and Hearing Disorders*, **50**, 288–289.

Kaufman, A.S. (1976) 'Verbal-performance IQ discrepancies on the WISC-R.' *Journal of Consulting and Clinical Psychology*, **44**, 739–744.

Kerr, A.I.G. (1984) 'Ear disorders; ear infections.' *The Physician*, **2**, 451–454.

Kimura, D. (1961) 'Cerebral dominance and the perception of verbal stimuli.' *Canadian Journal of Psychology*, **16**, 18–22.

—— (1967) 'Functional asymmetry of the brain in dichotic listening.' *Cortex*, **3**, 163–178.

King, R.R., Jones, C., Lasky, E. (1982) 'In retrospect: a fifteen year follow-up report of speech-language disordered children.' *Language, Speech and Hearing Services in Schools*, **13**, 24–32.

Kinsbourne, M. (1979) 'Language lateralisation and developmental disorders.' *In* Ludlow, C.L., Doran-Quine, M.E. (Eds) *The Neurological Bases of Language Disorders in Children: Methods and Directions for Research*. NINCDS Monograph No. 22.

Kirchner, D., Klatzky, R. (1985) 'Verbal rehearsal and memory in language disordered children.' *Journal of Speech and Hearing Research*, **28**, 556–565.

Klein, J.O. (1983) 'Epidemiology and natural history of otitis media.' *Pediatrics*, **71**, 639–640.

Laufer, M.Z. (1980) 'Temporal regularity in pre-speech.' *In* Murry, T., Murry, A. (Eds) *Infant Communication: Cry and Early Speech*. Houston: College Hill Press.

Lea, J. (1980) 'The association between rhythmic ability and language ability.' *In* Jones, F.M. (Ed.) *Language Disability in Children*. Lancaster: MTP Press.

Lehiste, I. (1972) 'The units of speech perception.' *In* Gilbert, J.H. (Ed.) *Speech and Cortical Functioning*. New York: Academic Press.

Lenneberg, E. (1976) *Biological Foundations of Language*. New York: Wiley.

Leonard, L. (1972) 'What is deviant language?' *Journal of Speech and Hearing Disorders*, **37**, 427–446.

Levi, G., Capozzi, F., Fabrizi, A., Sechi, E. (1982) 'Language disorders and prognosis for reading disabilities in developmental age.' *Perceptual and Motor Skills*, **54**, 1119–1122.

Lewis, N. (1976) 'Otitis media and linguistic incompetence.' *Archives of Otolaryngology*, **102**, 387–390.

Liberman, A.M., Cooper, F., Shankweiler, D.P., Studdert-Kennedy, M. (1967) 'Perception of the speech code.' *Psychological Review*, **74**, 431–461.

—— Mattingley, I.G. (1985) 'The motor theory of speech perception revised.' *Cognition*, **21**, 1–36.

Liles, B.Z., Watt, J.H. (1984) 'On the meaning of "language delay".' *Folia Phoniatrica*, **36**, 40–48.

Lindahl, E., Michelsson, K., Helenius, M., Parre, M. (1988) 'Neonatal risk factors and later neurodevelopmental disturbances.' *Developmental Medicine and Child Neurology*, **30**, 571–589.

Locke, J.L. (1969) 'Short-term memory, aural perception and experimental sound learning.' *Journal of Speech and Hearing Research*, **12**, 185–192.

—— Goldstein, J.I. (1971) 'Children's identification and discrimination of phonemes.' *British Journal of Disorders of Communication*, **6**, 107–112.

Lovell, K., Hoyle, H.W., Siddall, M.Q. (1968) 'A study of some aspects of the play and language of young children with delayed speech.' *Journal of Child Psychology and Psychiatry*, **9**, 41–50.

Low, J.A., Galbraith, R.S., Muir, D.W., Broekhoven, L.H., Wilkinson, J.W., Karchmer, E.J. (1985) 'The contribution of fetal-newborn complications to motor and cognitive deficits.' *Developmental Medicine and Child Neurology*, **27**, 578–587.

Lowe, A.D., Campbell, R.A. (1965) 'Temporal discrimination in aphasoid and normal children.' *Journal of Speech and Hearing Research*, **8**, 313–314.

Luchsinger, R. (1970) 'Inheritance of speech defects.' *Folia Phoniatrica*, **22**, 216–230.

Ludlow, C.L. (1980) 'Children's language disorders: recent research advances.' *Annals of Neurology*, **7**, 497–507.

Luick, A.H., Kirk, S.A., Agranowitz, A., Busby, R. (1982) 'Profiles of children with severe oral language disorders.' *Journal of Speech and Hearing Disorders*, **47**, 88–92.

Luria, A.R. (1966) *Higher Cortical Functions in Man*. New York: Basic.

—— Yudovich, F.I. (1956) *Speech in the Development of Mental Processes in the Child*. Harmondsworth: Penguin.

Lyons, J. (1972) *Chomsky*. London: Fontana/Collins.

McManus, I.C. (1985) *Handedness, Language Dominance and Aphasia: Genetic Model. Psychological Medicine; Monograph Supplement 8*. Cambridge: Cambridge University Press.

McReynolds, L.K. (1966) 'Operant conditioning for investigating speech sound discrimination in aphasic children.' *Journal of Speech and Hearing Research*, **9**, 519–528.

—— Kohn, J., Williams, G.C. (1975) 'Articulatory defective children's discrimination of their productive errors.' *Journal of Speech and Hearing Disorders*, **40**, 327–338.

Macken, M.A., Barton, D. (1980) 'The acquisition of the voicing contrast in English: the study of voice onset time in word-initial stop consonants.' *Journal of Child Language*, **7**, 41–74.

Mange, C.V. (1960) 'Relationships between selected auditory perceptual factors and articulation ability.' *Journal of Speech and Hearing Research*, **3**, 67–74.

Mann, V.A. (1984) 'Reading skill and language skill.' *Developmental Review*, **4**, 1–15.

—— Liberman, I.Y. (1984) 'Phonological awareness and short-term memory.' *Journal of Language Disabilities*, **17**, 592–599.

Marquardt, T.P., Saxman, J.H. (1972) 'Language comprehension and auditory discrimination in articulation deficient kindergarten children.' *Journal of Speech and Hearing Research*, **15**, 383–389.

Marsh, G., Friedman, M., Welch, V., Desberg, P. (1980) 'The development of strategies in spelling.' *In* Frith, U. (Ed.) *Cognitive Processes in Spelling*. London: Academic Press.

Marslen-Wilson, W.D., Welsh, A. (1978) 'Processing interactions and lexical access during word recognition in continuous speech.' *Cognitive Psychology*, **10**, 29–63.

Martin, J.A.M. (1980) 'Syndrome delineation in communication disorders.' *In* Hersov, L.A., Berger, M., Nichol, A.R. (Eds) *Language and Language Disorders in Childhood*. Oxford: Pergamon Press.

278

—— (1981) *Voice, Speech and Language in the Child: Development and Disorder*. New York: Springer.
Masland, R.L. (1981) 'Neurological aspects of dyslexia.' *In* Pavlidis, G.Th., Miles, T.R. (Eds) *Dyslexia Research and its Application to Education.* Chichester: Wiley.
Mellor, D.H. (1977) *A Study of Epilepsy in Childhood with Particular Reference to Behaviour Disorder.* University of Leeds: MD thesis.
—— (1980) 'Developmental language disorders: neurological and aetiological considerations.' *ICAA Conference: The Assessment and Remediation of Specific Language Disorders.* London: I CAN.
Menyuk, P. (1964) 'Comparison of grammar of children with functionally deviant and normal speech.' *Journal of Speech and Hearing Research*, **7**, 109–121.
—— (1979) 'Design factors in the assessment of language development in children with otitis media.' *Annals of Otology, Rhinology and Laryngology* (Suppl. 60), 78–87.
—— Looney, P.L. (1972) 'A problem of language disorder: length vs. structure.' *Journal of Speech and Hearing Research*, **15**, 264–279.
—— Menn, L., Silber, R. (1986) 'Early strategies for the perception and production of words and sounds.' *In* Fletcher, P., Garman, M. (Eds) *Language Acquisition, 2nd Edn.* Cambridge: Cambridge University Press.
Miller, G. (1956) 'The magical number seven plus or minus two: some limits on our capacity for processing information.' *Psychological Review*, **63**, 81–97.
Moffitt, T.E., Silva, P.A. (1987) 'WISC-R verbal and performance IQ discrepancy in an unselected cohort: clinical significance and longitudinal stability.' *Journal of Consulting and Clinical Psychology*, **55**, 768–774.
Monnin, L.M., Huntingdon, D.A. (1974) 'Relationship of articulatory defects to speech-sound identification.' *Journal of Speech and Hearing Research*, **17**, 352–366.
Morais, J., Allegria, J., Content, A. (1987) 'The relationship between segmental analysis and alphabetic literacy: an interactive view.' *Cahiers de Psychologie Cognitive*, **7**, 415–438.
Morgan, R. (1984) 'Auditory discrimination in speech-impaired and normal children as related to age.' *British Journal of Disorders of Communication*, **19**, 89–96.
Morley, M. (1965) *The Development and Disorders of Speech in Childhood.* Edinburgh: E. & S. Livingstone.
Morse, P. (1979) 'The infancy of infant speech perception: the first decade of research.' *Brain, Behaviour and Evolution*, **16**, 351–373.
Morris, J.M. (1966) *Standards and Progress in Reading.* Slough: NFER.
Morton, J. (1970) 'A functional model for memory.' *In* Norman, D.A. (Ed.) *Models of Human Memory.* New York: Academic Press.
Murphy, K.P. (1976) *In* Oyer, H.H. (Ed.) *Communication for the Hearing-handicapped.* Baltimore, MD: University Park Press.
Murray, L.A., Maliphant, R. (1982) 'Developmental aspects of the use of linguistic and graphemic information during reading.' *British Journal of Educational Psychology*, **52**, 155–169.
Mutton, D. (1982) 'Chromosome disorder in speech and language delay.' *Moor House School Research Bulletin*, **1**.
—— Lea, J. (1980) 'Chromosome studies of children with specific speech and language delay.' *Developmental Medicine and Child Neurology*, **22**, 588–594.
Nachshon, I. (1978) 'Handedness and dichotic listening to nonverbal features of speech.' *Perceptual and Motor Skills*, **47**, 1111–1114.
Naidoo, S. (1972) *Specific Dyslexia.* London: Pitman.
Needleman, H. (1977) 'Effect of hearing loss from early otitis media on speech and language development.' *In* Jaffe, B.F. (Ed.) *Hearing Loss in Children.* Baltimore, MD: University Park Press.
Neils, J., Aram, D.A. (1986a) 'Family history of children with developmental language disorders.' *Perceptual and Motor Skills*, **63**, 655–658.
—— —— (1986b) 'Handedness and sex of children with developmental language disorders.' *Brain and Language*, **28**, 53–65.
Neisser, U. (1967) *Cognitive Psychology.* New York: Appleton-Century-Crofts.
Neligan, G., Prudham, D. (1969a) 'Norms for four standard developmental milestones by sex, social class and place in family.' *Developmental Medicine and Child Neurology*, **11**, 413–422.
—— —— (1969b) 'Potential value of four early developmental milestones in screening children for

increased risk of later retardation.' *Developmental Medicine and Child Neurology*, **11**, 423–431.

Nellhaus, G. (1968) 'Head circumference from birth to eighteen years.' *Pediatrics*, **41**, 106–114.

Nice, M.M. (1918) 'Ambidexterity and delayed speech.' *Pedagogical Seminary and Journal of Genetics*, **25**.

Norusis, M.J. (1985) *SPSS-X Advanced Statistics Guide.* New York: McGraw-Hill.

Oakhill, J. (1984) 'Inferential and memory skills in children's comprehension of stories.' *British Journal of Educational Psychology*, **54**, 31–39.

Ojemann, G., Mateer, C. (1979) 'Human language cortex; localisation of memory, syntax and sequential motor-phoneme identification systems.' *Science*, **205**, 1401–1403.

Olson, G.M. (1973) 'Developmental changes in memory and the acquisition of language.' *In* Moore, T.E. (Ed.) *Cognitive Development and the Acquisition of Language.* New York: Academic Press.

Orton, S. (1937) *Reading, Writing and Speech Problems in Children.* New York: Norton.

Paden, E.P., Novak, M.A., Beiter, A.L. (1987) 'Predictors of phonological inadequacy in young children prone to otitis media.' *Journal of Speech and Hearing Disorders*, **52**, 232–242.

Paradise, J.L. (1981) 'Otitis media during early life: how hazardous to development? A critical review of the evidence.' *Pediatrics*, **68**, 869–873.

Pasamanick, B., Costantinou, F.K., Lilienfeld, A.M. (1956) 'Pregnancy experience and the development of childhood speech disorders.' *American Journal of Diseases of Children*, **91**, 113–118.

—— Knobloch, H. (1960) 'Brain damage and reproductive casualty.' *American Journal of Orthopsychiatry*, **30**, 298–305.

Paterson, M., Golding, J. (1986) 'Disorders of speech and language.' *In* Butler, N.R., Golding, J. (Eds) *From Birth to Five.* Oxford: Pergamon Press.

Paul, R., Cohen, D.J., Caparulo, B.K. (1983) 'A longitudinal study of patients with severe developmental disorders of language.' *Journal of the American Academy of Child Psychiatry*, **22**, 525–534.

Peters, A. (1979) 'Early syntax.' *In* Fletcher, P., Garman, M. (Eds) *Language Acquisition.* Cambridge: Cambridge University Press.

Petrie, I. (1975) 'Characteristics and progress of a group of language disordered children with severe receptive difficulties.' *British Journal of Disorders of Communication*, **10**, 123–133.

Piaget, J. (1926) *The Language and Thought of the Child.* London: Routledge Kegan Paul.

—— (1967) 'Language and thought from the genetic point of view.' *In* Adams, P. (Ed.) *Language in Thinking.* Harmondsworth: Penguin.

Pipe, M-E. (1987) 'Pathological left-handedness. Is it familial?' *Neuropsychologia*, **25**, 571–577.

Popay, J., Rimmer, L., Rossiter, C. (1983) *One Parent Families, Parents, Children and Public Policy.* London: Study Commission on the Family.

Porac, C., Coren, S. (1981) *Lateral Preferences and Human Behaviour.* New York: Springer.

Potter, F. (1982) 'The use of linguistic context: do good and poor readers use different strategies?' *British Journal of Educational Psychology*, **52**, 16–23.

Powers, M.H. (1971) 'Clinical and education procedures in functional disorders of articulation.' *In* Travis, L. E. (Ed.) *Handbook of Speech Pathology and Audiology.* New York: Appleton-Century-Crofts.

Prins, T.D. (1963) 'Relations among specific articulatory deviations and responses to a clinical measure of sound discrimination ability.' *Journal of Speech and Hearing Disorders*, **18**, 382–388.

Puckering, C., Rutter, M. (1987) 'Environmental influences on language development.' *In* Yule, W., Rutter, M. (Eds) *Language Development and Disorders. Clinics in Developmental Medicine, Nos 101/102.* London: Mac Keith Press with Blackwell Scientific; Philadelphia: J.B. Lippincott.

Quigley, S.P. (1978) 'Effects of early hearing impairment on normal language development.' *In* Martin, F.N. (Ed.) *Pediatric Neurology.* New York: Prentice Hall.

Rabbitt, P. (1986) 'Cognitive effects of mild deafness.' *Soundbarrier. The Journal of the Royal National Institute for the Deaf*, **9**, 6–8.

Rahko, T., Karma, P. (1989) 'Pure-tone hearing thresholds in otologically healthy 5-year-old children in Finland.' *Archives of Otorhinolaryngology*, **246**, 137–141.

Rapin, I. (1979) 'Conductive hearing loss effects on children's language and scholastic skills.' *Annals of Otology, Rhinology and Laryngology*, **88**, Suppl. 60.

—— (1982) *Children with Brain Dysfunction.* New York: Raven Press.

—— Wilson, B. (1978) 'Children with developmental language disability: neurological aspects and assessment.' *In* Wyke, M.A. (Ed.) *Developmental Dysphasia.* London: Academic Press.

—— Allen, D. (1983) 'Developmental language disorders: nosological considerations.' *In* Kirk, U. (Ed.) *Neuropsychology of Language, Reading and Spelling.* New York: Academic Press.

—— —— (1988) 'Syndromes in developmental dysphasia and adult aphasia.' *In* Plum, F. (Ed.) *Language, Communication and the Brain.* New York: Raven Press.

Rasmussen, T., Milner, B. (1977) 'The role of early left-brain injury in determining lateralisation of cerebral speech functions.' *Annals of the New York Academy of Sciences*, **299**, 355–369.

Ratcliffe, S.G. (1982) 'Speech and learning disorders in children with sex chromosome abnormalities.' *Developmental Medicine and Child Neurology*, **24**, 80–84.

Record, R.G., McKeown, T., Edwards, J.H. (1969) 'The relation of measured intelligence to birth order and maternal age.' *Annals of Human Genetics*, **33**, 61–69.

Rees, N. (1973) 'Auditory processing factors in language disorders: the view from Procrustes' bed.' *Journal of Speech and Hearing Disorders*, **38**, 304–315.

Reynolds, C.R., Gutkin, T.B. (1981) 'Test scatter on the WPPSI; normative analysis of the standardisation sample.' *Journal of Learning Disabilities*, **14**, 460–464.

Richman, N., Stevenson, J., Graham, P.J. (1982) *Pre-school to School: A Behavioural Study.* London: Academic Press.

Ripley, K. (1986) 'The Moor House School remedial programme: an evaluation.' *Child Language Teaching and Therapy*, **2**, 281–300.

—— (1987) 'Counselling children with specific speech and language disorders.' In *Proceedings of the First International Symposium on Specific Speech and Language Disorders in Children.* London: AFASIC.

Roberts, J., Sanyal, M., Burchinal, M., Collier, A., Ramey, C., Henderson, F. (1986) 'Otitis media in early childhood: relationship to later verbal and academic performance.' *Pediatrics*, **78**, 423–430.

Robinson, G.M., Solomon, D.J. (1974) 'Rhythm is processed by the speech hemisphere.' *Journal of Experimental Psychology*, **102**, 508–511.

Robinson, R. J. (1987) 'The causes of language disorder: an introduction and overview.' In *Proceedings of the First International Symposium on Specific Speech and Language Disorders in Children.* London: AFASIC.

Rosenthal, W.S. (1970) *Perception of Auditory Temporal Order as a Function of Selected Stimulus Features in a Group of Aphasic Children.* Stanford University: doctoral dissertation.

—— (1972) 'Auditory and linguistic interaction in developmental aphasia: evidence from two studies of auditory processing.' *In* Ingram, D. (Ed.) *Papers and Reports on Child Language Development*, **4**, 19–34.

Rutter, M. (1966) *Children of Sick Parents.* Oxford: Oxford University Press.

—— (1967) 'A children's behaviour questionnaire for completion by teachers: preliminary findings.' *Journal of Child Psychology and Psychiatry*, **8**, 1–11.

—— (1987) 'Developmental language disorders: some thoughts on causes and correlates.' In *Proceedings of the First International Symposium on Specific Speech and Language Disorders in Children.* London: AFASIC.

—— Graham, P., Yule, W. (1970) *A Neuropsychiatric Study in Choldhood. Clinics in Developmental Medicine, Nos 35/36.* London: SIMP with Heinemann Medical; Philadelphia: J.B. Lippincott.

—— Tizard, J., Whitmore, K. (1970) *Education, Health and Behaviour.* London: Longman.

—— Madge, N. (1976) *Cycles of Disadvantage.* London: Heinemann.

—— Lord, C. (1987) 'Language disorders associated with psychiatric disturbance.' *In* Yule, W., Rutter, M. (Eds) *Language Development and Disorders. Clinics in Developmental Medicine, Nos 101/102.* London: Mac Keith Press with Blackwell Scientific; Philadelphia: J.B. Lippincott.

Sak, R.J., Ruben, R.J. (1981) 'Recurrent middle ear effusion in childhood: implications of temporary auditory deprivation for language and learning.' *Annals of Otology, Rhinology and Laryngology*, **90**, 546–551.

Satz, P. (1972) 'Pathological left handedness: an explanatory model.' *Cortex*, **8**, 121–135.

—— (1973) 'Left-handedness and early brain insult: an explanation.' *Neuropsychologia*, **11**, 115–117.

Schery, T. (1985) 'Correlates of language development in language-disordered children.' *Journal of Speech and Hearing Disorders*, **50**, 73–83.

Schiff, N. (1985) 'The influence of deviant maternal input on the development of language during the preschool years.' *Journal of Speech and Hearing Research*, **22**, 581–593.

Schissel, R.J. (1980) 'The role of selected auditory skills in the misarticulation of "s", "r" and "th" by third grade children.' *British Journal of Disorders of Communication*, **15**, 129–139.

Schonell, F.J., Schonell, F.E. (1970) *Diagnostic and Attainment Testing.* Edinburgh: Oliver and Boyd.

Schwartz, M. (1988) 'Handedness, prenatal stress and pregnancy complications.' *Neuropsychologia*, **26**, 925–929.

Sergovich, F., Valentine, G.H., Chen, A.T.L., Kinch, R.A.H., Smout, M.S. (1969) 'Chromosome abberrations in 2159 consecutive newborn babies.' *New England Journal of Medicine*, **280**, 851–854.

Shah, N. (1981) 'Treatment of conductive deafness in children.' *In* Beagley, H.A. (Ed.) *Audiology and Audiological Medicine, Vol. 2.* Oxford: Oxford University Press.

Share, D.L., Silva, P.A. (1986) 'Classification of reading retardation.' *British Journal of Educational Psychology*, **56**, 32–39.

Sheridan, M. (1973) 'Children of seven years with marked speech defects.' *British Journal of Disorders of Communication*, **8**, 9–16

—— Peckham, C. (1973) 'Hearing and speech at seven.' *Special Education*, **62**, 16–20.

Shriberg, L., Smith, A.J. (1983) 'Phonological correlates of middle ear involvement in speech-delayed children: a methodological note.' *Journal of Speech and Hearing Research*, **26**, 293–297.

—— Kwiatkowski, J., Best, S., Hengst, J., Terselic-Weber, B. (1986) 'Characteristics of children with phonological disorders of unknown origin.' *Journal of Speech and Hearing Disorders*, **51**, 140–161.

Siegel, L.S., Cunningham, C.E., van der Spuy, H.I.J. (1985) 'Interactions of language delayed and normal preschool boys with their peers.' *Journal of Child Psychology and Psychiatry*, **26**, 77–83.

Silva, P.A., Satz, P. (1979) 'Pathological left handedness: evaluation of a model.' *Brain and Language*, **7**, 8–16.

—— Bradshaw, J. (1980) 'Some factors contributing to intelligence at age of school entry.' *British Journal of Educational Psychology*, **50**, 10–15.

—— Fergusson, D. (1980) 'Some factors contributing to language development in three year old children: a report from the Dunedin Multidisciplinary Child Development Study.' *British Journal of Disorders of Communication*, **15**, 205–214.

—— Kirkland, C., Simpson, A., Stewart, I.A., Williams, S.M. (1982*a*) 'Some developmental and behavioural characteristics of children with bilateral otitis media with effusion.' *Journal of Learning Disabilities*, **15**, 417–421.

—— Thomas, J., Williams, S.M. (1982*b*) 'A descriptive study of the socio-economic status and child development in Dunedin 5-year-olds.' *New Zealand Journal of Educational Studies*, **17**, 21–32.

—— Justin, C., McGee, R., Williams, S.M. (1984) 'Some developmental and behavioural characteristics of seven-year-old children with delayed speech development.' *British Journal of Disorders of Communication*, **19**, 147–154.

—— Williams, S., McGee, R. (1987) 'A longitudinal study of children with developmental language delay at age three: later intelligence, reading and behaviour problems.' *Developmental Medicine and Child Neurology*, **29**, 630–640.

Simon, C., Fourcin, A. (1978) 'Cross language study of speech pattern learning.' *Journal of the Acoustical Society of America*, **63**, 925–935.

Sinclair, C. (1971) 'Dominance patterns of young children: a follow-up study.' *Perceptual and Motor Skills*, **32**, 142.

Sipila, M., Pukander, J., Karma, P. (1987) 'Incidence of acute otitis media up to the age of one and a half years in urban infants.' *Acta Otolaryngologica*, **104**, 138–145.

Skinner, M.W. (1978) 'The hearing of speech during language acquisition.' *Otolaryngolic Clinics of North America*, **11**, 631–650.

Skuse, D.H. (1988) 'Extreme deprivation in early childhood.' *In* Bishop, D., Mogford, K. (Eds) *Language Development in Exceptional Circumstances.* Edinburgh: Churchill Livingstone.

Smith, N.V. (1973) *The Acquisition of Phonology: A Case Study.* Cambridge: Cambridge University Press.

Snyder, R.T., Pope, C. (1970) 'New norms for and an item analysis of the Wepman test at the first grade, six-year-level.' *Perceptual and Motor Skills*, **31**, 1007–1010.

Sommers, R., Meyer, W., Fenton, A. (1961) 'Pitch discrimination and articulation.' *Journal of Speech and Hearing Research*, **4**, 56–60.

Sonksen, P.M. (1979) *The Neuro-Developmental and Paediatric Findings Associated with Significant*

282

Disabilities of Language Development in Pre-School Children. University of London: MD thesis.
Sparrow, S., Satz, P. (1970) 'Dyslexia, laterality and neuropsychological development.' *In* Bakker, D.J., Satz, P. (Eds) *Specific Reading Disability.* Rotterdam: Rotterdam University Press.
Springer, S.P., Deutsch, G. (1985) *Left Brain, Right Brain. Revised Edn.* New York: W.H. Freeman.
Stark, R.E., Tallal, P. (1981) 'Selection of children with specific language deficits.' *Journal of Speech and Hearing Disorders,* **46**, 114–122.
—— Tallal, P., Kallman, C., Mellits, E.D. (1983) 'Cognitive abilities of language delayed children.' *Journal of Psychology,* **114**, 9–19.
—— Bernstein, L.E., Condino, R., Bender, M., Tallal, P., Catts, H. III, (1984) 'Four-year follow-up study of language impaired children.' *Annals of Dyslexia,* **34**, 49–68.
Stevenson, J., Richman, N., Graham, P. (1985) 'Behaviour problems and language abilities at three years and behavioural deviance at eight years.' *Journal of Child Psychology and Psychiatry,* **26**, 215–230.
Stewart, A. (1984) 'Severe perinatal hazards.' *In* Rutter, M. (Ed.) *Developmental Neuropsychiatry.* Edinburgh: Churchill Livingstone.
Subirana, A. (1969) 'Handedness and cerebral dominance.' *In* Vincken, P.J., Bruyn, G.W. (Eds) *Handbook of Clinical Neurology, Vol. 4.* Amsterdam: North Holland Publishing.
Tallal, P., Piercy, M. (1973) 'Defects of non-verbal auditory perception in children with developmental dysphasia.' *Nature,* **241**, 468–499.
—— —— (1978) 'Defects of auditory processing.' *In* Wyke, M. (Ed.) *Developmental Aphasia.* London: Academic Press.
—— Stark, R., Kallman, C., Mellits, D. (1980) 'Developmental dysphasia: relation between acoustic processing deficits and verbal processing.' *Neuropsychologia,* **18**, 273–284.
—— Ross, R., Curtiss, S. (1989a) 'Familial aggregation in specific language impairment.' *Journal of Speech and Hearing Disorders,* **54**, 167–173.
—— —— —— (1989b) 'Unexpected sex-ratios in families of language/learning-impaired children.' *Neuropsychologia,* **27**, 987–998.
Tanner, J.M. (1958) *Modern Trends in Paediatrics.* London: Butterworth.
Teele, D., Klein, J., Rosner, B. (1980) 'Epidemiology of otitis media in children.' *Annals of Otology, Rhinology and Laryngology,* **89**, Suppl. **68**, 5–6.
Tempest, B. (1986) 'Dyspraxia—an update.' In *Advances in Working with Language Disordered Children.* London: I CAN.
Templin, M. (1943) 'A study of sound discrimination ability of elementary school pupils.' *Journal of Speech Disorders,* **8**, 127–132.
Thompson, R.J., Cappelman, M.W., Zeitschel, K.A. (1979) 'Neonatal behaviour of infants of adolescent mothers.' *Developmental Medicine and Child Neurology,* **21**, 474–482.
Thomson, M.E. (1979) 'Laterality and reading attainment.' *In* Newton, M.J., Thomson, M.E., Richards, I.L. (Eds) *Readings in Dyslexia.* Wisbech: LDA.
Tomblin, J.B. (1989) 'Familial concentrations of developmental language impairment.' *Journal of Speech and Hearing Disorders,* **54**, 287–295.
Touwen, B.C.L. (1972) 'Laterality and dominance.' *Developmental Medicine and Child Neurology,* **14**, 747–755.
Travis, L.E., Rasmus, B. (1931) 'The speech sound discrimination ability of cases with functional disorders of articulation.' *Quarterly Journal of Speech,* **17**, 217–226.
Vellutino, F.R. (1979) *Dyslexia; Theory and Research.* Cambridge, MA: Erlbaum.
Washington, D.M., McBurney, A.K., Grunau, R.V.E. (1986) 'Communication skills'. *In* Dunn, H.G. (Ed.) *Sequelae of Low Birthweight: The Vancouver Study. Clinics in Developmental Medicine, Nos 95/96.* London: SIMP with Blackwell Scientific; Philadelphia: J.B. Lippincott.
Waterson, N. (1971) 'Child phonology: a prosodic view.' *Journal of Linguistics,* **7**, 179–211.
Wechsler, D. (1976) *WISC-R Manual (with British amendments).* Windsor: NFER.
Weiner, P.S. (1967) 'Auditory discrimination and articulation.' *Journal of Speech and Hearing Disorders,* **32**, 19–28.
—— (1974) 'A language-delayed child at adolescence.' *Journal of Speech and Hearing Disorders,* **39**, 202–212.
—— (1985) 'The value of follow-up studies.' *Topics in Language Disorders,* **5**, 78–92.
Wells, G.C., (1975) 'The contexts of children's early language experience.' *Educational Review,* **27**,

114–125.

—— (1986) 'Variations in child language.' *In* Fletcher, P., Garman, M. (Eds) *Language Acquisition, 2nd Edn*. Cambridge: Cambridge University Press.

—— Gutfreund, M. (1987) 'The conversational requirements for language learning.' *In* Yule, W., Rutter, M. (Eds) *Language Development and Disorders. Clinics in Developmental Medicine, Nos 101/102*. London: Mac Keith Press with Blackwell Scientific; Philadelphia: J.B. Lippincott.

Wepman, J.M. (1960) 'Auditory discrimination, speech and reading.' *Elementary School Journal*, **60**, 325–333.

Whittington, J.E., Richards, P.N. (1987) 'The stability of children's laterality prevalences and their relationship to measures of performance.' *British Journal of Educational Psychology*, **57**, 45–55.

Whorf, B.L. (1941) 'The relation of habitual thought and behaviour to language.' *In* Spier, L. (Ed.) *Language, Culture and Personality; Essays in Memory of Edward Sapir*. Utah: University of Utah Press.

Wiig, E., Semel, E.M. (1976) *Language Disabilities in Children and Adolescents*. Columbus, OH: Charles E. Merrill.

—— ——(1980) *Language Assessment and Intervention for the Learning Disabled*. Columbus, OH: Charles E. Merrill.

Wilson, B.C., Riscucci, D.A. (1986) 'A model for clinical-quantitative classification. Generation 1: application to language-disordered preschool children.' *Brain and Language*, **27**, 281–309.

Wolfus, B, Mascovitch, M., Kinsbourne, M. (1980) 'Subgroups of developmental language impairment.' *Brain and Language*, **10**, 152–171.

Wooster, A.D. (1970) 'Social and ethnic differences in understanding the spoken word.' *British Journal of Disorders of Communication*, **5**, 118–125.

Worster-Drought, C. (1974) 'Suprabulbar paresis.' *Developmental Medicine and Child Neurology*, **16** (Suppl. 30).

Yule, W., Rigley, L.V. (1982) 'Predicting future reading attainment from the WPPSI.' *Journal of Research in Reading*, **5**, 67–74.

Zangwill, O.L. (1960) *Cerebral Dominance and its Relation to Psychological Function*. Edinburgh: Oliver & Boyd.

—— (1978) 'The concept of developmental dysphasia.' *In* Wyke, M. (Ed.) *Developmental Dysphasia*. London: Academic Press.

Zinkus, P.W., Gottlieb, M.I. (1980) 'Patterns of perceptual and academic deficits related to early chronic otitis media.' *Pediatrics*, **66**, 246–253.

ASSESSMENTS

Anthony, A., Bogle, D., Ingram, T.T.S., McIsaacs, M.W. (1971) *Edinburgh Articulation Test.* Edinburgh: Churchill Livingstone.

Boehm, A.E. (1971) *Test of Basic Concepts.* New York: Psychological Corporation.

Bishop, D.V.M. (1983) *Test for Reception of Grammar.* Available from the author, Dept. of Psychology, University of Manchester.

Brimer, M.A., Dunn, L.M. (1962) *English Picture Vocabulary Test.* Bristol: Bristol Educational Evaluation Enterprises.

Burt (Revised) Spelling Test (1974) Available from Hodder and Stoughton, Sevenoaks, Kent.

Carrow, E. (1973) *Test of Auditory Comprehension of Language.* Boston, MA: Teaching Resources Corporation.

Crystal, D., Fletcher, P., Garman, M. (1976) *The Grammatical Analysis of Language Disability. A Procedure for Assessment and Remediation.* London: Edward Arnold.

Dunn, L., Dunn, L., Whetton, C., Pintillie, D. (1982) *British Picture Vocabulary Scale.* Windsor: NFER-Nelson.

Elliott, C.D., Murray, D.J., Pearson, L.S. (1983) *British Ability Scales, Revised Edn.* Windsor: NFER-Nelson.

German, D. (1986) *Test of Word Finding.* Texas: DLM Teaching Resources.

Kirk, S.A., McCarthy, J., Kirk, W.D. (1968) *The Illinois Test of Psycholinguistic Abilities.* Urbana: University of Illinois Press.

Neale, M.D. (1966) *Neale Analysis of Reading Ability, 2nd Edn.* Basingstoke: Macmillan Education.

Renfrew, C.E. (1966) *The Action Picture Test.* Available from the author at North Place, Old Headington, Oxford.

—— (1969) *The Bus Story: a Test of Continuous Speech.* Available from the author at North Place, Old Headington, Oxford.

—— (1972) *Word-Finding Vocabulary Scale.* Available from the author at North Place, Old Headington, Oxford.

Reynell, J. (1969) *Developmental Language Scales.* Windsor: NFER-Nelson.

—— (1977) *Developmental Language Scales (Revised).* Windsor: NFER-Nelson.

Schonell, F.J. *Graded Word Reading Test & Graded Word Spelling Test.* Edinburgh: Oliver & Boyd.

Scottish Council for Research in Education. (1976) *The Burt Word Reading Test (1974 Revision).* Sevenoaks, Kent: Hodder and Stoughton.

Southgate, V. (1976) *Southgate Group Reading Tests 1 and 2.* Sevenoaks, Kent: Hodder and Stoughton.

Vernon, P.E. (1977) *Graded Word Spelling Test.* Sevenoaks, Kent: Hodder and Stoughton.

Wechsler, D. (1949) *Wechsler Intelligence Scale for Children (WISC).* Windsor: NFER-Nelson. (No longer available.)

—— (1967) *Wechsler Preschool and Primary Scale of Intelligence (WPPSI).* Windsor: NFER-Nelson.

—— (1976) *Wechsler Intelligence Scale for Children—Revised (WISC-R).* Windsor: NFER-Nelson.

Wepman, J.M. (1958) Auditory Discrimination Test. Chicago: Language Research Associates.

INDEX

287